Clinical Advances in Implant Dentistry

Clinical Advances in Implant Dentistry

Editor: Preston Bailey

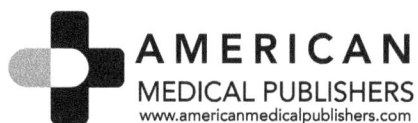

AMERICAN
MEDICAL PUBLISHERS
www.americanmedicalpublishers.com

AMERICAN
MEDICAL PUBLISHERS
www.americanmedicalpublishers.com

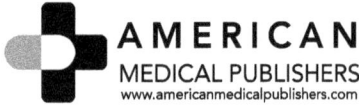

Cataloging-in-Publication Data

Clinical advances in implant dentistry / edited by Preston Bailey.
    p. cm.
Includes bibliographical references and index.
ISBN 978-1-63927-051-4
1. Dental implants. 2. Dentistry, Operative. 3. Dentures. 4. Implants, Artificial.
5. Mouth--Surgery. I. Bailey, Preston.
RK667.I45 I47 2022

617.693--dc23

American Medical Publishers,
41 Flatbush Avenue,
1st Floor, New York,
NY 11217, USA

ISBN 978-1-63927-051-4 (Hardback)

Contents

Permissions

List of Contributors

Index

Preface

The main aim of this book is to educate learners and enhance their research focus by presenting diverse topics covering this vast field. This is an advanced book which compiles significant studies by distinguished experts in the area of analysis. This book addresses successive solutions to the challenges arising in the area of application, along with it; the book provides scope for future developments.

Dentistry is a discipline of medicine that focuses on the diagnosis, prevention and treatment of diseases and disorders of the oral cavity, oral mucosa, and related structures and tissues. Implant dentistry is the branch of dentistry that includes a surgical component that interfaces with the bone of the jaw to support a dental prosthesis such as a crown, bridge, denture and facial prosthesis. The primary use of implant dentistry is to support a dental prosthesis. Osseointegration is the biological process behind modern dental implants. In osseointegration, materials like titanium form an intimate bond to the bone. Risks and complications related to implant therapy are excessive bleeding, infection, failure to osseointegrate, peri-implantitis, etc. The health of the person receiving the treatment, health of the tissues in the mouth and the drugs which affect the chances of osseointegration, are some factors on which the success or the failure of the dental implant depends. This book contains some path-breaking studies in the field of implant dentistry. It strives to provide a fair idea about this discipline and to help develop a better understanding of the latest advances within this field. This book is a resource guide for experts as well as students.

It was a great honour to edit this book, though there were challenges, as it involved a lot of communication and networking between me and the editorial team. However, the end result was this all-inclusive book covering diverse themes in the field.

Finally, it is important to acknowledge the efforts of the contributors for their excellent chapters, through which a wide variety of issues have been addressed. I would also like to thank my colleagues for their valuable feedback during the making of this book.

Editor

Interfacial biomechanical properties of a dual acid-etched versus a chemically modified hydrophilic dual acid-etched implant surface: an experimental study in Beagles

Rainde Naiara Rezende de Jesus[1,2], Eunice Carrilho[2], Pedro V. Antunes[3], Amílcar Ramalho[3], Camilla Christian Gomes Moura[4], Andreas Stavropoulos[1]* and Darceny Zanetta-Barbosa[5]

Abstract

Background: The high survival clinical success rates of osseointegration are requisites for establishing a long-term biomechanical fixation and load-bearing potential of endosseous oral implants. The objective of this preclinical animal study was to evaluate the effect of surface microtopography and chemistry on the early stages of biomechanical rigidity with a sandblasted, dual acid-etched surface, with or without an additional chemical modification (SAE-HD and SAE, respectively), in the tibia of Beagle dogs.

Methods: Two pairs of implants, with the same macrogeometry but different surface technology ((a) dual acid-etched surface treatment with hydrochloric and sulfuric acid followed by microwave treatment and insertion in isotonic saline solution to increase hydrophilicity (SAE-HD) (test, $n = 12$) and (b) dual acid-etched surface (SAE) (control, $n = 12$)), were installed bilaterally in the proximal tibia of six Beagle dogs. In order to determine the effect of surface modification on biomechanical fixation, a test protocol was established to assess the torque and a complete set of intrinsic properties. Maximum removal torque (in N cm) was the primary outcome measure, while connection stiffness (N cm/rad) and removal energy ($\times 10^{-2}$J) were the secondary outcome measures and were assessed after 2 and 4 weeks in vivo. A general linear statistical model was used and performed for significant differences with the one-way ANOVA followed by Tukey post hoc test ($P < 0.05$).

Results: The removal torque values did not reveal significant statistical differences between SAE-HD and SAE implants at any observation times ($P = 0.06$). Although a slight increase over time could be observed in both test and control groups. SAE-HD showed higher removal energy at 4 weeks ($999.35 \pm 924.94 \times 10^{-2}$ J) compared to that at 2 weeks ($421.94 \pm 450.58 \times 10^{-2}$ J), while SAE displayed lower values at the respective healing periods ($P = 0.16$). Regarding connection stiffness, there were no significant statistical differences neither within the groups nor over time. There was a strong, positive monotonic correlation between removal torque and removal energy ($= 0.722$, $n = 19$, $P < 0.001$).

(Continued on next page)

* Correspondence: andreas.stavropoulos@mah.se
[1]Department of Periodontology, Faculty of Odontology, Malmö University, Carl Gustafs väg 34, 205-06 Malmö, Sweden
Full list of author information is available at the end of the article

(Continued from previous page)

Conclusions: In this study, no significant differences were observed between the specific hydrophilic (SAE-HD) and hydrophobic (SAE) surfaces evaluated, in terms of biomechanical properties during the early osseointegration period.

Keywords: Biomaterial, Dental implant, Removal torque, Removal energy, Connection stiffness, Implant roughness, Wettability, Dogs, New methodology assessment for implants

Background

The progressive evolution of oral implant surface technology (i.e., micro to nanotopography and chemical composition) [1, 2], implant macrogeometry, surgical procedures [3–5], and loading protocols [6–8] has resulted in high survival and clinical success rates [9]. Accordingly, chemically active micro and nanostructured implant surfaces, presenting moderate surface roughness (R_a/S_a values between 1 and 2 µm), enhance host-to-implant interactions [10–12] and have been shown to shorten the period needed for time-critical functional implant loading (i.e., so-called immediate or early loading) [13–15].

Recent in vitro analyses support the concept that hydrophilic surfaces upregulate the expression of angiogenic factors, activate the production of anti-inflammatory factors, and downregulate the expression of pro-inflammatory cytokines by osteoblasts [16] and macrophage-like cells [17, 18], and regulate osteogenic differentiation and maturation of mesenchymal stem cells (MSCs) [10, 19, 20] and human osteoblast-like cells [21–23], increasing osteogenesis and decreasing osteoclastogenesis [11, 23, 24]. Furthermore, higher surface energy and hydrophilicity is demonstrated to induce faster bone-to-implant contact (%BIC) and bone density, both in preclinical in vivo experiments [25–27] and in patients [7, 28, 29]. Indeed, higher biomechanical stability as expression of primary and secondary bone anchorage is recorded following hydrophilic implant placement [26, 30].

Particularly, a superhydrophilic moderately rough titanium (Ti) implant surface (contact angle less than 5°) has been suggested to play a critical role during the early healing period [27] and establishment of a successful osseointegration [31] in preclinical in vivo studies. The microarchitecture and density of the trabecular bone formed around oral implants, characterized by a high ratio of metabolic activity and remodeling, is one of the main determinants of interfacial shear strength, mechanical resistance, and adaptation to overloading stress [32]. The potential of chemically modified superhydrophilic implant surfaces to enhance osteogenic differentiation and increase early bone apposition onto the implant may shorten the implant stability drop, occurring due to bone remodeling during the first few weeks of implantation [13].

Consequently, such microstructured surface technology may lessen the healing (non-loading) period and allow more readily immediate or early functional implant loading in patients with reduced bone density. Nevertheless, there is lack of knowledge regarding the intrinsic biomechanical aspects of osseointegration related to this specific implant surface technology (i.e., removal torque, removal energy, and connection stiffness) during the initial osseointegration process.

Evaluation of biological effects and biomechanical properties of innovative technologies in the field of implant dentistry in preclinical animal models, prior to translational research, complies with standard regulations [33]. Thus, the aim of this preclinical animal study was to evaluate the effect of surface microtopography and chemistry on the biomechanical properties of implants with a sandblasted, dual acid-etched surface, with or without an additional chemical modification (SAE-HD[1] and SAE,[2] respectively), during the early stages of osseointegration in the tibia of Beagle dogs. Specifically, we hypothesized that a chemically active implant surface presenting superhydrophilicity generates higher interfacial shear strength in comparison to a hydrophobic surface, expressed as higher maximum removal torque, removal energy, and connection stiffness.

Methods

The present preclinical in vivo study is reported according to the Animal Research: Reporting of In Vivo Experiments (ARRIVE) guidelines, in regard with relevant items [33]. The animal experimental protocol was approved by the Bioethics Committee for Animal Experimentation (CEUA, protocol no. 098/10) at the Federal University of Uberlândia and followed the normative guidelines of the National Council for Animal Control and Experimentation (CONCEA), constituent of the Ministry of Science, Technology and Innovation (MCTI), Law no. 11.794, 08/19/2008, Brazil. The in vivo part of the study was conducted between November 2012 and January 2013.

Experimental units

Twenty-four commercially pure Ti implants (10 mm × 4 mm, $L \times \emptyset$) with a moderately rough surface, produced by means of sandblasting and dual acid-etching with hydrochloric and sulfuric acid were used in the present study. Implants in the control group were only sandblasted and dual acid-etched (SAE; $n = 12$). In the test group, after sandblasting and dual acid etching, implants received proprietary technology treatment, including microwave treatment and insertion in isotonic saline solution resulting in significantly increased hydrophilicity (SAE-HD; $n = 12$). These specific implant surfaces exhibit the following 3D surface roughness parameters for SAE and SAE-HD, respectively: S_a 1.44 μm ± 1.15 and 1.26 μm ± 0.17; S_z 14.57 μm ± 1 and 16.20 μm ± 7.8; S_{dr} 1.51 and 1.21%; S_{ds} 658.67 $1/mm^2$ ± 27.42 and 643.33 $1/mm^2$ ± 37.74; and S_{sk} −0.51 and −0.43 [27]. The chemical composition of the different surfaces was examined by X-ray photoelectron spectroscopy (XPS). The atomic percentage values of carbon were 49 and 17, and 22 and 59 of oxygen in SAE and SAE-HD groups, respectively. The surface energy and wettability was investigated by means of a static contact angle analysis by means of the sessile drop technique [34] applying simulated body fluid (SBF) solution. SAE-HD disks reveal a superhydrophilic behavior (contact angle < 5°), whereas SAE surfaces display superhydrophobic properties (contact angle > 90°).

The implants present similar macrodesign with an external hexagon connection system and cylindrical body containing double triangular threads with high potential for bone compression recommended for type III and IV bone, commercially available as Titamax Ti Ex®. Neodent®[3] supplied all implants.

Animal model

Six male Beagle dogs (~ 1.5 years old), weighting between 13 and 15 kg, were used in the present study. All animals were acclimatized in the experimental animal care facility of Federal University of Uberlândia for 2 weeks previously to the experimental procedures and randomly pair-housed in standard shelters (1×1.5 m kennel) to allow environmental enrichment (i.e., variety of toys, daily group play sessions, resistance running, and training) at the ambient temperature of 22 °C, under controlled humidity and 12-h circadian rhythm. The diet consisted of hard pellet and water ad libitum. The animal caretakers were blind to the experimental groups. The level of pain, distress, or suffering was daily assessed during the observation period to ensure the welfare of the animals. Aiming to guarantee selection blindness during the experimental allocation, the groups were systematically coded by a third person and the first implant to be placed in each tibia was randomly assigned. Sample size was calculated based on information in previous studies using the dog tibia model to allow evaluation of possible differences in bone-to-implant contact between groups. The surgical procedures and

the histological/histomorphometrical outcomes of the study have been reported elsewhere [31].

Briefly, two pairs of implants (10 mm × 4 mm, $L \times \varnothing$) from each of the experimental groups were placed under copious sterile saline irrigation and with a torque of about 45 N cm (last drill 3.5 mm $\varnothing$) in each proximal tibia of the animals (total no. of implants 48). Implants were placed with an alternating fashion in terms of medio-distal positioning with the first group chosen at random and surgeries were staged between left and right tibia to provide 2 and 4 weeks of healing times, i.e., 12 implants per group and per observation time. The first implant was inserted ca. 2 cm below the femoral-tibial-patellar joint line at the central medial-lateral portion of the proximal tibiae (Fig. 1). The following implants were placed in a distal direction with inter-implant distances of 1 cm along the central region of the bone until the tibia patellar joint. Implants were furnished with cover screws and then soft tissues were sutured in layers for primary intention healing. Postoperative pain and infection control was provided for 7 days. The animals were euthanized under sedation with an anesthesia overdose, and the upper third of the tibias was retrieved. The specimens were fixed in 10% buffered formalin solution and half of them were allocated to histomorphometric analysis and the other half to biomechanical analysis, reported herein.

Assessment of interfacial biomechanical properties

To assess the biomechanical strength of the bone-implant interface, the following parameters were assessed: (a) maximum removal torque (N cm) (primary outcome measure), obtained during the unscrewing process (primary outcome measure); (b) connection stiffness (N cm/rad), corresponding to the ratio between

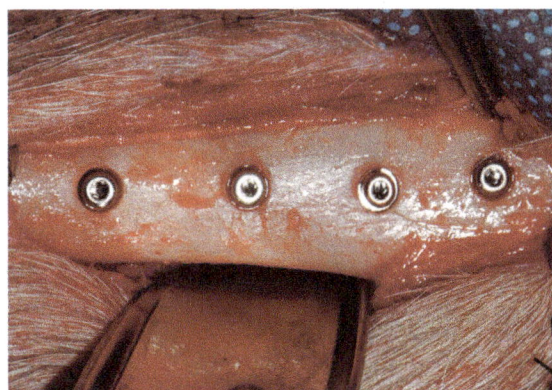

Fig. 1 Two pairs of implants (10 mm × 4 mm, $L \times \varnothing$) from each of the experimental groups were placed in each tibia with an alternating fashion in terms of medio-distal positioning regarding the group, but with the first group chosen at random. Implants were placed with an inter-implant distance of 1 cm

removal torque and angular displacement (secondary outcome measure); and (c) removal energy ($\times 10{-}2$ J), corresponding to the energy (workload) necessary to completely unscrew the implant, (secondary outcome measure).

The removal torque test was conducted on a Shimadzu universal testing machine.[4] This equipment was adapted in order to determine the referred properties (Fig. 2a, b). A horizontal shaft, supported by two ball bearings, with Allen keys socket on one end and a rotation sensor on the other end, was connected with a steel string to the mobile span of the Shimadzu universal testing machine, in such a way that the linear motion was converted to a rotational motion. The dog's tibia bone block containing the implant was placed in alignment and inside the Allen keys socket and fixed with an adjustable clamp, in order not to rotate during the test. The upper span speed, at which the string was attached, was adjusted to produce a shaft rotation speed of 0.005 rad/s. During the test, both torque (N cm) and angular displacement (rad) were acquired using a sampling rate of 10 samples/s (Fig. 3a, b). In order to calculate the connection stiffness (N cm/rad), the tangent method was applied to the data after obtaining the linear correlation coefficient (R^2) compared to the secant method, revealing the absence of mathematical discrepancy between the application of both methods (Fig. 4).

Calibration of one blinded examiner (R.N.R.J) and repeated measurements for data reproducibility was performed under supervision and prior to performing the removal torque test and respective calculation of connection stiffness.

Statistical analysis
A general linear statistical model with torque, energy, and stiffness as dependent variables and implant surface and time in vivo as independent variables was used at 95% level of significance and performed by one-way ANOVA followed by Tukey's post hoc test. The Spearman rank correlation test was taken in order to test the association concerning the investigated dependent variables. Since sample size calculation, as already mentioned, was made to allow evaluation of possible differences in bone-to-implant contact between groups, a post hoc analysis was performed to define the minimum detectable difference between groups regarding the parameters assessed herein, with a power of 80% and an alpha error of 0.05%. The IBM® SPSS® Statistics software[5] was used.

Results
No remarkable events were observed during the surgical procedures and the subsequent healing period. The relative biomechanical performance of both experimental implant surfaces is illustrated in a representative graph of removal torque versus angular displacement. The removal torque, removal energy, and connection stiffness values are described in terms of mean, standard deviation, and 95% confidence interval for mean in Fig. 5. The results of one-way ANOVA variance and Tukey's post hoc test values of the variables for SAE-HD and SAE implant at 2 and 4 weeks postoperatively ($n = 6$) are demonstrated in Table 1.

The removal torque values (N cm) did not reveal significant statistical differences between SAE-HD and SAE implants at any observation period ($P = 0.06$), but a slight increase over time could be observed in both test and control groups (Fig. 5a). Removal torque at 2 weeks was 60.18 ± 24.12 and 54.00 ± 29.91 N cm, and at 4 weeks was 88.11 ± 14.96 and 79.05 ± 14.59 N cm for SAE-HD and SAE implants, respectively (Fig. 5b). SAE-HD showed higher removal energy [J] at 4 weeks (9.99 ± 9.25) compared to 2 weeks (4.22 ± 4.50), while SAE displayed lower values at corresponding healing times (5.21 ± 1.49 vs. 2.83 ± 2.49, respectively) ($P = 0.16$). Regarding connection stiffness (N cm/rad), SAE showed lower values at 2 weeks (462.57 ± 507.75) compared with 4 weeks of healing (689.01 ± 496.28), however not

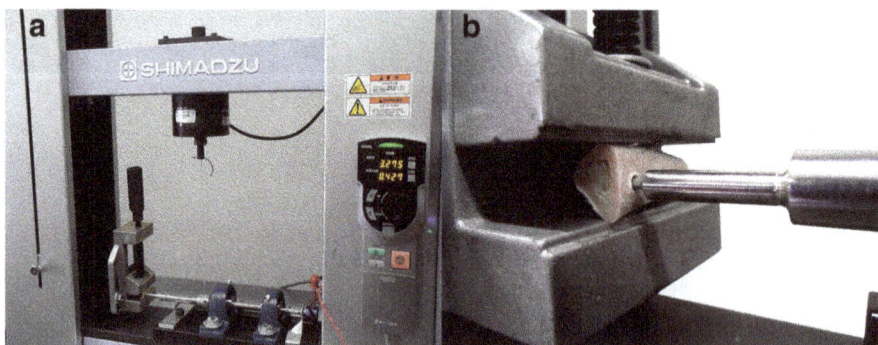

Fig. 2 Adaptation of Shimadzu universal testing machine for performing removal torque test of dental implants. **a** General view. **b** Assembly detail of connection between Allen keys socket and the implant placed in the tibia

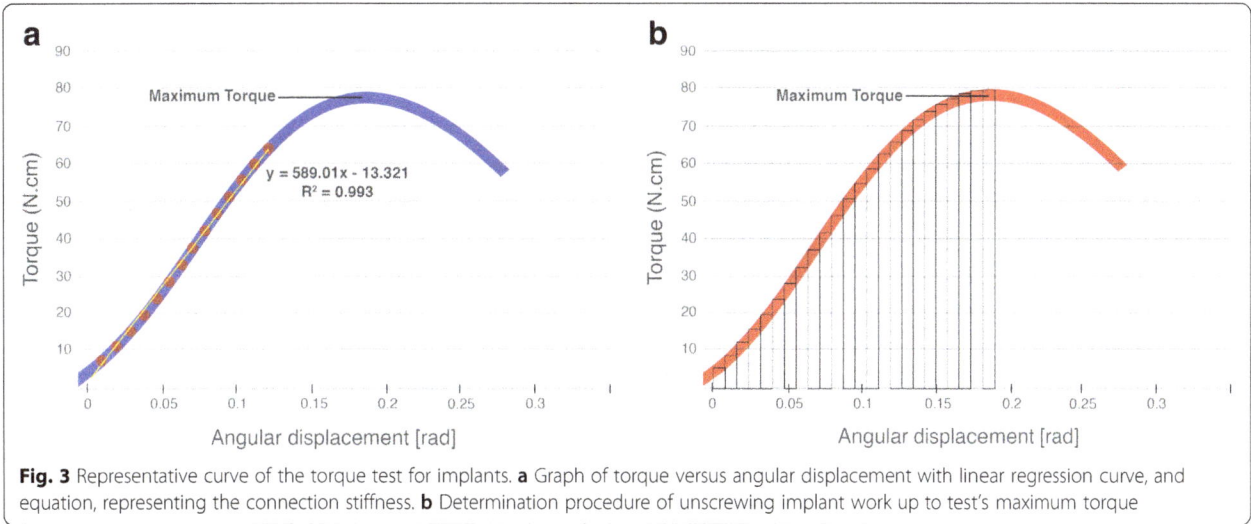

Fig. 3 Representative curve of the torque test for implants. **a** Graph of torque versus angular displacement with linear regression curve, and equation, representing the connection stiffness. **b** Determination procedure of unscrewing implant work up to test's maximum torque

statistically significant (Fig. 5c). SAE-HD disclosed similar results at 2 and 4 weeks (652.98 ± 111.26 vs. 661.56 ± 369.28, respectively) without statistically significant differences neither between the groups, nor over time ($P = 0.76$).

A Spearman's correlation test was run to determine the connection between maximum removal torque, removal energy, and connection stiffness values (Table 2) during the interfacial strength assessment. There was a strong, positive monotonic correlation between removal torque and removal energy ($=0.722$, $n = 19$, $P < 0.001$). However, there was no evidence of positive correlation between removal torque and connection stiffness ($=0.352$, $n = 24$, $P = 0.092$). Moreover, a negative correlation between removal energy and connection stiffness was observed ($=-0.91$, $n = 19$, $P = 0.710$).

Discussion

Improving surface wettability aims to increase the implant surface area achieving most favorable protein adsorption and cellular adhesion and thereby to positively regulate the biological response at the initial osseointegration process. Thus, the superior potential of superhydrophilic surfaces in enhancing osseointegration at early stages of bone formation may also enhance their load-bearing capacity and biomechanical resistance.

In the present study, both SAE-HD implants and SAE implants showed relatively high amounts of maximum removal torque values at both observation times. In contrast, the SAE-HD implants showed relatively high values in removal energy compared with SAE implants at both 2 and 4 weeks. Specifically, the test group presented consistently higher values (about 100% higher) in

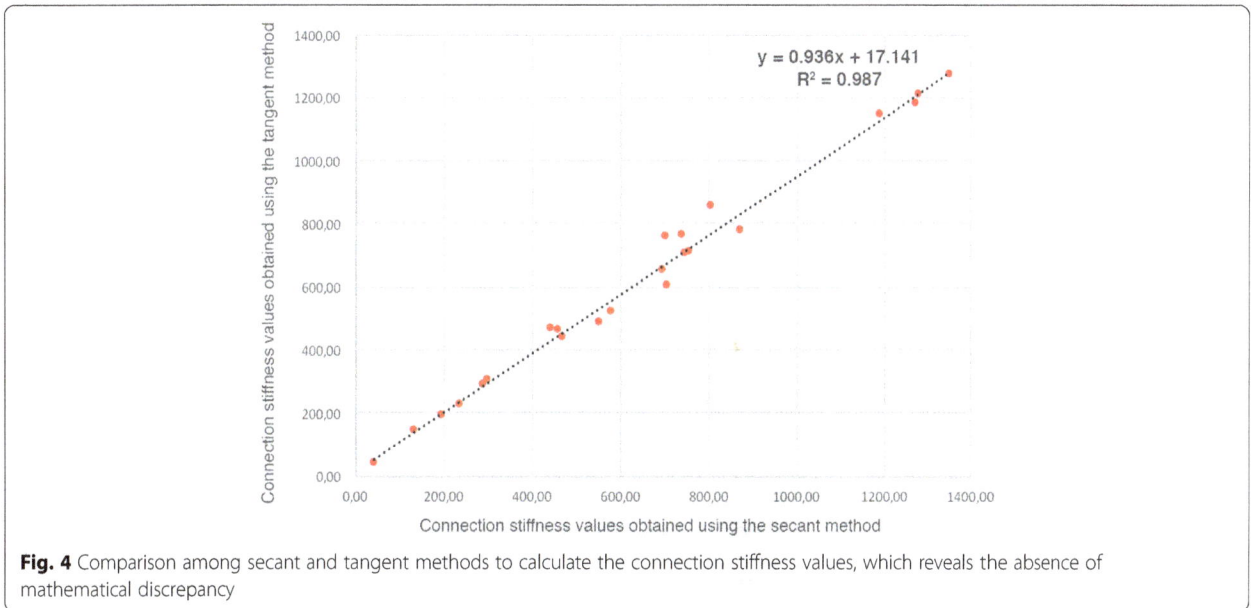

Fig. 4 Comparison among secant and tangent methods to calculate the connection stiffness values, which reveals the absence of mathematical discrepancy

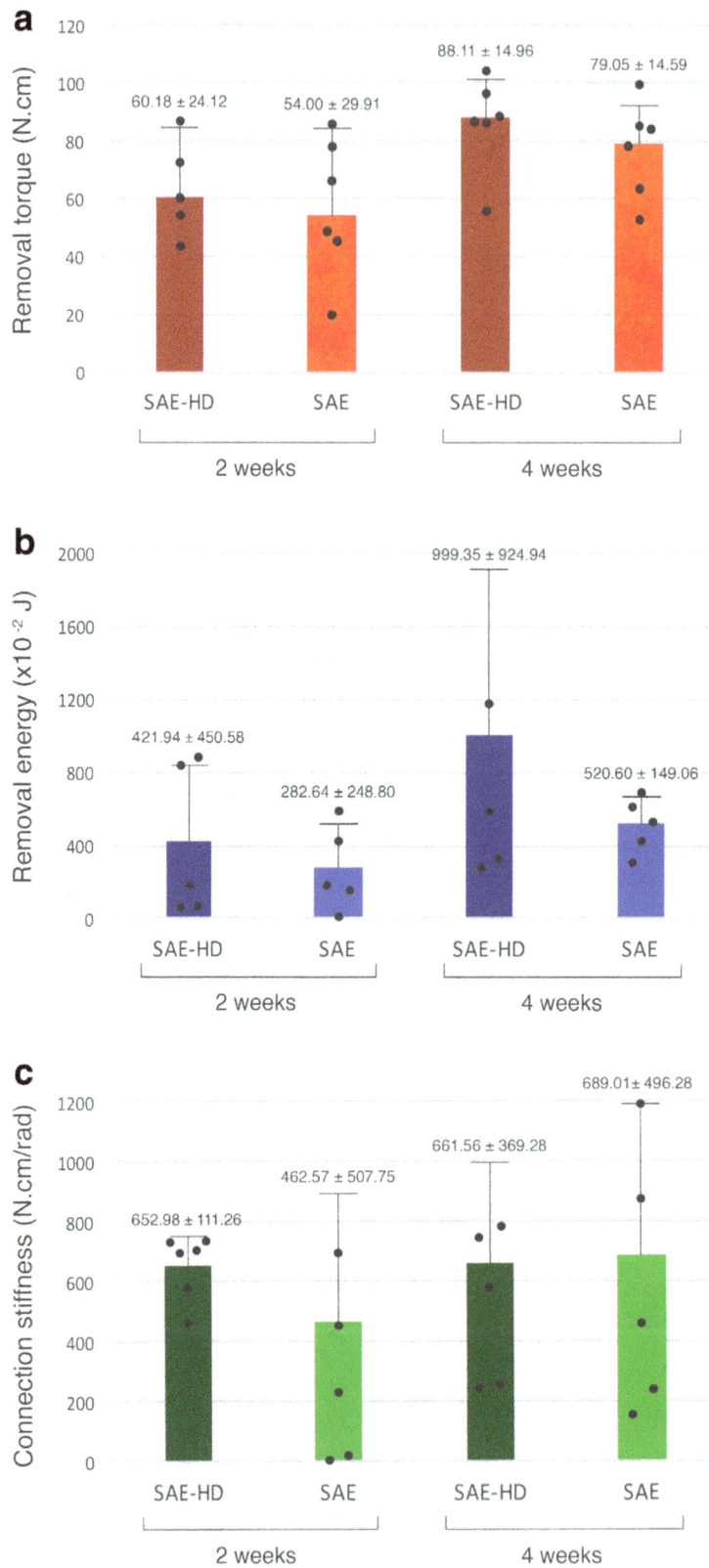

Fig. 5 Mean and standard deviation of the biomechanical data at both observation periods ($P > 0.05$). **a** Removal torque. **b** Removal energy. **c** Connection stiffness

Table 1 One-way ANOVA variance and Tukey's post hoc test values of removal torque (N cm), removal energy [N cm/rad (0.01 J)], and connection stiffness [N cm/rad] for SAE-HD and SAE implants at 2 and 4 weeks postoperatively ($n = 6$; $P < 0.05$)

		Sum of squares	df	Mean square	F	Sig. (P value)
Removal torque	Between groups	4572.571	3	1524.190	3.186	0.06
	Within groups	9569.095	21	478.455		
	Total	14,141.666	24			
Removal energy	Between groups	1,245,769.635	3	415,256.545	1.677	0.16
	Within groups	3,715,217.914	16	247,681.194		
	Total	4,960,987.549	19			
Connection stiffness	Between groups	193,886.351	3	64,628.784	0.396	0.76
	Within groups	3,264,332.301	18	163,216.615		
	Total	3,458,218.652	21			

removal energy compared with the control group at both observation times. Further, SAE-HD implants showed high values in connection stiffness already after 2 weeks of healing, while SAE implants required 4 weeks of healing to reach a similar level. Thus, despite the fact that the differences between the two groups were not significant for any of the evaluated parameters or observation times, the results seem to indicate that differences in surface properties between SAE-HD and SAE implants, somehow influenced osseointegration and intrinsic properties of shear strength. Indeed, greater removal torque values and interfacial stiffness for hydrophilic implants (modSLA)[1] between 2 and 4 weeks, in comparison with SLA[2], have been previously reported [35]. In this study [35], performed in the anterior maxilla of miniature pigs, hydrophilic implants revealed, on average, 8–21 and 9–14% significantly higher removal torque and interfacial stiffness values, respectively, than those of the SLA implants. Due to the remodeling process, the biomechanical parameters decreased with time for both implant surfaces, reflecting the developing biological stability.

It has been previously reported the existence of a correlation between removal torque and %BIC values [26],

although the nature of these parameters differs from one another (three-dimensional versus most often two-dimensional parameter) [36]. Indeed, the lack of differences between the groups herein reflect well the results of the histomorphometric analysis of the other half of implants in the present study, reported elsewhere [31]. In particular, similar amounts of osseointegration in terms of %BIC and bone density were observed in both groups (SAE-HD vs. SAE) at each observation time, and there were no statistically significant differences regarding the respective parameters between the two observations times [31]. In contrast, Sartoretto et al. [27] demonstrated that Acqua® implants (Neodent®), which present similar technology as the SAE-HD implants, resulted in accelerated osseointegration when placed in tibia of rabbits after 2 weeks of healing, compared with implants with the Neoporos® surface, which in turn presents similar technology with the SAE surface. The difference between the study of de Jesus et al. [31] and Sartoretto et al. [27] in terms of the impact of surface technology on histomorphometric osseointegration parameters may be due to anatomical and/or biological differences in the experimental

Table 2 Spearman rank correlation coefficient values between removal torque (N cm), removal energy [N cm/rad (0.01 J)], and connection stiffness [N cm/rad] for SAE-HD and SAE implants at 2 and 4 weeks postoperatively ($n = 6$; $P < 0.01$)

			Removal torque	Removal energy	Connection stiffness
Spearman's rho	Removal torque	Coefficient	1.000	0.722	0.352
		Sig. (two-tailed)		0.000	0.092
		N	24	24	24
	Removal energy	Coefficient	0.722	1.000	(−) 0.091
		Sig. (two-tailed)	0.000		0.710
		N	19	19	19
	Connection stiffness	Coefficient	0.352	(−) 0.091	1.000
		Sig. (two-tailed)	0.092	0.710	
		N	21	21	21

models employed. In this context, although there is no scientific support regarding the optimal experimental model to evaluate aspects of osseointegration, the dog is one of the most commonly used animal platforms [36]. The mandible of dogs is the most frequent location; however, a high percentage of studies on implant integration have used extra-oral implant sites, including the tibia [37]. It is suggested that due to its anatomy, with a large lumen and relatively low trabecular density [38], it possesses high discriminating potential regarding the impact of implant surface technologies to enhance osseointegration. Furthermore, the tibia allows placement of a larger number of implants comparing with the mandible, thus allowing the use of fewer animals and/or multiple types of comparisons/tests (e.g., biomechanical and histological evaluation).

On the other hand, lack of significant differences between the two groups in the present experiment could be due to the fact that the effect of hydrophilicity, in terms of accelerating bone healing and osseointegration, was unfolded before the first evaluation time-point of 2 weeks, i.e., during the very early healing period. Consistently, pre-clinical investigations show the potential of chemically modified surfaces to rapidly modulate the host-to-implant response upon prompt adsorption of blood proteins [20, 22]. In a recent study reported by Vasak et al. [39], hydrophilic implants (SLActive[a]) strengthened the apposition of newly formed bone at the very early healing period between 5 and 10 days in the intra-oral model of minipigs, even though they did not reveal significant statistical differences in comparison to hydrophobic surfaces (SLA). Clinically, a systematic review of human histological studies on molecular aspects of osseointegration [29] has shown that moderately rough implant surfaces with high hydrophilicity enhance molecular processes related to osseointegration during the early stages of wound healing. Similar clinical studies assessed the degree of new bone-to-implant contact (%NBIC) around SLActive implants in comparison to SLA placed in the mandibular retromolar region in man during the early stages of osseointegration [28, 40]. The authors reported a progressive increase in %NBIC around both implants, whereas chemically active surfaces disclosed higher values at 2 and 4 weeks compared with SLA, no longer observed after 6 weeks of osseointegration.

Studies including biomechanical analysis of osseointegration are usually assessing maximum removal torque. Although this parameter is important, use of a single parameter appears not sufficient for a complete biomechanical assessment of osseointegration. Herein, connection stiffness, reflecting the rigidity (i.e., the stability of the implant under load), and removal energy, reflecting the overall energy (workload) necessary to loosen the bone-to-implant connection, were additionally assessed. It is suggested that the use of these three parameters in a complementary manner is essential for complete evaluation of the biomechanical properties of implants. Indeed, two different osseointegrated implants can have the same maximum removal torque, but distinct connection stiffness; similarly, they may show the same removal energy but perform in a very distinct fashion and show distinct connection stiffness and maximum removal torque. To the best of the authors' knowledge, this is the first original research reporting removal energy as an intrinsic removal torque property in relation to connection stiffness during biomechanical assessment of hydrophilic implants; however, removal energy has already been used assessing mini-implants with hydrophobic surfaces [41].

In fact, the observed lack of differences between the groups could be attributed to the relatively low number of specimens per group. According to the observed data herein, applying a high power (80%) with the present sample size would had revealed a relatively large difference in removal torque equivalent to 43% between the experimental groups. Regarding removal energy and connection stiffness, this difference would had been equal to 71 and 34%, respectively. In addition, a significant difference may not had been achieved due to the nature of the specimens. Biological material properties vary greatly from organism to organism and even in the same animal. Therefore, in future studies when using the presented methodology, a greater number of specimens must be considered. This will evidence a superior discrimination capacity. Nonetheless, the current methodology is far more reliable than the use of a single parameter methodology.

Conclusions

No significant differences were observed between the specific hydrophilic (SAE-HD) and hydrophobic (SAE) surfaces evaluated in this study, in terms of biomechanical properties during the early osseointegration period.

Endnotes

[1]Chemically modified sandblasted, large grit, and acid-etched surfaces

[2]Sandblasted, large grit, and acid-etched surfaces

[3]Neodent, Rua Benjamin Lins, 742, Curitiba, PR 80420–100, Brazil

[4]Shimadzu Corporation, Nishinokyo Kuwabara-cho, Nakagyo-ku, Kyoto 604–8511, Japan

[5]IBM Corporation v.23, 1 New Orchard Road, Armonk, New York 10, 504–1722, USA

Acknowledgements
The assistance of fifth-year dental students of the Federal University of Uberlândia in surgeries, including auscultation, and other practicalities is highly appreciated.

Funding
The Brazilian Federal Agency for Support and Evaluation of Graduate Education (CAPES research fellow, Full PhD Program, process no. 0975-14.1) provided funding and Neodent® (Curitiba, PR, Brazil) produced the titanium implants. None of the funding institutions influenced the study design and data collection, analysis, and interpretation or the manuscript writing process.

Authors' contributions
RNRJ participated in the study concept and design and performed the animal operations, biomechanical test, and data analysis and interpretation. EC, PVA, and AR contributed to define the test protocol and performed the biomechanical test and data analysis. CCGM and DZ participated in the study concept and design and performed the animal operations and data analysis. AS contributed to data analysis, interpretation, and drafting of the manuscript. All authors have contributed to and/or critically revised the manuscript and given approval to the final version of the manuscript.

Competing interests
Rainde Naiara Rezende de Jesus, Eunice Carrilho, Pedro V. Antunes, Amílcar Ramalho, Camilla Christian Gomes Moura, Andreas Stavropoulos, and Darceny Zanetta-Barbosa declare that they have no competing interests.

Author details
[1]Department of Periodontology, Faculty of Odontology, Malmö University, Carl Gustafs väg 34, 205-06 Malmö, Sweden. [2]IBILI, Faculty of Medicine, University of Coimbra, Av. Bissaya Barreto, Bloco de Celas, 3000-075 Coimbra, Portugal. [3]CEMUC, Mechanical Engineering Department, University of Coimbra, Pinhal de Marrocos, 3030-788 Coimbra, Portugal. [4]Department of Endodontics, Faculty of Odontology, Federal University of Uberlândia, Av Pará 1720, Bloco4LB, Campus Umuarama, Uberlândia, Minas Gerais 38405-900, Brazil. [5]Department of Oral and Maxillofacial Surgery and Implantology, Faculty of Odontology, Federal University of Uberlândia, Av Pará 1720, Bloco4LB, Campus Umuarama, Uberlândia, Minas Gerais 38405-900, Brazil.

References
1. Cochran DL, Jackson JM, Jones AA, Jones JD, Kaiser DA, Taylor TD, et al. A 5-year prospective multicenter clinical trial of non-submerged dental implants with a titanium plasma-sprayed surface in 200 patients. J Periodontol. 2011; 82(7):990–9. https://doi.org/10.1902/jop.2011.100464.
2. Wallkamm B, Ciocco M, Ettlin D, Syfrig B, Abbott W, Listrom R, et al. Three-year outcomes of Straumann Bone Level SLActive dental implants in daily dental practice: a prospective non-interventional study. Quintessence Int. 2015;46(7):591–602. https://doi.org/10.3290/j.qi.a34076.
3. Baires-Campos FE, Jimbo R, Bonfante EA, Fonseca-Oliveira MT, Moura C, Zanetta-Barbosa D, et al. Drilling dimension effects in early stages of osseointegration and implant stability in a canine model. Med Oral Patol Oral Cir Bucal. 2015;20(4):471–9.
4. Blanco J, Alvarez E, Munoz F, Linares A, Cantalapiedra A. Influence on early osseointegration of dental implants installed with two different drilling protocols: a histomorphometric study in rabbit. Clin Oral Implants Res. 2011; 22(1):92–9. https://doi.org/10.1111/j.1600-0501.2010.02009.
5. Jimbo R, Tovar N, Anchieta RB, Machado LS, Marin C, Teixeira HS, et al. The combined effects of undersized drilling and implant macrogeometry on bone healing around dental implants: an experimental study. Int J Oral Maxillofac Surg. 2014;43(10):1269–75. https://doi.org/10.1016/j.ijom.2014.03.017.
6. Marković A, Čolić S, Šćepanović M, Mišić T, Đinić A, Bhusal DS. A 1-year prospective clinical and radiographic study of early-loaded bone level implants in the posterior maxilla. Clin Implant Dent Relat Res. 2015;17(5): 1004–13. https://doi.org/10.1111/cid.12201.
7. Nicolau P, Korostoff J, Ganeles J, Jackowski J, Krafft T, Neves M, et al. Immediate and early loading of chemically modified implants in posterior jaws: 3-year results from a prospective randomized multicenter study. Clin Implant Dent Relat Res. 2013;15(4):600–12. https://doi.org/10.1111/j.1708-8208.2011.00418.

8. Romanos G, Grizas E, Laukart E, Nentwig GH. Effects of early moderate loading on implant stability: a retrospective investigation of 634 implants with platform switching and Morse-tapered connections. Clin Implant Dent Relat Res. 2016;18(2):301–9. https://doi.org/10.1111/cid.12314.
9. Karabuda ZC, Abdel-Haq J, Arısan V. Stability, marginal bone loss and survival of standard and modified sand-blasted, acid-etched implants in bilateral edentulous spaces: a prospective 15-month evaluation. Clin Oral Implants Res. 2011;22(8):840–9. https://doi.org/10.1111/j.1600-0501.2010.02065.
10. Wall I, Donos N, Carlqvist K, Jones F, Brett P. Modified titanium surfaces promote accelerated osteogenic differentiation of mesenchymal stromal cells in vitro. Bone. 2009;45(1):17–26. https://doi.org/10.1016/j.bone.2009.03.662.
11. Mamalis AA, Markopoulou C, Vrotsos I, Koutsilirieris M. Chemical modification of an implant surface increases osteogenesis and simultaneously reduces osteoclastogenesis: an in vitro study. Clin Oral Implants Res. 2011;22(6):619–26. https://doi.org/10.1111/j.1600-0501.2010.02027.
12. Lotz EM, Olivares-Nasarrete R, Berner S, Boyan BD, Schwartz Z. Osteogenic response of human MSCs and osteoblasts to hydrophilic and hydrophobic nanostructured titanium implant surfaces. J Biomed Mater Res A. 2016; 104(12):3137–48. https://doi.org/10.1002/jbm.a.35852.
13. Chambrone L, Shibli JA, Mercurio CE, Cardoso B, Preshaw PM. Efficacy of standard (SLA) and modified sandblasted and acid-etched (SLActive) dental implants in promoting immediate and/or early occlusal loading protocols: a systematic review of prospective studies. Clin Oral Implants Res. 2015;26(4): 359–70. https://doi.org/10.1111/clr.12347.
14. Heinemann F, Hasan I, Bourauel C, Biffar R, Mundt T. Bone stability around dental implants: treatment related factors. Ann Anat. 2015;199:3–8. https://doi.org/10.1016/j.aanat.2015.02.004.
15. Hinkle RM, Rimer SR, Morgan MH, Zeman P. Loading of titanium implants with hydrophilic endosteal surface 3 weeks after insertion: clinical and radiological outcome of a 12-month prospective clinical trial. J Oral Maxillofac Surg. 2014;72(8):1495–502. https://doi.org/10.1016/j.joms.2014.04.016.
16. Hyzy SL, Olivares-Navarrete R, Hutton DL, Tan C, Boyan BD, Schwartz Z. Microstructured titanium regulates interleukin production by osteoblasts, an effect modulated by exogenous BMP-2. Acta Biomater. 2013;9(3):5821–9. https://doi.org/10.1016/j.actbio.2012.10.030.
17. Hamlet S, Alfarsi M, George R, Ivanovski S. The effect of hydrophilic titanium surface modification on macrophage inflammatory cytokine gene expression. Clin Oral Implants Res. 2012;23(5):584–90. https://doi.org/10.1111/j.1600-0501.2011.02325.
18. Hotchkiss KM, Ayad NB, Hyzy SL, Boyan BD, Olivares-Navarrete R. Dental implant surface chemistry and energy alter macrophage activation in vitro. Clin Oral Implants Res. 2017;28(4):414–23. https://doi.org/10.1111/clr.12814.
19. Rosa AL, Kato RB, Castro Raucci LMS, Teixeira LN, de Oliveira FS, Bellesini LS, et al. Nanotopography drives stem cell fate toward osteoblast differentiation through α1β1 integrin signaling pathway. J Cell Biochem. 2014;115(3):540–8. https://doi.org/10.1002/jcb.24688.
20. Boyan BD, Cheng A, Olivares-Navarrete R, Schwartz Z. Implant surface design regulates mesenchymal stem cell differentiation and maturation. Adv Dent Res. 2016;28(1):10–7. https://doi.org/10.1177/0022034515624444.
21. Mamalis AA, Silvestros SS. Analysis of osteoblastic gene expression in the early human mesenchymal cell response to a chemically modified implant surface: an in vitro study. Clin Oral Implants Res. 2011;22(5):530–7. https://doi.org/10.1111/j.1600-0501.2010.02049.
22. Kato RB, Roy B, De Oliveira FS, Ferraz EP, De Oliveira PT, Kemper AG, et al. Nanotopography directs mesenchymal stem cells to osteoblast lineage through regulation of microRNA-SMAD-BMP-2 circuit. J Cell Physiol. 2014; 229(11):1690–6. https://doi.org/10.1002/jcp.24614.
23. Zhao G, Schwartz Z, Wieland M, Rupp F, Geis-Gerstorfer J, Cochran DL, et al. High surface energy enhances cell response to titanium substrate microstructure. J Biomed Mater Res A. 2005;74((1):49–58. https://doi.org/10.1002/jbm.a.30320.
24. Bang SM, Moon HJ, Kwon YD, Yoo JY, Pae A, Kwon IK. Osteoblastic and osteoclastic differentiation on SLA and hydrophilic modified SLA titanium surfaces. Clin Oral Implants Res. 2014;25(7):831–7. https://doi.org/10.1111/clr.12146.
25. Buser D, Broggini N, Wieland M, Schenk RK, Denzer AJ, Cochran DL, et al. Enhanced bone apposition to a chemically modified SLA titanium surface. J Dent Res. 2004;83(7):529–33. https://doi.org/10.1177/154405910408300704.
26. Gottlow J, Barkarmo S, Sennerby L. An experimental comparison of two different clinically used implant designs and surfaces. Clin Implant Dent Relat Res. 2012;14(Suppl 1):204–12. https://doi.org/10.1111/j.1708-8208.2012.00439.
27. Sartoretto SC, Alves AT, Resende RF, Calasans-Maia J, Granjeiro JM, Calasans-Maia MD. Early osseointegration driven by the surface chemistry

and wettability of dental implants. J Appl Oral Sci. 2015;23(3):279–87. https://doi.org/10.1590/1678-775720140483.

28. Lang NP, Salvi GE, Huynh-Ba G, Ivanovski S, Donos N, Bosshardt DD. Early osseointegration to hydrophilic and hydrophobic implant surfaces in humans. Clin Oral Implants Res. 2011;22(4):349–56. https://doi.org/10.1111/j.1600-0501.2011.02172.

29. Shanbhag S, Shanbhag V, Stavropoulos A. Genomic analyses of early peri-implant bone healing in humans: a systematic review. Int J Implant Dent. 2015;1(1):5. https://doi.org/10.1186/s40729-015-0006-2.

30. Guler AU, Sumer M, Duran I, Sandikci EO, Telcioglu NT. Resonance frequency analysis of 208 Straumann dental implants during the healing period. J Oral Implantol. 2013;39(2):161–7. https://doi.org/10.1563/AAID-JOI-D-11-00060.

31. de Jesus RNR, Stavropoulos A, Oliveira MTF, Soares PBF, Moura CCG, Zanetta-Barbosa D. Histomorphometric evaluation of a dual acid-etched vs. a chemically modified hydrophilic dual acid-etched implant surface. An experimental study in dogs. Clin Oral Implants Res. 2017;28(5):551–7. https://doi.org/10.1111/clr.12833.

32. Frost HM. Skeletal structural adaptations to mechanical usage (SATMU): 1. Redefining Wolff's law: the bone modeling problem. Anat Rec. 1990;226(4): 403–13.

33. Berglundh T, Stavropoulos A; Working Group 1 of the VIII European Workshop on Periodontology. Preclinical in vivo research in implant dentistry. Consensus of the eighth European workshop on periodontology J Clin Periodontol 2012; 39 Suppl 12:1–5. doi: https://doi.org/10.1111/j.1600-051X.2011.01827.

34. Sawase T, Jimbo R, Baba K, Shibata Y, Ikeda T, Atsuta M. Photo-induced hydrophilicity enhances initial cell behavior and early bone apposition. Clin Oral Implants Res. 2008;19(5):491–6. https://doi.org/10.1111/j.1600-0501.2007.01509.

35. Ferguson SJ, Broggini N, Wieland M, de Wild M, Rupp F, Geis-Gerstorfer J, et al. Biomechanical evaluation of the interfacial strength of a chemically modified sandblasted and acid-etched titanium surface. J Biomed Mater Res A. 2006;78((2):291–7. https://doi.org/10.1002/jbm.a.30678.

36. Marin C, Granato R, Suzuki M, Gil JN, Piattelli A, Coelho PG. Removal torque and histomorphometric evaluation of bioceramic grit-blasted/acid-etched and dual acid-etched implant surfaces: an experimental study in dogs. J Periodontol. 2008;79(10):1942–9. https://doi.org/10.1902/jop.2008.080106.

37. Stadlinger B, Pourmand P, Locher MC, Schulz MC. Systematic review of animal models for the study of implant integration, assessing the influence of material, surface and design. J Clin Periodontol. 2012;39(Suppl 12):28–36. https://doi.org/10.1111/j.1600-051X.2011.01835.

38. Pearce AI, Richards RG, Milz S, Schneider E, Pearce SG. Animal models for implant biomaterial research in bone: a review. Eur Cell Mater. 2007;13:1):1–10.

39. Vasak C, Busenlechner D, Schwarze UY, Leitner HF, Munoz Guzon F, Hefti T, et al. Early bone apposition to hydrophilic and hydrophobic titanium implant surfaces: a histologic and histomorphometric study in minipigs. Clin Oral Implants Res. 2014;25(12):1378–85. https://doi.org/10.1111/clr.12277.

40. Bosshardt DD, Salvi GE, Huynh-Ba G, Ivanovski S, Donos N, Lang NP. The role of bone debris in early healing adjacent to hydrophilic and hydrophobic implant surfaces in man. Clin Oral Implants Res. 2011;22(4): 357–64. https://doi.org/10.1111/j.1600-0501.2010.02107.

41. Kim S, Lee S, Cho I, Kim S, Kim T. Rotational resistance of surface-treated mini-implants. Angle Orthod. 2009;79(5):899–907. https://doi.org/10.2319/090608-466.1.

2

The influence of implant–abutment connection on the screw loosening and microleakage

Katsuhiro Tsuruta, Yasunori Ayukawa* ⓘ, Tatsuya Matsuzaki, Masafumi Kihara and Kiyoshi Koyano

Abstract

Background: There are some spaces between abutment and implant body which can be a reservoir of toxic substance, and they can penetrate into subgingival space from microgap at the implant–abutment interface. This penetration may cause periimplantitis which is known to be one of the most important factors associated with late failure. In the present study, three kinds of abutment connection system, external parallel connection (EP), internal parallel connection (IP), and internal conical connection (CC), were studied from the viewpoint of microleakage from the gap between the implant and the abutment and in connection with the loosening of abutment screw.

Methods: We observed dye leakage from abutment screw hole to outside through microgap under the excessive compressive and tensile load and evaluated the anti-leakage characteristics of these connection systems.

Results: During the experiment, one abutment screw for EP and two screws for IP, out of seven samples in each group, were fractured. After the 2000 cycles of compressive tensile loadings, removal torque value (RTV) of abutment screw represented no statistical differences among three groups. Standard deviation was largest in the RTV of EP and smallest in that of CC. The results of microleakage of toluidine blue from implant–abutment connection indicated that microleakage generally increased as loading procedure progressed.

The amount of microleakage was almost plateau at 2000 cycles in CC, but still increasing in other two groups. The value of microleakage greatly scattered in EP, but the deviation of that in CC is significantly smaller. At 500 cycles of loading, there were no significant differences in the amount of microleakage among the groups, but at 1000, 1500, and 2000 cycles of loading, the amount of microleakage in CC was significantly smaller than that in IP. Throughout the experiment, the amount of microleakage in EP was largest, but no statistical difference was indicated due to the high standard deviation.

Conclusions: Within the limitation of the present study, CC was stable even after the loading in the RTV of abutment screw and it prevented microleakage from the microgap between the implant body and the abutment, among the three tested connections.

Keywords: Implant–abutment connection, Microleakage, Microgap, Screw loosening, Toluidine blue, Non-axial load

* Correspondence: ayukawa@dent.kyushu-u.ac.jp
Section of Implant and Rehabilitative Dentistry, Division of Oral
Rehabilitation, Faculty of Dental Science, Kyushu University, 3-1-1 Maidashi,
Higashi-ku, Fukuoka 8128582, Japan

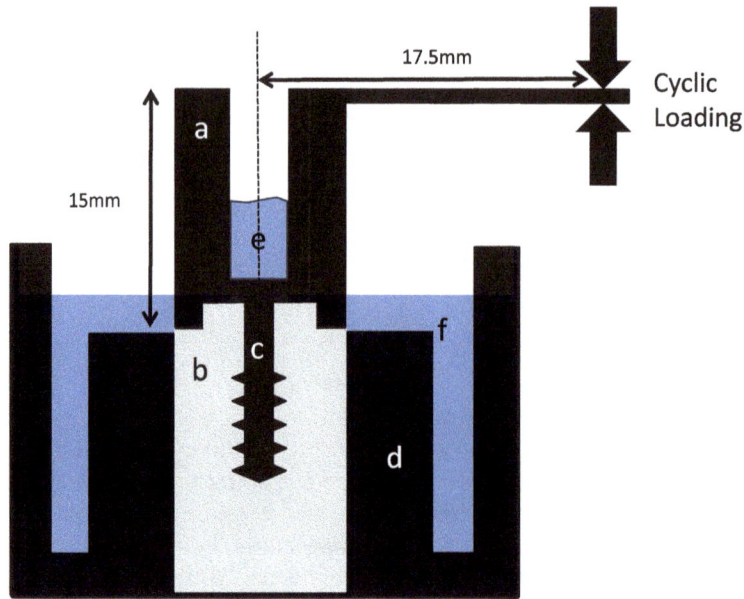

Fig. 1 A scheme of experimental assembly. a: Abutment and superstructure; b: implant body; c: abutment screw; d: steel mold; e: toluidine blue solution; and f: water

Background

Although promising outcome of implant therapy has been reported, periimplantitis which is known to be one of the most important factors associated with late failure [1] is a serious complication and expected to overcome to obtain successful outcome. It is known that there are some spaces between abutment and implant body which can be a reservoir of microorganisms and other toxic substance [2], and they can penetrate into subgingival space from microgap located at the implant–abutment interface. This is believed to impact to periimplant inflammation [3]. Thus, many kinds of implant–abutment connection have been proposed to minimize the microgap [4].

Implant–abutment connection can be divided into three types, external parallel connection (EP), internal parallel connection (IP), and conical connection which has the friction between the implant and the abutment (CC). Nobel Biocare has implant systems with these three kinds of implant–abutment connections, and these connection systems are popular even in other manufacturers and they also employ one or some of these connection systems. These systems have a lot of pros and cons and should be selected depending on the dentists' demand.

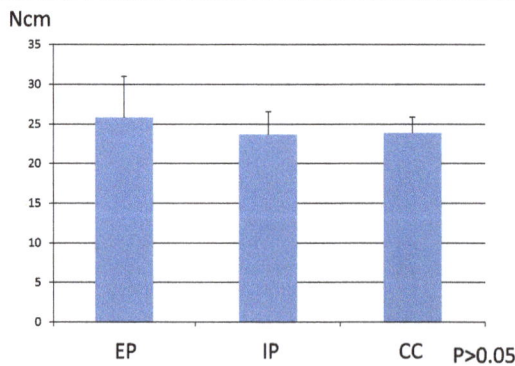

	External(SG)	Internal parallel (REP)	Conical connection (CC)
Removal torque	25.83	23.70	23.88
S.D.	5.19	2.86	1.98

Fig. 2 Removal torque of abutment screw after 2000-cycle loading

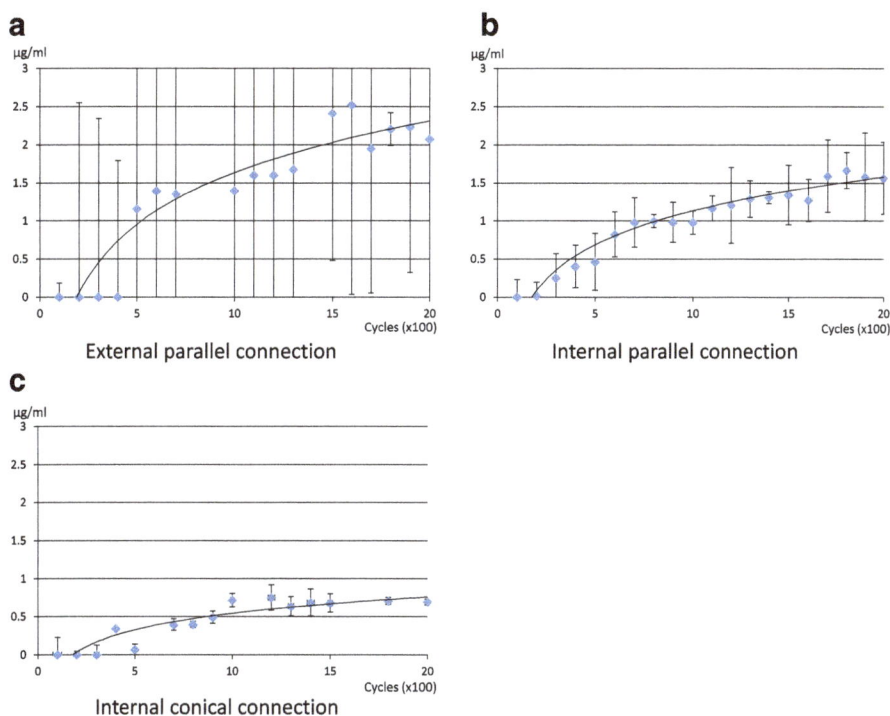

Fig. 3 a Microleakage from external parallel connection implant–abutment connection. Vertical bars indicate standard deviation. **b** Microleakage from internal parallel connection implant–abutment connection. Vertical bars indicate standard deviation. **c** Microleakage from internal conical connection implant–abutment connection. Vertical bars indicate standard deviation

In the present study, we would like to consider these three kinds of connection system from the point of view of microleakage from the gap between the implant and the abutment and in connection with the loosening of abutment screw. We herewith performed the investigation of dye leakage from abutment screw hole to outside through microgap under the excessive cyclic load applied to cantilever superstructure. Cantilever model could simulate non-axial offset loading applied to implant–abutment complex, and toluidine blue solution was used to measure the extravasation from the gap at the implant–abutment interface.

Methods

Three kinds of Nobel Biocare implants were employed in the present study, namely, Nobel SpeedyGroovy WP 5.0×15 mm (EP), Nobel Replace WP 5.0×15 mm (IP), and Nobel Parallel CC RP 5.0×15 mm (CC) ($n = 7$ each) (Nobel Biocare, Kloten, Switzerland). Implant–abutment connections are external, internal parallel, and internal and conical connection, respectively. Implant was embedded into steel mold and fixed with epoxy resin (Araldite®, Nichiban, Tokyo, Japan). A superstructure with cantilever (height 15 mm; length 20 mm from the center of access hole) was fabricated using Au–Pt alloy (Degudent LTG, Degudent, Hanau-Wolfgang, Germany) and fixed with abutment screw with fastening torque recommended by the manufacturer (35 Ncm), using torque wrench (Nobel Biocare). Five hundred microliter of water was poured into steel mold, the surface of water located, to small extent, superior to microgap. Then, 50 µl of 0.05% toluidine blue solution was poured at the access hole (Fig. 1).

This assembly was set in a universal test machine (Autograph AS-1S, Shimadzu, Kyoto, Japan), and load was applied to the cantilever, at 17.5 mm distance from the center of access hole.

As one cycle, one compressive and tensile loads (10 N each) was applied per 1 s and 2000 cycles of loading was done. Before starting load application and every 100 cycles, 100 µl solutions were collected from pool and absorbance at 627 nm was measured using a spectrophotometer (Biospec-mini, Shimadzu). Every 500 cycles, the amount of microleakage was statistically compared using Student t test with Bonferroni correction for multiple comparisons. After the completion of 2000-cycle loading, removal torque value (RTV) of abutment screw was measured.

Results

During the experiment, one (EP) and two (IP) abutment screws out of seven samples were fractured. In this case, abutment screw was changed to new one and experimental procedure was re-run.

a

μg/ml

b

μg/ml

c

μg/ml

d

μg/ml

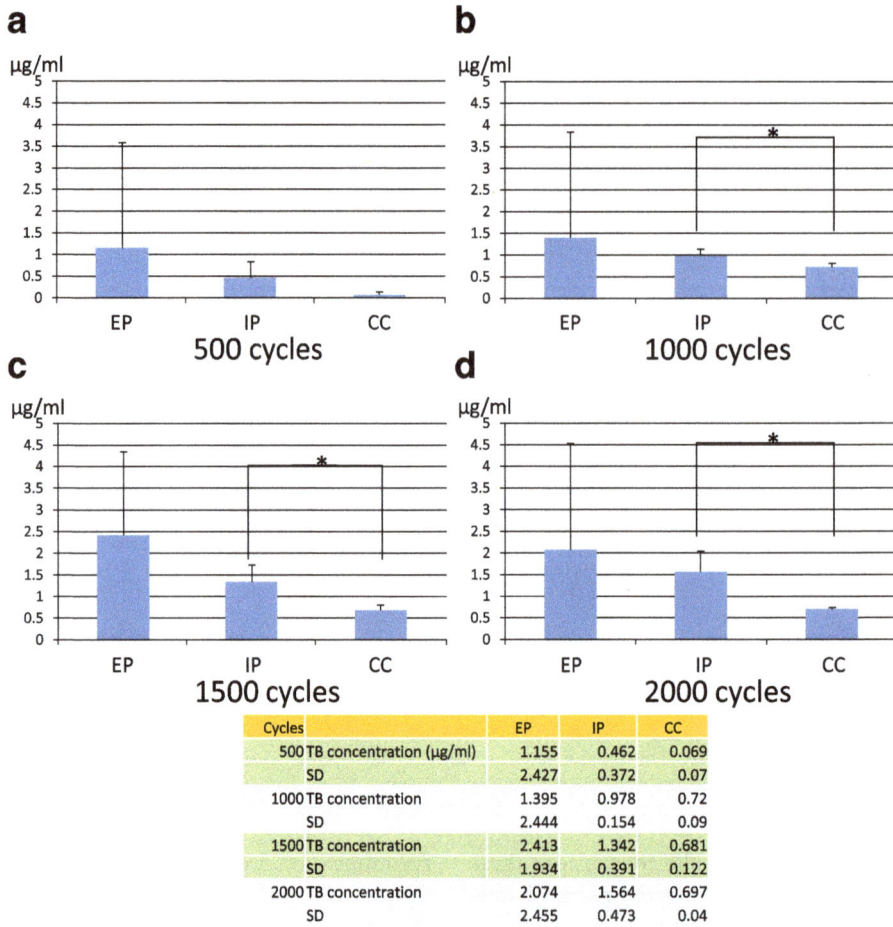

Cycles		EP	IP	CC
500	TB concentration (μg/ml)	1.155	0.462	0.069
	SD	2.427	0.372	0.07
1000	TB concentration	1.395	0.978	0.72
	SD	2.444	0.154	0.09
1500	TB concentration	2.413	1.342	0.681
	SD	1.934	0.391	0.122
2000	TB concentration	2.074	1.564	0.697
	SD	2.455	0.473	0.04

Fig. 4 a Microleakage of toluidine blue from implant–abutment connection at 500 cycles of loading. No statistical difference is indicated ($P > 0.05$). **b** Microleakage of toluidine blue from implant–abutment connection at 1000 cycles of loading. **c** Microleakage of toluidine blue from implant–abutment connection at 1500 cycles of loading. **d** Microleakage of toluidine blue from implant–abutment connection at 2000 cycles of loading. EP external parallel connection, IP internal parallel connection, CC internal conical connection. Asterisk indicates statistically significant difference ($P < 0.05$)

RTV of abutment screw after 2000-cycle loading

After the 2000 cycles of compressive tensile loadings, RTV of abutment screw was measured. There were no statistical differences in the RTV among three groups. Standard deviation was largest in the RTV of EP and smallest in that of CC (Fig. 2).

Microleakage of toluidine blue from implant–abutment connection

All groups indicated that microleakage generally increased as loading procedure progressed (Fig. 3) and logarithmic trendline could be drawn, with R^2 values of 0.854 in EP, 0.924 in IP, and 0.847 in CC. The amount of microleakage was almost plateau at 2000 cycles in CC group (Fig. 3c), but still increasing in other two groups (Fig. 3a, b). The value of microleakage greatly scattered in EP groups (Fig. 3a), but the deviation of that in CC group is significantly smaller (Fig. 3c).

At 500 cycles of loading, there were no significant differences in the amount of microleakage among the groups (Fig. 4a), But at 1000, 1500, and 2000 cycles of loading, the amount of microleakage in CC group was significantly smaller than that in IP group (Fig. 4b–d). There were no statistical differences between EP and other groups in every measurement (Fig. 4).

Discussion

In the present study, cyclic tensile and compressive loading were applied to cantilever superstructure. In the clinical situation, both compressive and tensile force was exerted to implant-supported prosthesis, but no previous study has discussed the microleakage using model study under this situation. In case of conical connection, compressive force may have promoted a higher penetration of the abutments into implant body, which may eliminate microgap [5]. But in the clinical situation, tensile force may also be applied to abutment–implant interface as indicated above; the model employed in the present study may be pertinent.

Some previous model studies which measured the extent of microleakage from implant–abutment interface employed microorganisms [6–9]. These studies focused on bacteria itself using visible solution cloudiness test [6], scanning electron microscopy [7], bacteria viability test [8], or checkerboard DNA–DNA hybridization method [9] and did not mentioned about the bacterial toxin. Toluidine blue employed in the present study can easily be measured using absorptiometry and it was reported to be similar to bacterial toxins in its molecular size [5]. In addition, trend in microleakage was reportedly similar between bacterial leakage model and dye leakage model [10].

In the present study, removal toque of abutment screw after the cyclic loading showed no statistically significant difference among the groups. Generally, conical abutment is believed to be better in fit and stability than non-conical connection [11]. One possibility of this discrepancy may be due to the deformation of abutment screw. Actually, implant–abutment connection after the removal of abutment screw was still tight in CC group, but they were easily divided in other two groups. This may indicate that implant–abutment connection in CC group was almost sound and intact after the loading. In contrast, in EP and IP groups, abutment screw may be deformed which lead to the increase of RTV of abutment screw. The fracture of abutment screws in EP and IP groups may support this speculation. In addition, axial force is strongly affected by the interfacial friction coefficient [12]. In the present study, interfacial friction was supposed to be largest in CC group because the contact area between implant body and abutment was smallest in EP group and both EP and IP groups had parallel walls at the interface with gaps and voids [13, 14]. This may be one reason for the larger standard deviation of RTV in both EP and IP groups.

In the present study, chronological increase of the amount of microleakage was observed in all three groups. This is in consistent with previous studies [5, 13, 15, 16]. Sigmoid curves of microleakage in all groups meant that the amount of leakage was large at the early stage of loading. This was in agreement with previous reports. Harder et al. reported that bacterial toxin leak occurred within 5 min of incubation using in vitro experimental model study, even without application of loading [15, 16].

The comparison of microleakage among the groups at every 500-cycle load indicated that there were no significant differences among the groups at 500-cycle loading but were statistically significant differences in those between IP and CC groups. The reason for microleakage in EP group having no significant differences indicated

between EP and IP or CC groups may be due to the largeness of standard deviation in the value of EP group.

The limitation of the present study was the number of samples. We believed the sample number (seven in each group) was sufficient to obtain the trends of microleakage, but it may be better to investigate using large number of samples to analyze the nature of microleakage at the implant–abutment interface in detail. Another limitation was that the fastening torque applied to screw was not necessarily accurate. To mimic clinical situation, we used dedicated beam-type toque wrench delivered from manufacturer. According to the previous studies, the wrench of Nobel Biocare only reportedly demonstrated the target torque value falling within the 95% confidence interval for the true population mean among four kinds of wrenches [17]. In addition, significantly lower deviations of torque values for beam-type wrenches were reported than for coil and toggle-style wrenches [18]. But toque wrench still has an inaccuracy because the scale printed on the wrench is not fine and it seems to be inappropriate to apply precise torque value. In the present study, we used new torque wrench, but in the clinical settings, variability of toque value may expand because torque wrench is repeatedly used, with sterilization procedure, which decrease the accuracy [19].

Conclusions

Within the limitation of the present study, after the offset cyclic tensile and compressive loading, the amount of microleakage from implant–abutment interface was smaller in conical connection than in internal parallel connection.

Funding
The experiment was done by self-funding.

Authors' contributions
YA contributed to the establishment of the concept of this work, data acquisition and analysis, drafting the paper, and final approval of the work. KT contributed to the establishment of the concept of this work, data acquisition and analysis, drafting the paper, and final approval of the work. TM contributed to the data acquisition and analysis, drafting the paper, and final approval of the work. MK contributed to the data acquisition and analysis, drafting the paper, and final approval of the work. KK contributed to the data acquisition and analysis, drafting the paper, and final approval of the work.

Competing interests
Katsuhiro Tsuruta, Yasunori Ayukawa, Tatsuya Matsuzaki, Masafumi Kihara, and Kiyoshi Koyano declare that they have no competing interests.

References
1. Sakka S, Baroudi K, Nassani MZ. Factors associated with early and late failure of dental implants. J Investig Clin Dent. 2012;3:258–61.
2. Tallarico M, Canullo L, Caneva M, Ozcan M. Microbial colonization at the implant-abutment interface and its possible influence on periimplantitis: a systematic review and meta-analysis. J Prosthodont Res. 2017;61:233–41.

3.   Sasada Y, Cochran DL. Implant-abutment connections: a review of biologic consequences and peri-implantitis implications. Int J Oral Maxillofac Implants. 2017;32:1296–307.

4.   Liu Y, Wang J. Influences of microgap and micromotion of implant-abutment interface on marginal bone loss around implant neck. Arch Oral Biol. 2017;83:153–60.

5.   da Silva-Neto JP, Prudente MS, Dantas TS, Senna PM, Ribeiro RF, das Neves FD. Microleakage at different implant-abutment connections under unloaded and loaded conditions. Implant Dent. 2017;26:388–92.

6.   Aloise JP, Curcio R, Laporta MZ, Rossi L, da Silva AM, Rapoport A. Microbial leakage through the implant-abutment interface of Morse taper implants in vitro. Clin Oral Implants Res. 2010;21:328–35.

7.   Dibart S, Warbington M, Su MF, Skobe Z. In vitro evaluation of the implant-abutment bacterial seal: the locking taper system. Int J Oral Maxillofac Implants. 2005;20:732–7.

8.   Silva-Neto JP, Prudente MS, Carneiro Tde A, Nobilo MA, Penatti MP, Neves FD. Micro-leakage at the implant-abutment interface with different tightening torques in vitro. J Appl Oral Sci. 2012;20:581–7.

9.   do Nascimento C, Barbosa RE, Issa JP, Watanabe E, Ito IY, de Albuquerque Junior RF. Use of checkerboard DNA-DNA hybridization to evaluate the internal contamination of dental implants and comparison of bacterial leakage with cast or pre-machined abutments. Clin Oral Implants Res. 2009;20:571–7.

10. Piattelli A, Scarano A, Paolantonio M, Assenza B, Leghissa GC, Di Bonaventura G, et al. Fluids and microbial penetration in the internal part of cement-retained versus screw-retained implant-abutment connections. J Periodontol. 2001;72:1146–50.

11. Schmitt CM, Nogueira-Filho G, Tenenbaum HC, Lai JY, Brito C, Doring H, et al. Performance of conical abutment (Morse Taper) connection implants: a systematic review. J Biomed Mater Res A. 2014;102:552–74.

12. Egol KA, Kubiak EN, Fulkerson E, Kummer FJ, Koval KJ. Biomechanics of locked plates and screws. J Orthop Trauma. 2004;18:488–93.

13. Tsuge T, Hagiwara Y, Matsumura H. Marginal fit and microgaps of implant-abutment interface with internal anti-rotation configuration. Dent Mater J. 2008;27:29–34.

14. Scarano A, Valbonetti L, Degidi M, Pecci R, Piattelli A, de Oliveira PS, et al. Implant-abutment contact surfaces and microgap measurements of different implant connections under 3-dimensional X-ray microtomography. Implant Dent. 2016;25:656–62.

15. Harder S, Dimaczek B, Acil Y, Terheyden H, Freitag-Wolf S, Kern M. Molecular leakage at implant-abutment connection—in vitro investigation of tightness of internal conical implant-abutment connections against endotoxin penetration. Clin Oral Investig. 2010;14:427–32.

16. Harder S, Quabius ES, Ossenkop L, Kern M. Assessment of lipopolysaccharide microleakage at conical implant-abutment connections. Clin Oral Investig. 2012;16:1377–84.

17. Britton-Vidal E, Baker P, Mettenburg D, Pannu DS, Looney SW, Londono J, et al. Accuracy and precision of as-received implant torque wrenches. J Prosthet Dent. 2014;112:811–6.

18. Neugebauer J, Petermoller S, Scheer M, Happe A, Faber FJ, Zoeller JE. Comparison of design and torque measurements of various manual wrenches. Int J Oral Maxillofac Implants. 2015;30:526–33.

19. Stroosnijder E, Gresnigt MM, Meisberger EW, Cune MS. Loss of accuracy of torque wrenches due to clinical use and cleaning procedure: short communication. Int J Prosthodont. 2016;29:253–5.

3D-evaluation of the maxillary sinus in cone-beam computed tomography

Julia Luz[1]*[iD], Dominique Greutmann[1], Daniel Wiedemeier[2], Claudio Rostetter[1], Martin Rücker[1] and Bernd Stadlinger[1]

Abstract

Background: There are few studies measuring the dimensions of the maxillary sinus, being mostly based on computed tomography imaging and rarely being based on cone-beam computed tomography (CBCT). The aim of this study was to measure the 3D osseous and soft tissue defined volume and surface area of the maxillary sinus. Further, possible associations with patient-specific and sinus-related variables were evaluated.

Methods: A total of 128 maxillary sinuses in 64 patients were analyzed using cone-beam computed tomography data. Surface area and volume of the osseus maxillary sinuses as well as of the remaining pneumatized cavities in cases of obliterated sinuses were calculated by the implant planning software SMOP (Swissmeda AG, Baar, Switzerland). Further, patient-specific general variables such as age, gender, and dentition state as well as sinus-related factors including apical lesions, sinus pathologies, and number of teeth and roots communicating with the maxillary sinus were recorded.

Results: For osseus bordered sinuses, mean surface area was 39.7 cm^2 and mean volume 17.1 cm^3. For the remaining pneumatized cavities, mean surface area was 36.4 cm^2 and mean volume 15 cm^3. The calculated mean volume of obliterated sinuses (42.2% of all sinuses were obliterated) was 5.1 cm^3. Further, an association between the obliterated volume and the presence of pathologies was detected. Male patients showed a significantly higher mean osseus volume compared to female patients. No association was apparent between a patient's age or dentition state and sinus volume, nor for communicating tooth roots and sinus pathologies or unilateral opacity and apical radiolucency. There was also no significant association between bilateral obliterated sinuses and the scan date being in autumn/winter.

Conclusions: The present study showed that the CBCT is suitable for the evaluation of the maxillary sinus. The implant planning software SMOP and its included volume measuring tool are valuable for the analysis of the maxillary sinus, and possible relations with the dentition can be analyzed.

Keywords: Cone-beam computed tomography, CBCT, Digital imaging, Maxillary sinus, Volumetric analysis

Background

The precise assessment of the maxillary sinus is important in oral and maxillofacial surgery in cases of traumatology, sinusitis, and dental implantology. After the introduction of cone-beam computed tomography (CBCT) in dental medicine in 1998 [1], the number of clinicians using CBCTs increased constantly. Whereas in 2004, there were only three CBCTs registered in Switzerland, the current number exceeds 600. The CBCT has become an important diagnostic tool in dental medicine due to its high resolution and its possibility to limit imaging to specific areas of interest. Various specialties in dental medicine like oral and maxillofacial surgery and endodontics increasingly utilize CBCT imaging.

In general dentistry, however, panoramic imaging is still more popular than CBCT. The advantages of panoramic imaging are less radiation, less costs, and its suitability for primary diagnostics. The advantages of CBCT on the other hand are a high image quality of high-contrast structures, no geometric distortion, and no superimposition of surrounding anatomical structures [2].

The aim of this study was to examine the suitability of a volume measuring tool, being included in the implant planning software SMOP (Swissmeda AG, Baar,

* Correspondence: julia.hoehn@zzm.uzh.ch
[1]Clinic of Cranio-Maxillofacial and Oral Surgery, University of Zurich, University Hospital Zurich, Zurich, Switzerland
Full list of author information is available at the end of the article

Switzerland), for the measurement of the 3D shape of the maxillary sinus. Next, this tool was used to measure the volume and surface of the maxillary sinuses. To the best of our knowledge, there is currently no study measuring the osseus and mucosal borders in CBCTs on a 3D level for the analysis of volume reduction due to obliteration. By measuring the osseus and mucosal bordered volume (remaining pneumatized cavity), not only the volume of the obliteration could be calculated, but also possible association between sinus obliteration and the dentition state as well as with the presence of periapical radiolucencies and foreign bodies could be analyzed. Further, possible associations between these measured sinus volumes and patient-specific general variables such as age and gender were evaluated.

Methods

In the present study, 64 CBCT images (128 maxillary sinuses), taken between 1 January 2013 and 31 December 2013 at the Department of Cranio-Maxillofacial and Oral Surgery at the University of Zurich, were included. The inclusion criterion of each CBCT scan was the presence of two complete maxillary sinuses; the osseus borders of both sinuses had to be entirely visible.

The scans were performed using a KaVo 3D eXam CBCT (Biberach, Germany). The settings were 5.0 mA and 120 kV, with a voxel size of 0.125, 0.25, 0.3, or 0.4 mm (exposure time 26.9 s for 0.3/0.4 voxel size or 26.9 s for 0.125/0.25 voxel size). The field of view (FOV) ranged between a height of 10–13.3 cm (patient-adjusted) with a constant diameter of 16 cm.

For the measurement of the maxillary sinus volume, the CBCT images were imported as DICOM files into SMOP, an implant planning software (Swissmeda AG, Baar, Switzerland). This software allows the calculation of volumes (mm^3) and surfaces (mm^2) of a 3D object (e.g., maxillary sinus) by interpolating closed curves.

Using this tool, the volume of each maxillary sinus was calculated by drawing parallel-oriented closed curves in the same coronal plane. Volume measurements were performed in a standardized manner. First, the most posterior and anterior part of each maxillary sinus was defined by placing a curve each in the coronal plane. Next, the space between the two curves was divided into equally sized slices of 2 mm by placing further curves. As a result, a single sinus consisted of 15–25 curves (depending upon the size of the maxillary cavity), having an intercurve distance of 2 mm (Fig. 1).

Some CBCT scans showed sinus cavities that were radiographically partially or fully obliterated indicating a swelling of the mucosa or a sinus pathology. In order to calculate the exact volume of this obliteration, two measurements were performed: first, the sinus volume within the osseus borders was measured by placing the curves on these osseus boundaries. Second, in cases of

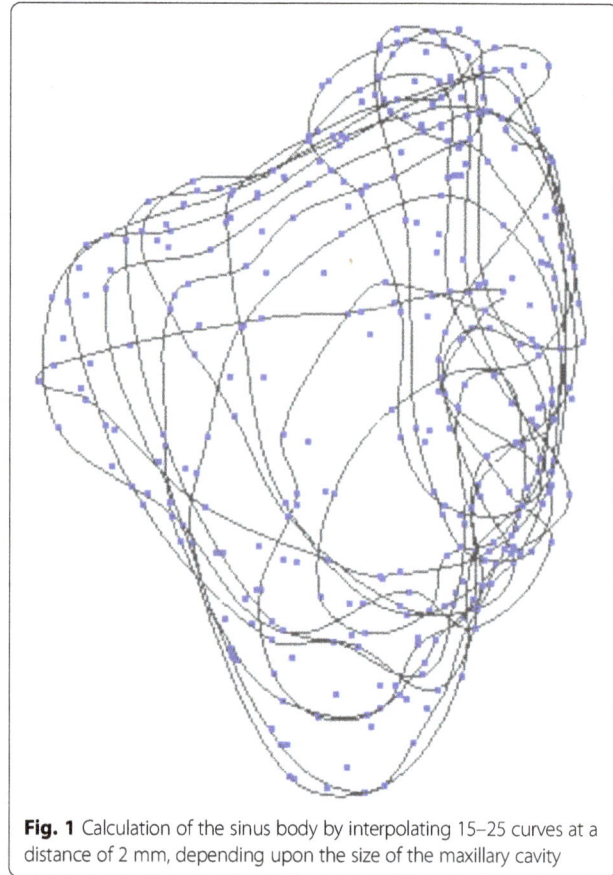

Fig. 1 Calculation of the sinus body by interpolating 15–25 curves at a distance of 2 mm, depending upon the size of the maxillary cavity

obliteration, the curves were placed on the mucous borders within the osseus maxillary sinus, measuring the remaining pneumatized cavity. Next, subtracting the two volumes, the obliterated sinus volume was calculated (Figs. 2 and 3).

Patient-specific variables like gender, date of birth, and date of CBCT were recorded. The date of the CBCT image was further divided into either being in autumn/winter (1 January 2013–19 March 2013; 22 September 2013–31 December 2013) or spring/summer (20 March 2013–21 September 2013). The maxillary sinus was classified into obliterated or nonobliterated. It was also documented if there was a unilateral or bilateral obliteration in the CBCT image. Obliterated cavities were further classified using the following radiographic findings: absence of alteration (0), mucosal thickening (1), sinus polyp (2), complete obliteration (3), mucosal thickening and periapical radiolucency (4), foreign body (5), mucosal thickening and foreign body (6), and nonspecific obliteration (7, partial obliteration, not being defined by the previous criteria). Due to the close relationship between the posterior teeth (premolars, molars) and the maxillary sinus, the teeth starting at the first premolar were recorded as either present or missing, along with the presence or absence of endodontic treatment. Additionally, the number

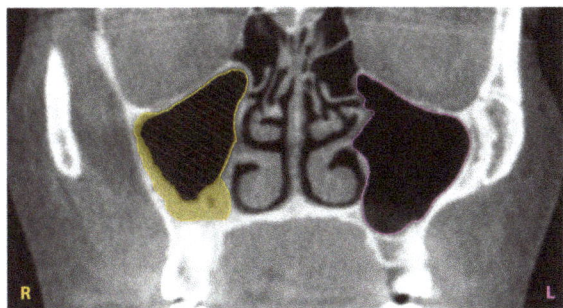

Fig. 2 View from the coronal plane. The marked curves define the osseus and mucous boundaries of the maxillary sinuses. The hatched surface illustrates the measured remaining pneumatized cavity of an obliterated sinus and the filled (yellow) surface highlights the calculated obliterated volume

of teeth and roots communicating with the maxillary sinus and any apical radiolucency was documented.

Statistical analysis

The data was primarily analyzed descriptively. The analysis was performed on two different datasets depending on the main question: either on a sinus level consisting of 128 maxillary sinuses or on a patient level consisting of the respective 64 patients. In cases where sinus-level information was associated with patient-level characteristics (presence of pathology vs. obliterated volume, presence of apical radiolucency vs. obliterated volume, presence of pathology vs. number of communicating roots, dentition status vs. osseus sinus volume), one sinus per patient was randomly chosen for the analysis in order to not violate assumptions of independency for the Wilcoxon rank sum and Kruskal-Wallis tests.

For patient-level analysis, the association between a patient's age and the presence of obliteration was analyzed using logistic regression and patient's age vs. the mean osseus sinus volume was assessed using linear regression. The Wilcoxon rank sum test was used to investigate if there is an association between the mean osseus sinus volume and gender. Differences between osseus sinus volumes on the left and right side of a patient were assessed with the Wilcoxon signed-rank test. Fisher's exact test was used to assess possible associations between bilateral obliteration and the date of the CBCT scan (season of the year) as well as between unilateral obliteration and apical radiolucency. The significance level α was set to 0.05 for all analyses. Calculations were performed using R [3].

Results

Sinus-level analysis

In total, 128 maxillary sinuses were analyzed. The mean surface area was found to be 39.7 cm^2 and the mean volume 17.1 cm^3. The mean surface area of the remaining pneumatized cavities of obliterated sinuses was found to be 36.4 cm^2 and the mean volume 15 cm^3 (Table 1). 42.2% of all sinuses showed an obliteration, and the mean volume of the obliterated sinuses was 5.1 cm^3. If there was an obliteration, on average, 27% of the maxillary sinus was obliterated, and overall, the obliterations ranged between 1 and 95%. The dentition state (edentulous, partly edentulous, or dentate posterior region) had no influence on the size of the osseus sinus volume (Fig. 4, $p = 0.52$).

A total of 73 maxillary sinuses showed unimpaired conditions (57.0%), and 55 showed a pathology (43%). Out of these 55 patients showing a pathology, 30 had a mucosal thickening (23.4%), 17 had a sinus polyp (13.3%), one showed a complete obliteration (0.8%), four had a mucosal thickening and a periapical radiolucency (3.1%), one had a foreign body (0.8%), one had a mucosal thickening and a foreign body (0.8%), and one had a nonspecific opacification (0.8%) (Table 2). Moreover, 20 out of the 55 recorded pathologies were seen in women (36.4%) and 35 in men (63.6%).

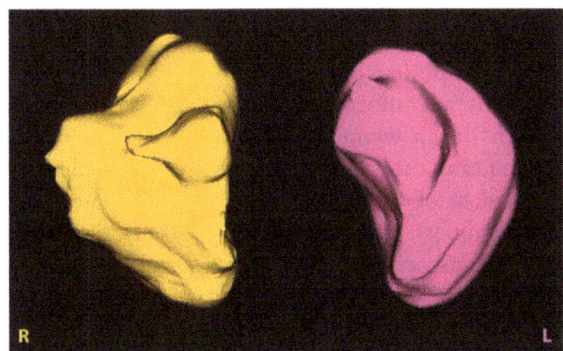

Fig. 3 3D view of osseus sinus volumes. Surface area (cm^2) and volume (cm^3) were calculated by the software

Table 1 Mean, median minimum, maximum, and standard deviation of the surface in square centimeter and volume in cubic centimeter of the osseus maxillary sinuses and the remaining pneumatized cavities in cases of obliterated sinuses as well as mean, median, minimum, maximum, and standard deviation of the calculated obliterated sinus volume in cubic centimeter

	Mean	Median	Minimum	Maximum	SD
Osseus sinus surface area (cm^2)	39.7	39.7	19.1	56.0	7.8
Osseus sinus volume (cm^3)	17.1	16.8	4.0	28.9	4.8
Remaining pneumatized sinus surface area (cm^2)	36.4	36.9	15.3	55.8	8.7
Remaining pneumatized sinus volume (cm^3)	15.0	15.2	0.8	28.0	4.8
Obliterated sinus volume (cm^3)	5.1	3.5	0.1	26.8	4.7

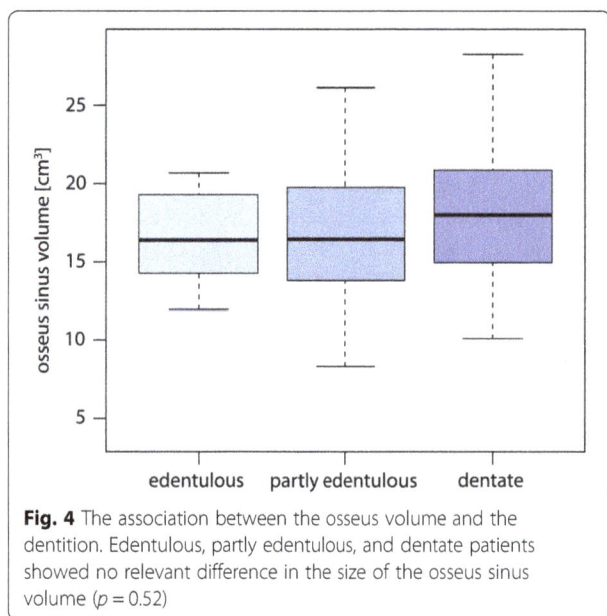

Fig. 4 The association between the osseus volume and the dentition. Edentulous, partly edentulous, and dentate patients showed no relevant difference in the size of the osseus sinus volume ($p = 0.52$)

The presence of a pathology significantly ($p < 0.001$) increased the obliterated volume of a maxillary sinus (Fig. 5). Apical radiolucency, on the other hand, did not increase the obliterated volume of the maxillary sinus ($p = 0.32$). There was also no association between the presence of pathology and the number of communicating roots with the maxillary sinus ($p = 0.62$).

Patient-level analysis

In total, 64 patients were analyzed. Patients had a mean age of 46.2 years. Out of 64 patients, 38 were female (59.4%) and 26 were male (40.6%). Fifty-five patients (85.9%) were dentate or partially dentate and 9 edentulous (14.1%). Fifteen patients (23.4%) had endodontic treatment on at least one tooth in the posterior region of the upper jaw starting from the first premolar. The frequency of teeth communicating with at least one maxillary sinus was 34.4% (22 patients). More than half of the patients (54.7%) had at least one partially or fully obliterated sinus. Out of these 35 patients, 16 had a unilateral obliteration of the maxillary

Table 2 Frequency of pathologies in 128 maxillary sinuses

Frequency of pathologies	n	(%)
Absence of alteration	73	(57.0)
Mucosal thickening	30	(23.4)
Sinus polyp	17	(13.3)
Complete opacity	1	(0.8)
Mucosal thickening and periapical radiolucency	4	(3.1)
Foreign body	1	(0.8)
Mucosal thickening and foreign body	1	(0.8)
Nonspecific opacification	1	(0.8)

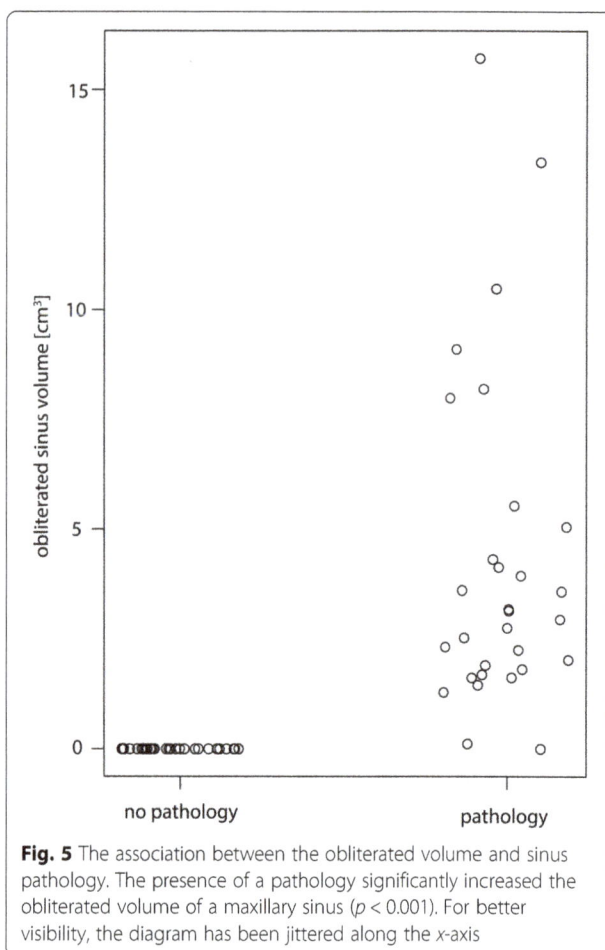

Fig. 5 The association between the obliterated volume and sinus pathology. The presence of a pathology significantly increased the obliterated volume of a maxillary sinus ($p < 0.001$). For better visibility, the diagram has been jittered along the x-axis

sinus (25%) and 19 had a bilateral obliteration (29.7%). Apical radiolucencies were present in 11 patients (17.2%).

No relationship was observed between a patient's age and the presence of partial or complete obliteration of at least one maxillary sinus (Fig. 6, $p = 0.92$). Patient's age and the mean osseus sinus volume were also not associated significantly (Fig. 7, $p = 0.20$). Both maxillary sinuses (osseus borders) of each patient were quite similar in size (mean difference between left and right 0.5 cm^3), yet statistically significant with slightly larger volumes on the left side ($p = 0.045$). Men were found to have a statistically significant higher mean osseus volume (19.0 cm^3) than women (15.5 cm^3) (Fig. 8, $p = 0.007$). No significant association between bilateral obliteration and the date of the CBCT scan (autumn/winter versus spring/summer) could be found ($p = 0.41$). Further, no significant association between unilateral obliterated sinuses and apical radiolucencies was found ($p = 1$).

Discussion

The aim of this study was to analyze volume parameters of the maxillary sinus based on CBCT data. Further,

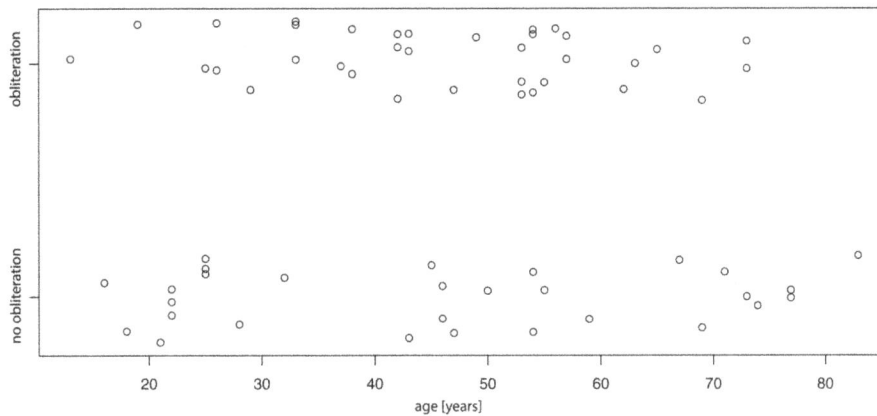

Fig. 6 No statistical significant association between a patient's age and the presence of obliteration of at least one maxillary sinus was found ($p = 0.92$). For better visibility, the diagram has been jittered along the y-axis

neighboring anatomical structures and related pathologies were recorded. Overall, the applied volume software used in this study allowed the calculation of the surface area and volume of maxillary sinuses.

In clinics, the radiographic evaluation of the maxillary sinus is obligatory prior to for example sinus floor elevation. Based on this image, the risk for sinus floor elevation and implant placement can be evaluated. The CBCT data can be further used for later implant placement, using guided techniques. CBCT has been proven to be a valuable tool for the analysis of the maxillary sinus as long as the information provided exceeds the radiological risks [4, 5]. Moreover, its accuracy has been proven [6, 7]. Using CBCT images, anatomical structures may be measured in terms of distances as well as volumes.

Sinus-level analysis

In this study, the measurements were performed using the SMOP volume software. This software was used earlier by another group for the analysis of the 3D shape of nasopalatine duct cysts [8]. The present study measured both the sinus volume within the osseus borders and the remaining pneumatized sinus volume in cases of obliteration. For the osseus bordered sinus, the measured mean sinus volume was 17.1 cm^3, the minimum 4.0 cm^3, and the maximum value 28.9 cm^3. These measurements are quite comparable to the results of other studies [9, 10]. With regard to sinus obliteration, various studies suggest a potential relationship between periapical lesions and mucosal irritation of the maxillary sinus [11–13]. Brook [14] showed that 10–12% of all cases of maxillary sinusitis were caused by teeth. In this study, no association between apical radiolucencies in the upper jaw and sinus obliteration was found. However, it should be mentioned that this study was not designed to observe this relation. In a study, analyzing this association, Nunes et al. [15] selected patients with periapical lesions for a comparison to a group without periapical lesions. Analyzing sinus abnormalities, they showed a relation between periapical lesions and sinus obliteration. Another aspect is the possible

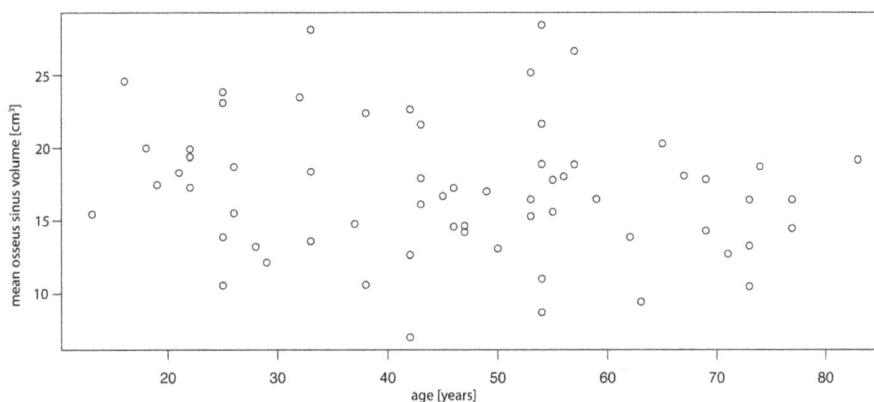

Fig. 7 The association between the mean osseus sinus volume and age. No significant association between these parameters was found ($p = 0.2$)

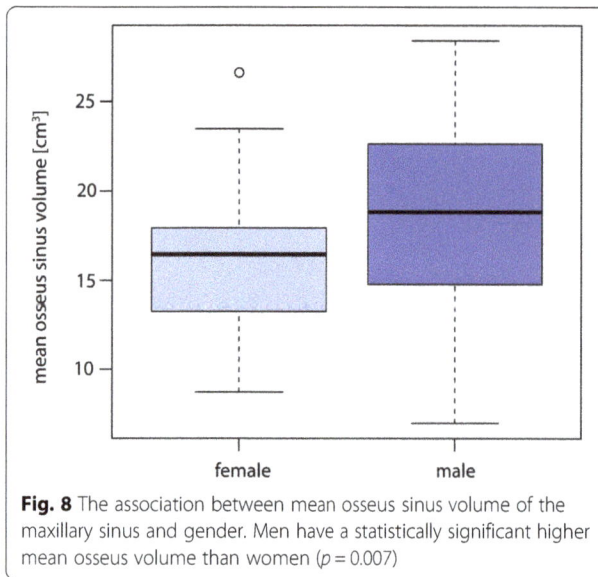

Fig. 8 The association between mean osseus sinus volume of the maxillary sinus and gender. Men have a statistically significant higher mean osseus volume than women ($p = 0.007$)

association between sinus obliteration and the time of the year. In contrast to other studies [16–18], the present study showed no seasonal differences in the presence of obliteration of the maxillary sinus.

Velasco-Torres et al. [19] showed a larger sinus volume for dentate patients compared to edentulous and partially edentulous patients. This may be explained through the loss of posterior teeth in the maxilla, leading to the reduction of mechanical stimulation of the maxillary sinus. As a consequence, the sinus could expand (pneumatization) due to increased pressure and ostoclastic activity of the Schneiderian membrane [7, 20–23]. Another factor of influence may be bone resorption following tooth loss [24]. In the present study, however, no significant association between the sinus volume and the state of dentition could be found.

Patient-level analysis

The results of this study showed a statistically significant smaller mean osseus sinus volume in women compared to men, confirming previous findings [19, 25, 26]. Comparing the bilateral situation, the study showed that both maxillary sinuses (osseus borders) of each participant had similar osseus volumes (mean difference between left and right 0.5 cm^3), thus confirming previous studies [9, 27–30]. Also confirming other studies [29, 30], the results show no association between the participant's age and the maxillary sinus volume. This is in contradiction to Velasco-Torres et al., who showed an increase in sinus volume with the patient's age [19].

A limitation of this study is the analysis of the influence of variable parameters on the dimensions of the sinus, which would have benefitted of a larger study size. Moreover, an examination of data deviation and identification of potential data outliers would have been possible.

Conclusions

The present study showed the volume software to be a suitable tool for the measurement of the dimensions of the maxillary sinus. The results show that the osseus volume of the maxillary sinus varies on the base of gender and that the obliterated volume varies on the base of a present pathology. No statistically significant association between the patient's age and the sinus volume or a present sinus pathology, the scan date (winter/autumn) and a sinus pathology, communicating roots and sinus pathologies, or unilateral obliteration and apical radiolucencies could be found.

Funding
This study was conducted without external funding.

Authors' contributions
BS and JL designed the study. BS was responsible for the approval of the study protocol and the final manuscript. JL performed the radiological analysis and was responsible for the preparation of the manuscript. DG performed the data acquisition and the measurements and was responsible for the preparation of the manuscript. DW performed the statistical analysis. MR edited the manuscript. CR designed the application for ethical approval and edited the manuscript. All authors read and approved the final manuscript.

Authors' information
JL and CR are residents at the Clinic of Cranio-Maxillofacial and Oral Surgery, University of Zurich, University Hospital Zurich, Switzerland.
DG is a master student at the Center of Dental Medicine, University of Zurich, Zurich, Switzerland.
MR is the Chairman of the Clinic for Cranio-Maxillofacial and Oral Surgery, University of Zurich, University Hospital Zurich, Zurich, Switzerland.
DW is the statistician at the Center of Dental Medicine, University of Zurich, Switzerland.
BS is the Chief of Service of the Clinic for Cranio-Maxillofacial and Oral Surgery, University of Zurich, University Hospital Zurich, Zurich, Switzerland.

Competing interests
Julia Luz, Dominique Greutmann, Daniel Wiedmeier, Claudio Rostetter, Martin Rücker, and Bernd Stadlinger declare that they have no competing interests.

Author details
[1]Clinic of Cranio-Maxillofacial and Oral Surgery, University of Zurich, University Hospital Zurich, Zurich, Switzerland. [2]Statistical Services, Center of Dental Medicine, University of Zurich, Zurich, Switzerland.

References

1. Mozzo P, Procacci C, Tacconi A, Martini PT, Andreis IAB. A new volumetric CT machine for dental imaging based on the cone-beam technique: preliminary results. Eur Radiol. 1998;8(9):1558–64.
2. Price JB, Thaw KL, Tyndall DA, Ludlow JB, Padilla RJ. Incidental findings from cone beam computed tomography of the maxillofacial region: a descriptive retrospective study. Clin Oral Implants Res. 2012;23(11):1261–8.
3. Team RC. A language and environment for statistical computing. R Foundation for Statistical Computing, 2015; Vienna, Austria 2016.
4. Chau AC, Fung K. Comparison of radiation dose for implant imaging using conventional spiral tomography, computed tomography, and cone-beam computed tomography. Oral Surg Oral Med Oral Pathol Oral Radiol Endod. 2009;107(4):559–65.
5. Loubele M, Jacobs R, Maes F, Denis K, White S, Coudyzer W, et al. Image quality vs radiation dose of four cone beam computed tomography scanners. Dento Maxillo Facial Radiology. 2008;37(6):309–18.

6. Pinsky HM, Dyda S, Pinsky RW, Misch KA, Sarment DP. Accuracy of three-dimensional measurements using cone-beam CT. Dento Maxillo Facial Radiology. 2006;35(6):410–6.

7. Tolstunov L, Thai D, Arellano L. Implant-guided volumetric analysis of edentulous maxillary bone with cone-beam computerized tomography scan. Maxillary sinus pneumatization classification. J Oral Implantol. 2012; 38(4):377–90.

8. Suter VG, Warnakulasuriya S, Reichart PA, Bornstein MM. Radiographic volume analysis as a novel tool to determine nasopalatine duct cyst dimensions and its association with presenting symptoms and postoperative complications. Clin Oral Investig. 2015;19(7):1611–8.

9. Fernandes CL. Volumetric analysis of maxillary sinuses of Zulu and European crania by helical, multislice computed tomography. J Laryngol Otol. 2004; 118(11):877–81.

10. Jun BC, Song SW, Park CS, Lee DH, Cho KJ, Cho JH. The analysis of maxillary sinus aeration according to aging process; volume assessment by 3-dimensional reconstruction by high-resolutional CT scanning. Otolaryngology Head Neck Surgery. 2005;132(3):429–34.

11. Mehra P, Murad H. Maxillary sinus disease of odontogenic origin. Otolaryngol Clin N Am. 2004;37(2):347–64.

12. Mehra P, Jeong D. Maxillary sinusitis of odontogenic origin. Curr Allergy Asthma Rep. 2009;9(3):238–43.

13. Lee KC, Lee SJ. Clinical features and treatments of odontogenic sinusitis. Yonsei Med J. 2010;51(6):932–7.

14. Brook I. Sinusitis of odontogenic origin. Otolaryngology Head Neck Surgery. 2006;135(3):349–55.

15. Nunes CA, Guedes OA, Alencar AH, Peters OA, Estrela CR, Estrela C. Evaluation of periapical lesions and their association with maxillary sinus abnormalities on cone-beam computed tomographic images. J Endod. 2016;42(1):42–6.

16. Beaumont C, Zafiropoulos G-G, Rohmann K, Tatakis DN. Prevalence of maxillary sinus disease and abnormalities in patients scheduled for sinus lift procedures. J Periodontol. 2005;76(3):461–7.

17. Tarp B, Fiirgaard B, Christensen T, Jensen JJ, Black FT. The prevalence and significance of incidental paranasal sinus abnormalities on MRI. Rhinology. 2000;38(1):33–8.

18. Casamassimo PS, Lilly GE. Mucosal cysts of the maxillary sinus: a clinical and radiographic study. Oral Surgery Oral Medicine Oral Pathology. 1980;50(3): 282–6.

19. Velasco-Torres M, Padial-Molina M, Avila-Ortiz G, Garcia-Delgado R, O'Valle F, Catena A, et al. Maxillary sinus dimensions decrease as age and tooth loss increase. Implant Dent. 2017;26(2):288–95.

20. Sharan A, Madjar D. Maxillary sinus pneumatization following extractions: a radiographic study. Int J Oral Maxillofac Implants. 2008;23(1):48–56.

21. Barak MM, Lieberman DE, Hublin JJ. A Wolff in sheep's clothing: trabecular bone adaptation in response to changes in joint loading orientation. Bone. 2011;49(6):1141–51.

22. Chappard D, Basle MF, Legrand E, Audran M. Trabecular bone microarchitecture: a review. Morphologie. 2008;92(299):162–70.

23. Lang NP, Lindhe J. Clinical periodontology and implant dentistry, vol. 2. Set: John Wiley & Sons; 2015.

24. Hamdy RM, Abdel-Wahed N. Three-dimensional linear and volumetric analysis of maxillary sinus pneumatization. J Adv Res. 2014;5(3):387–95.

25. Unruh AM. Gender variations in clinical pain experience. Pain. 1996;65(2–3): 123–67.

26. Mohlhenrich SC, Heussen N, Peters F, Steiner T, Holzle F, Modabber A. Is the maxillary sinus really suitable in sex determination? A three-dimensional analysis of maxillary sinus volume and surface depending on sex and dentition. Journal of Craniofacial Surgery. 2015;26(8):e723–6.

27. Ariji Y, Kuroki T, Moriguchi S, Ariji E, Kanda S. Age changes in the volume of the human maxillary sinus: a study using computed tomography. Dento Maxillo Facial Radiology. 1994;23(3):163–8.

28. Ariji Y, Ariji E, Yoshiura K, Kanda S. Computed tomographic indices for maxillary sinus size in comparison with the sinus volume. Dento Maxillo Facial Radiology. 1996;25(1):19–24.

29. Uchida Y, Goto M, Katsuki T, Akiyoshi T. A cadaveric study of maxillary sinus size as an aid in bone grafting of the maxillary sinus floor. J Oral Maxillofac Surg. 1998;56(10):1158–63.

30. Uchida Y, Goto M, Katsuki T, Soejima Y. Measurement of maxillary sinus volume using computerized tomographic images. Int J Oral Maxillofac Implants. 1998;13(6):811–8.

4

Impact of surgical management in cases of intraoperative membrane perforation during a sinus lift procedure: a follow-up on bone graft stability and implant success

Benedicta E. Beck-Broichsitter[1*], Dorothea Westhoff[2], Eleonore Behrens[2], Jörg Wiltfang[2] and Stephan T. Becker[2]

Abstract

Background: Until now, sinus floor elevation represents the gold standard procedure in the atrophic maxilla in order to facilitate dental implant insertion. Although the procedure remains highly predictive, the perforation of the Schneiderian membrane might compromise the stability of the augmented bone and implant success due to chronic sinus infection. The aim of this retrospective cohort study was to show that a membrane tear, if detected and surgically properly addressed, has no influence on the survival of dental implants and bone resorption in the augmented area.

Methods: Thirty-one patients with 39 perforations could be included in this evaluation, and a control group of 32 patients with 40 sinus lift procedures without complications were compared regarding the radiographically determined development of bone level, peri-implant infection, and implant loss.

Results: Implant survival was 98.9% in the perforation group over an observation period of 2.7 ($\pm$ 2.03) years compared to 100% in the control group after 1.8 ($\pm$ 1.57) years. The residual bone level was significantly lower in the perforation group ($p = 0.05$) but showed no difference direct postoperatively ($p = 0.7851$) or in the follow-up assessment ($p = 0.2338$). Bone resorption remained not different between both groups ($p = 0.945$). A two-stage procedure was more frequent in the perforation group ($p = 0.0003$) as well as peri-implantitis ($p = 0.0004$).

Conclusions: Within the limits of our study, the perforation of the Schneiderian membrane did not have a negative impact on long-term graft stability or the overall implant survival.

Keywords: Sinus floor elevation, Intraoperative complication, Perforation, Schneiderian membrane, Implant survival

Background

Sinus floor elevation procedures have become a predictable and successful treatment, performed when the maxillary alveolar ridge is atrophied and the bone height is not sufficient for primary implantation. If the postoperative course remains uneventful, the outcome is highly predictable [1–3]. However, complications may have a negative impact on the overall treatment success. As a common complication, perforation of the Schneiderian membrane occurs in 12 to 44% of cases depending on

the literature [2, 4–6], with an average of 20 to 25% [7–9] in all cases due to septa morphological aspects of the membrane or other pathologic conditions; the perforation itself represents the major intraoperative complication despite common complications, such as postoperative infection [5, 10].

Still, it is not completely clear to what extent these complications influence implant survival or might impact the augmented material in the sinus. To evaluate the impact of early-onset complications during implant insertion on the implant success, Becker et al. published a follow-up study evaluating the first year after a sinus lift procedure [11], which did not reveal a negative impact on implant survival after an observation period of

* Correspondence: benedicta.beck-broichsitter@charite.de
[1]Department of Oral and Maxillofacial Surgery, Charité–University Medical Center Berlin, Augustenburger Platz 1, 13353 Berlin, Germany
Full list of author information is available at the end of the article

162 days. In contrast to these results, a study by Nolan et al. retrospectively re-assessed a total of 359 sinus augmentation procedures with a perforation rate of 41.8% (150 patients) at least 1 year after implant loading and reported a graft failure rate of 6.7%, in which 70.8% of membranes were perforated. In a study by Sakkas et al. [12], membrane tear (perforation rate 10.8%) was slightly not significantly associated with postoperative complications in 105 sinus lift procedures. A highly significant connection was shown in a study by Schwartz-Arad et al. [5], but these complications reportedly had no impact on implant survival.

In this retrospective study, the patient cohort with perforations of the Schneiderian membrane from the previously reported study [11] was re-evaluated to specifically assess local bone remodeling and resorption processes in the augmented area, signs of chronic infection of the sinus, and implant survival compared to a group of patients without a membrane tear over a longer time period. We hypothesize that if detected and properly handled surgically or with an adequate adaption of the surgical protocol, a perforation of the Schneiderian membrane would not endanger the outcome parameters of stable bone augmentation and promotion of signs of peri-implant disease and implant loss.

Methods
Patient recruitment
In accordance with the WMA Declaration of Helsinki—Ethical Principles for Medical Research Involving Human Subjects, approval was given by the local ethics committee of the Christian-Albrechts-University in Kiel (AZ 132/10). All patients gave informed written consent to participate.

A total of 201 sinus floor elevation procedures, which were performed from 2005 to 2006 in the Department of Oral and Maxillofacial Surgery of the University Hospital of Kiel, were primarily included in this retrospective cohort study. Within this cohort, 41 perforations (20.4%) of the Schneiderian membrane in 33 patients (21 female, 12 male) occurred. One patient was deceased, and one patient did not engage in the follow-up offered by the department. After exclusion of these two patients, a total of 31 patients aged 60.86 (± 11.21) years with 39 perforations were available to participate in regular recall examinations with an average observation time of 2.69 years (± 2.04 years). According to this study group, 32 patients with 40 sinus lift procedures without perforations aged 58.76 years (± 9.43) were randomized from the cohort to represent the control group (average observation time 2.14 years ± 1.85 years). Patients were recruited from the established recall system in the department. Requirements of inclusion were engagement in at least three follow-up visits after dental implantation

and receiving dental implants in the department, if a two-stage procedure was performed. The inclusion rate of patients in the control group was 33.28%. In total, 56.16% of patients (54 patients) within the control group had not completed the follow-up visits for various reasons (relocation, impairment because of age, follow-up performed elsewhere) and therefore were excluded. Sixteen patients received implants in other private practices (16.64%), and 2 patients were deceased.

Medical record assessment
The manufacturer and position of implants were previously extracted from surgical reports in the medical record, as were in-house treated implant failures and consecutive explanation procedures. Vertical bone augmentation was additionally classified dependent on donor site (none/linea obliqua/iliac crest/scapula).

Implant therapy
Three different oral and maxillofacial surgeons performed the sinus lift procedure with an external approach according to comparable surgical standards and inserted all implants examined in this study in a submerged protocol with uncovering after 3–4 months due to the manufacturer's surgical recommendations. Specifically, a total of 35 external sinus floor elevations were performed through a bone window in the facial aspect of the maxillary sinus. The internal sinus lift approach was applied once. In four patients, sinus floor elevation was accompanied with a LeFort I osteotomy or in one case with a reconstruction of the maxilla after tumor surgery. Preexisting defects were assumed due to trauma or previous surgical interventions in three operation sites.

For sinus floor augmentation including defects of less than 2 cm^3, bone filter material and bone substitute [13, 14] were applied. If the defect exceeded 2 cm^3, only autologous bone was used.

Perforations up to a diameter of 5 mm in size were covered with a BioGide membrane (Geistlich, Wolhusen, Switzerland), and perforations beyond a diameter of 5 mm up to 10 mm were additionally stitched with resorbable sutures (Vicryl 6-0, Ethicon, Norderstedt, Germany) while larger defects led to termination of the procedure. Only in exceptional cases were perforations left untreated or sealed with fibrin glue.

Implants were either placed in a one-stage procedure accompanied with the sinus floor elevation or in a two-stage procedure if primary stability might not be achieved due to the bone being present.

Patients received antibacterial mouth rinse, systemic antibiotics, nose drops, and inhalants from 7 to 10 days beginning directly after the operation. Sutures were removed 7 to 10 days after the surgical procedure. All patients were instructed how to maintain appropriate

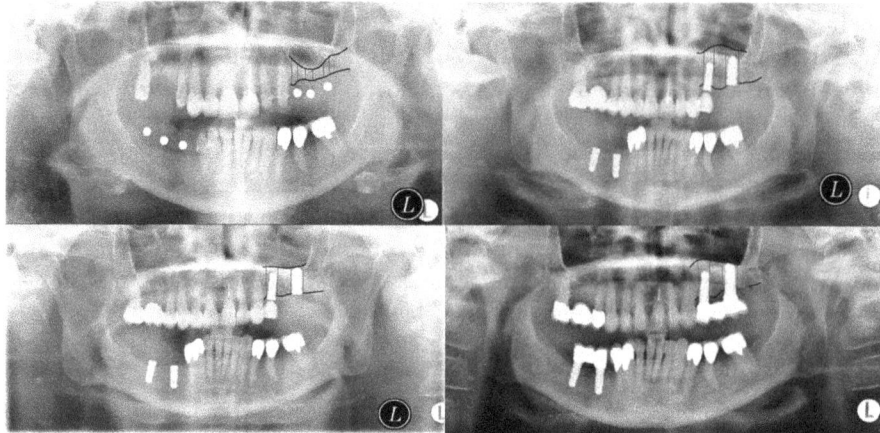

Fig. 1 Bone levels after sinus floor elevation

oral hygiene directly after surgical intervention and were re-instructed after the uncovering procedure and during recall sessions. Patients were further asked to join for regular recall examinations after prosthodontic rehabilitation and thereafter each year. Six months after sinus floor elevation, panoramic radiographs were made.

Clinical assessment

One independent oral and maxillofacial surgeon performed the clinical follow-up examinations according to a standardized protocol. A peri-implant probing including probing pocket depths and recessions on four sites of each implant was assessed as was bleeding on probing (BOP) to determine the status of oral hygiene objectively. Signs of gingivitis and pus suppuration were also recorded. The criteria of peri-implantitis were based on those published by Ong et al. [15]: peri-implant probing depth ≥ 5 mm and bleeding on probing and/or suppuration and radiographic bone loss ≥ 2.5 mm.

Based on panoramic radiographs, marginal bone levels were measured on the distal and mesial sites of each implant. Bone loss was calculated based on the known implant length and the radiographic magnification

factors accordingly. Distances were measured to the nearest millimeter. Bone levels after sinus floor elevation were compared to bone levels in follow-up (Fig. 1).

The implant success rate was defined as the absence of patients' complaints and objective signs of peri-implant inflammation (bleeding on probing, peri-implantitis, dehiscence defects, and implant stability).

Statistical assessment

Statistical data analyses were performed using GraphPad Prism version 6.0 (GraphPad Software, La Jolla, CA, USA). Descriptive statistics (mean value, standard deviation, and percentage distribution) were calculated, and the data were checked for Gaussian distribution applying the Shapiro-Wilk test. Comparisons between the groups with and without perforation were assessed with non-parametric statistic testing (Mann-Whitney-U-Wilcoxon). Fisher's exact test was applied for combinations of factors, and implant survival was displayed in a Kaplan-Meier plot. Multiple comparisons according to Tukey were applied in cases of further subdivision of the

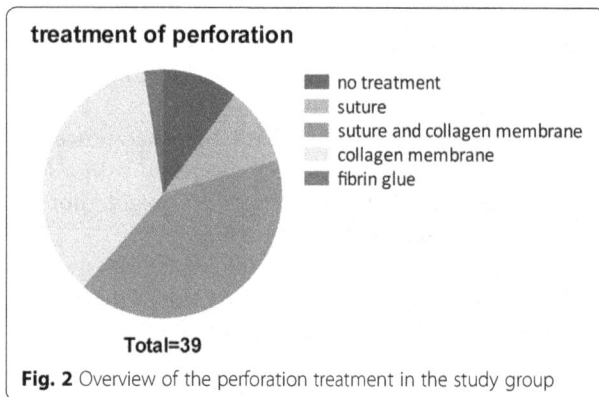

treatment of perforation

- no treatment
- suture
- suture and collagen membrane
- collagen membrane
- fibrin glue

Total=39

Fig. 2 Overview of the perforation treatment in the study group

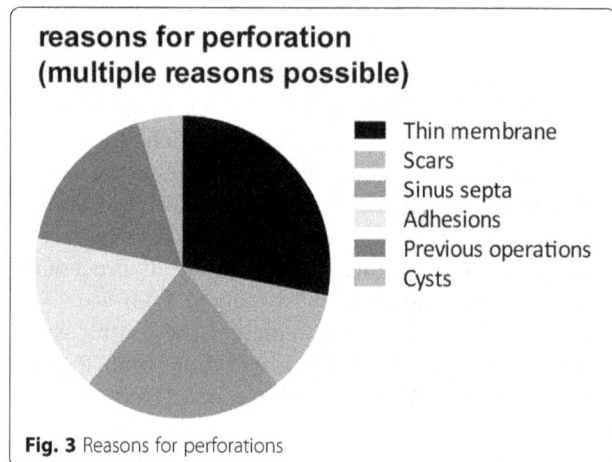

reasons for perforation (multiple reasons possible)

- Thin membrane
- Scars
- Sinus septa
- Adhesions
- Previous operations
- Cysts

Fig. 3 Reasons for perforations

Table 1 Distribution of implant positions

Implant position	3		4		5		6		7		8	
Perforation group	7	7.6%	23	25.0%	27	29.4%	30	32.6%	5	5.4%	0	0%
Control group	9	10.8%	20	24.1%	25	30.1%	21	25.3%	7	8.4%	1	1.2%

datasets. If the probability of error was less than 5%, the result was presented as statistically significant.

Results

Descriptive statistical evaluation

Perforation group

The mean control interval was 2.69 (± 2.03) years. At the time of the follow-up examination, the average age was 59.95 (± 11.82) years.

In the remaining collective of 31 patients (96.97%; 12 males (37.54%) and 19 females (59.43%)), a total of 92 implants were inserted. The overview of perforation treatment in the study group is given in Fig. 2, and Fig. 3 depicts the reasons for perforations. Eleven implants (11.96%) were inserted in a one-stage procedure, whereas the remaining 81 implants (88.04%) were inserted in a second surgical intervention. One implant (1.09%) had to be removed due to wound infection 3 months after implant insertion. After a 6-month healing period, the implant could be successfully replaced.

Many implants were purchased from Nobel Biocare with a total of 33 (35.87%), followed by Camlog with 24 (26.09%), Straumann with 18 (19.57%), Ankylos with 10 (10.87%), and Frialit with 5 implants (5.43%). The Astra implant system was applied twice (2.17%).

Twelve implants showed a probing depth above 3 mm; bleeding on probing was positive in 7 implants, and 6 implants showed signs of peri-implantitis or patients had previously had peri-implant surgery.

Control group

The patients' (16 female, 15 male) mean age included in this group was 59.32 years (± 11.34 years) with a mean observation period of 1.80 years (± 1.57 years).

A total of 83 implants were inserted, of which 30 implants were inserted in a one-stage procedure and 53 in a two-stage procedure. No implant had to be removed during the observation period.

Forty-two implants were purchased from Camlog (50.6%), followed by Nobel Biocare with 22 implants

(26.51%), Straumann with 18 implants (21.69%), and one Astra implant (1.2%). No signs of inflammation or peri-implantitis were detected in the clinical examinations.

Group comparison

The preferred implant positions in both groups are depicted in Table 1, showing a homogenous distribution when comparing both groups. Table 2 provides an overview of bone graft origin. In the control group, the majority of procedures (65.1%) did not require an additional bone graft, whereas 59.8% of surgical interventions required iliac crest in the perforation group.

The initial bone level differed significantly ($p = 0.05$) between both groups with a median value of 5.69 mm in the study group and 3.87 mm in the control group (Fig. 4). A Mann-Whitney-U-Wilcoxon test revealed no significant difference between bone level postoperatively ($p = 0.7851$; median value control group 17.40 mm; median value perforation group 16.91 mm), in follow-up ($p = 0.2238$; median value control group 13.88 mm; median value perforation group 13.31 mm), or for bone resorption ($p = 0.9455$, median value study/perforation group 3.45 mm; Fig. 5). The data are further summarized in Table 3.

Groups were further subdivided and separated at an initial bone level of 4 mm, above which the sinus lift procedure is considered a relative indication for achievement of primary stability [16]. Regarding the height of augmented sinus floor postoperatively, a multiple comparison analysis revealed a significant difference between the groups. The adjusted p values of multiple comparisons are depicted in Table 4. Interestingly, only two group comparisons revealed a relevant difference. Multiple comparisons of bone resorption in subgroups did not reveal a statistically significant difference ($p = 0.1418$).

Fisher's exact test revealed a statistically significant difference of proportions of one-stage versus two-stage procedures due to the presence of perforation ($p = 0.0003$; Table 5) and a significantly higher trend for peri-implantitis in patients with perforation ($p = 0.0004$; Table 6).

Table 2 Origin of bone graft

Origin of bone graft	No bone graft		Linea obliqua		Iliac crest		Scapula flap	
Perforation group	15	16.3%	22	23.9%	55	59.8%	0	0%
Control group	54	65.1%	11	13.3%	13	15.7%	5	6.02%

bone level preoperatively

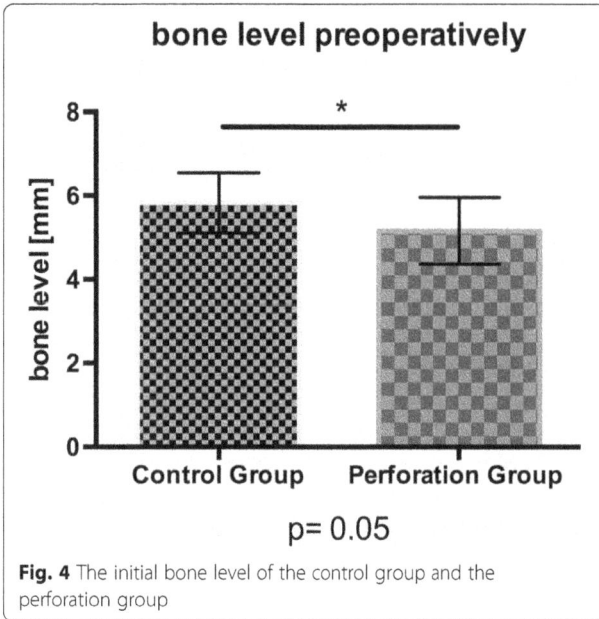

Fig. 4 The initial bone level of the control group and the perforation group

Discussion

The aim of this retrospective cohort study was to evaluate the impact of intraoperative perforations of the Schneiderian membrane during sinus floor elevation on the stability of the augmented area and its influence on osseointegration after implant insertion. Therefore, we could re-assess a patient cohort of originally 34 patients with 41 perforations and compare their outcome with a control group of patients with sinus floor elevation but without membrane tear, offering a long-term perspective over a range of 1.8 years in the control group to 2.7 years in the study group.

bone resorption in follow-up

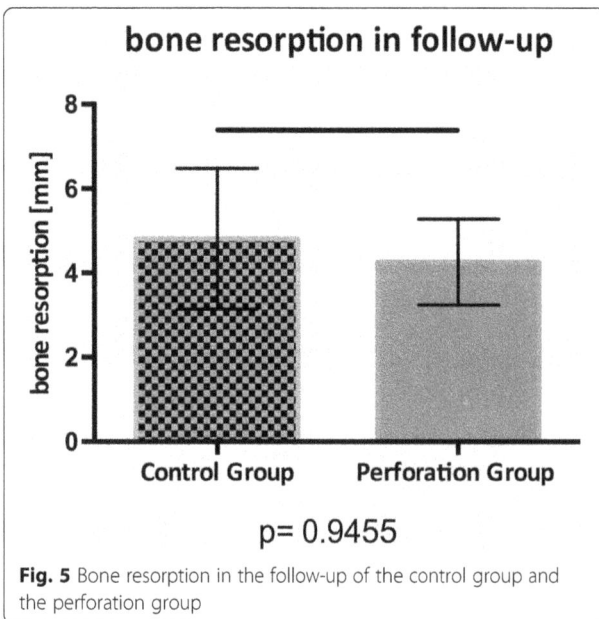

Fig. 5 Bone resorption in the follow-up of the control group and the perforation group

Although the height of the alveolar crest differed significantly, the total postoperative height of augmented and residual bone was on a comparable level allowing for sufficient elevation of the sinus floor to insert dental implants independently of a perforation. This fact remains reassuring as the latter represents the mostly common complication with a reported variation of 10 to 44% [5, 6, 8, 12, 17–23].

In this context, the surgical experience and the tissue quality, e.g., scarring due to previous procedures or local inflammation, might lead to a high probability of Schneiderian membrane perforation [16, 22, 24, 25] with anatomical variations, such as sinus septa or thin, vulnerable membrane textures [4, 16, 22, 24, 25]. Some studies have suggested contraindication of sinus floor elevation in patients with anatomical variations such as septa or mucosal swelling [8]. As our results did not indicate any negative impact of membrane tear on the augmented sinus, the results of Nolan et al., including a total of 359 sinus floor augmentations, indicated that graft failure occurred in 6.7% of all procedures and was significantly correlated ($p = 0.0028$) with membrane perforation. Compared to our evaluation, where procedures were, without exception, performed by attending physicians, the perforation rate was twice as high (21 vs. 41%). Surgical experience was ruled out as an influencing factor, as membrane perforations were equally distributed in cases treated by attending physicians compared to those performed by residents [6]. Another reason for the different findings might be due to the differences between the numbers of compared membrane tears (39 perforations vs. 150 perforations), as both evaluations were performed retrospectively.

One implant was lost in the perforation group due to early-onset peri-implantitis, whereas all implants in the control group were still in place. As we had previously prospectively reported on the first 6 months after dental implantation in this cohort [11], there was no further impact of membrane perforation on implant loss for at least 12 to 24 months in this retrospective evaluation. The appearance of peri-implantitis was more often observed in patients who experienced a procedure with an intraoperative perforation. However, this finding might be because the control group did not fully represent the patients without membrane perforation as only one third engaged in a sufficient follow-up. The reduced time span of the patients' observation time in the control group might be due to the lack of postoperative complications in this group who did have follow-up examinations in the department. Therefore, we cannot conclude whether there is or is not an impact based on the results in our study cohort. Sakkas et al. reported no impact of membrane perforation on the overall implant within a 1-year evaluation [12], whereas Proussaefs et al. reported a decreased implant survival in two-stage procedures and membrane tear compared

Table 3 Data summary of bone level development

	Bone level preoperatively		Bone level postoperatively		Bone level follow-up		Bone resorption	
	Perforation group	Control group	Perforation group	Control group	Perforation group	Control group	Perforation group	Control group
Median value	3.87	5.69	16.91	17.40	13.31	13.88	3.45	3.45
Standard deviation	3.79	3.32	5.06	6.04	2.39	4.02	4.84	7.64
p value	0.05		0.7851		0.2235		0.9455	

to intact membranes (69.56 vs. 100%) [10], as did a study published by Khoury [7].

In our study, bone resorption in the augmented area did not differ significantly between sinus lifting procedures with or without perforations. It is now widely accepted that following initial bone remodeling after an augmentation procedure followed by a dental implantation, bone loss within the following 3 years with implants in the interproximal space should be less than 0.5 mm in radiographic evaluations [26, 27]. Consistent with the results of Sakkas et al., there was no impact of bone graft origin or postoperative complications in patients with perforation of the Schneiderian membrane [12], similar to a study by Moreno Vazquez et al., which also did not find a correlation between complications, graft failure, and membrane perforation, assessing 8 years postoperatively [24]. In contrast to these studies, Proussaefs et al. reported a significant negative impact of membrane tear on bone formation in the sinus, more soft tissue formation, and less contact of graft particles to the residual bone [10].

The surgical management in cases of a membrane perforation might also influence the overall postoperative outcome and complications. Although the sinus lifting procedure has been established for many years now, there are no evidence-based guidelines for perforation closure or indications to interrupt the procedure. To date, most existing studies recommend sealing smaller sizes of perforations with membranes (collagen, demineralized laminar bone) or fibrin glue. Additional resorbable sutures in cases of larger perforations are advisable if a complete closure of the perforation is feasible [5, 8, 28]

but have not been shown to be superior as the coverage of larger perforations with membranes alone were shown to be effective [9, 12, 28, 29]. A lateral approach in sinus lifting might be obligatory to securely detect and therefore treat a perforation. In the primary assessment of the study, four procedures had to be terminated due to an extensive perforation, thin mucosa, or a retention cyst. After waiting 6 months, the procedure was repeated without any complications [11]. Other studies also recommend interrupting the procedure, when the repair does not seem to be sufficiently possible [7, 17].

In this study, a one-stage procedure was significantly less likely to result in membrane perforation. Implant insertion was immediately performed only if the estimated residual bone quality ensured high primary stability, which was consistent with a study by Cha et al. [3]. Residual bone height between 1 to 3 mm was not favorable for immediate implant insertion after sinus floor elevation with a lateral approach [16]. Therefore, the surgeon should be aware that a two-stage approach includes the risk of further complications relating to the surgical procedure itself. A recently published study revealed a significantly higher risk for soft-tissue complications in cases of a second procedure [30].

Due to the retrospective nature of this study, the management in cases of perforation did not follow a standardized protocol. Most of the studies regarding the outcome after membrane tear rely on retrospectively acquired data, and similar to in our study, with an inhomogeneous study cohort with different approaches in cases of perforation, there were different augmentation procedures, including grafts and grafting material, one- and two-stage procedures and different types of dental implants. Based on our data and regarding the limitations within the design of this study, we might conclude that a perforation of the Schneiderian membrane, if

Table 4 Multiple comparisons of subgroups: postoperative bone level

Adjusted p values multiple comparison	Control group bone level < 4 mm		
Control group bone level > 4 mm	0.0453	Control group bone level > 4 mm	
Perforation group bone level < 4 mm	0.3174	0.7586	Study group bone level < 4 mm
Perforation group bone level > 4 mm	0.0203	0.9679	0.5144

Table 5 Fisher's exact test: surgical strategy dependent on membrane perforation ($p = 0.0003$)

	One-stage procedure	Two-stage procedure
Perforation group	11	81
Control group	30	53

Table 6 Fisher's exact test: incidence of peri-implant disease after sinus lifting procedure with and without membrane perforation ($p = 0.0004$)

	Peri-implantitis	No peri-implantitis
Perforation group	12	80
Control group	0	83

recognized and properly addressed, does not necessarily endanger or negatively impact the stability of the augmented bone or implant survival. To systematically assess the impact of membrane perforation on the augmented sinus and implant survival, prospective studies and higher case numbers should be considered in the future.

Conclusions

In conclusion, and within the limits of its retrospective nature, our study implies that in cases of intraoperative perforation of the Schneiderian membrane, a consequent surgical assessment and treatment might avoid complications regarding graft stability and implant survival. Two-stage procedures might be appropriate if primary stability does not seem to be achievable. Augmentation of the sinus floor might be possible even in cases of perforation. A negative impact on the bone graft itself or on remodeling processes in follow-up could not have been shown, but prospective long-term studies should be performed to deliver reliable data on the impact of membrane perforation on graft stability and implant survival.

Funding
This study was not funded.

Authors' contributions
BEBB made substantial contributions to the conception and design and analysis and interpretation of data and drafting the manuscript and revising it critically for important intellectual content. BEBB gave final approval of the version to be published and agreed to be accountable for all aspects of the work in ensuring that questions related to the accuracy or integrity of any part of the work are appropriately investigated and resolved. DW contributed to the acquisition of data and revising the manuscript critically for important intellectual content. DW gave final approval of the version to be published and agreed to be accountable for all aspects of the work in ensuring that questions related to the accuracy or integrity of any part of the work are appropriately investigated and resolved. EB made substantial contributions to the conception and design of the study and revising the manuscript critically for important intellectual content. EB gave final approval of the version to be published and agreed to be accountable for all aspects of the work in ensuring that questions related to the accuracy or integrity of any part of the work are appropriately investigated and resolved. JW made substantial contributions to the conception and design and revising the manuscript critically for important intellectual content. JW gave final approval of the version to be published and agreed to be accountable for all aspects of the work in ensuring that questions related to the accuracy or integrity of any part of the work are appropriately investigated and resolved. STB made substantial contributions to the conception and design and revising the manuscript critically for important intellectual content. STB gave final

approval of the version to be published and agreed to be accountable for all aspects of the work in ensuring that questions related to the accuracy or integrity of any part of the work are appropriately investigated and resolved.

Competing interests
The authors Benedicta Beck-Broichsitter, Dorothea Westhoff, Eleonore Behrens, Jörg Wiltfang, and Stephan T. Becker declare that there are no existing competing interests concerning this collaborative work.

Author details
[1]Department of Oral and Maxillofacial Surgery, Charité–University Medical Center Berlin, Augustenburger Platz 1, 13353 Berlin, Germany. [2]Department of Oral and Maxillofacial Surgery, Schleswig-Holstein University Hospital, Arnold-Heller-Straße 3, Haus 26, 24105 Kiel, Germany.

References
1. Wiltfang J, Schultze-Mosgau S, Nkenke E, Thorwarth M, Neukam FW, Schlegel KA. Onlay augmentation versus sinuslift procedure in the treatment of the severely resorbed maxilla: a 5-year comparative longitudinal study. Int J Oral Maxillofac Surg. 2005;34(8):885–9.
2. Pikos MA. Maxillary sinus membrane repair: report of a technique for large perforations. Implant Dent. 1999;8(1):29–34.
3. Cha HS, Kim A, Nowzari H, Chang HS, Ahn KM. Simultaneous sinus lift and implant installation: prospective study of consecutive two hundred seventeen sinus lift and four hundred sixty-two implants. Clin Implant Dent Relat Res. 2014;16(3):337–47.
4. Pommer B, Ulm C, Lorenzoni M, Palmer R, Watzek G, Zechner W. Prevalence, location and morphology of maxillary sinus septa: systematic review and meta-analysis. J Clin Periodontol. 2012;39(8):769–73.
5. Schwartz-Arad D, Herzberg R, Dolev E. The prevalence of surgical complications of the sinus graft procedure and their impact on implant survival. J Periodontol. 2004;75(4):511–6.
6. Nolan PJ, Freeman K, Kraut RA. Correlation between Schneiderian membrane perforation and sinus lift graft outcome: a retrospective evaluation of 359 augmented sinus. J Oral Maxillofac Surg. 2014;72(1):47–52.
7. Khoury F. Augmentation of the sinus floor with mandibular bone block and simultaneous implantation: a 6-year clinical investigation. Int J Oral Maxillofac Implants. 1999;14(4):557–64.
8. van den Bergh JP, ten Bruggenkate CM, Disch FJ, Tuinzing DB. Anatomical aspects of sinus floor elevations. Clin Oral Implants Res. 2000;11(3):256–65.
9. Wannfors K, Johansson B, Hallman M, Strandkvist T. A prospective randomized study of 1- and 2-stage sinus inlay bone grafts: 1-year follow-up. Int J Oral Maxillofac Implants. 2000;15(5):625–32.
10. Proussaefs P, Lozada J, Kim J, Rohrer MD. Repair of the perforated sinus membrane with a resorbable collagen membrane: a human study. Int J Oral Maxillofac Implants. 2004;19(3):413–20.
11. Becker ST, Terheyden H, Steinriede A, Behrens E, Springer I, Wiltfang J. Prospective observation of 41 perforations of the Schneiderian membrane during sinus floor elevation. Clin Oral Implants Res. 2008;19(12):1285–9.
12. Sakkas A, Konstantinidis I, Winter K, Schramm A, Wilde F. Effect of Schneiderian membrane perforation on sinus lift graft outcome using two different donor sites: a retrospective study of 105 maxillary sinus elevation procedures. GMS Interdisc Plast Reconstr Surg DGPW. 2016;5:Doc11.
13. Springer IN, Terheyden H, Geiss S, Harle F, Hedderich J, Acil Y. Particulated bone grafts—effectiveness of bone cell supply. Clin Oral Implants Res. 2004; 15(2):205–12.
14. Barone A, Crespi R, Aldini NN, Fini M, Giardino R, Covani U. Maxillary sinus augmentation: histologic and histomorphometric analysis. Int J Oral Maxillofac Implants. 2005;20(4):519–25.
15. Ong CT, Ivanovski S, Needleman IG, Retzepi M, Moles DR, Tonetti MS, et al. Systematic review of implant outcomes in treated periodontitis subjects. J Clin Periodontol. 2008;35(5):438–62.
16. Felice P, Pistilli R, Piattelli M, Soardi E, Barausse C, Esposito M. 1-stage versus 2-stage lateral sinus lift procedures: 1-year post-loading results of a multicentre randomised controlled trial. Eur J Oral Implantol. 2014; 7(1):65–75. Spring
17. Timmenga NM, Raghoebar GM, Boering G, van Weissenbruch R, et al. J Oral Maxillofac Surg. 1997;55(9):936–9. discussion 40

18. Wiltfang J, Schultze-Mosgau S, Merten HA, Kessler P, Ludwig A, Engelke W. Endoscopic and ultrasonographic evaluation of the maxillary sinus after combined sinus floor augmentation and implant insertion. Oral Surg Oral Med Oral Pathol Oral Radiol Endod. 2000;89(3):288–91.

19. Barone A, Santini S, Sbordone L, Crespi R, Covani U. A clinical study of the outcomes and complications associated with maxillary sinus augmentation. Int J Oral Maxillofac Implants. 2006;21(1):81–5.

20. Silva FM, Cortez AL, Moreira RW, Mazzonetto R. Complications of intraoral donor site for bone grafting prior to implant placement. Implant Dent. 2006;15(4):420–6.

21. Timmenga NM, Raghoebar GM, Liem RS, van Weissenbruch R, Manson WL, Vissink A. Effects of maxillary sinus floor elevation surgery on maxillary sinus physiology. Eur J Oral Sci. 2003;111(3):189–97.

22. Pikos MA. Maxillary sinus membrane repair: update on technique for large and complete perforations. Implant Dent. 2008;17(1):24–31.

23. Shlomi B, Horowitz I, Kahn A, Dobriyan A, Chaushu G. The effect of sinus membrane perforation and repair with Lambone on the outcome of maxillary sinus floor augmentation: a radiographic assessment. Int J Oral Maxillofac Implants. 2004;19(4):559–62.

24. Moreno Vazquez JC, Gonzalez de Rivera AS, Gil HS, Mifsut RS. Complication rate in 200 consecutive sinus lift procedures: guidelines for prevention and treatment. J Oral Maxillofac Surg. 2014;72(5):892–901.

25. Johansson LA, Isaksson S, Lindh C, Becktor JP, Sennerby L. Maxillary sinus floor augmentation and simultaneous implant placement using locally harvested autogenous bone chips and bone debris: a prospective clinical study. J Oral Maxillofac Surg. 2010;68(4):837–44.

26. Lang NP, Jepsen S. Implant surfaces and design (Working Group 4). Clin Oral Implants Res. 2009;20(Suppl 4):228–31.

27. Abrahamsson I, Berglundh T. Effects of different implant surfaces and designs on marginal bone-level alterations: a review. Clin Oral Implants Res. 2009;20(Suppl 4):207–15.

28. van den Bergh JP, ten Bruggenkate CM, Krekeler G, Tuinzing DB. Maxillary sinusfloor elevation and grafting with human demineralized freeze dried bone. Clin Oral Implants Res. 2000;11(5):487–93.

29. Aimetti M, Romagnoli R, Ricci G, Massei G. Maxillary sinus elevation: the effect of macrolacerations and microlacerations of the sinus membrane as determined by endoscopy. Int J Periodontics Restorative Dent. 2001;21(6):581–9.

30. Esquivel-Upshaw J, Mehler A, Clark A, Neal D, Gonzaga L, Anusavice K. Peri-implant complications for posterior endosteal implants. Clin Oral Implants Res. 2015;26(12):1390–6.

5

Case report on managing incomplete bone formation after bilateral sinus augmentation using a palatal approach and a dilating balloon technique

Tobias K. Boehm

Abstract

Background: Patients with resorbed edentulous alveolar ridges in the posterior maxilla often require lateral window sinus augmentation procedures prior to implant placement. Lateral window sinus augmentation procedures can produce incomplete bone augmentation as consequence of surgical and healing complications producing unusual and complex sinus anatomy. Although incomplete bone formation after sinus augmentation has been described in a previous case reports, this is the first case report that describes grafting these compromised sites prior to implant placement.

Case presentation: A 65-year-old male patient with no known medical conditions presented with severe chronic localized periodontitis and a combined periodontal-endodontic lesion affecting three first molars. Initial ridge preservation and lateral window sinus augmentation resulted in incomplete bone formation and complex sinus floor anatomy on both right and left sides. A dilating balloon technique on one side and a palatal approach on the other side were utilized for additional sinus augmentation using particulate allograft and resorbable collagen membranes. Healing was uneventful, and implants could be placed and restored at all sites. Periodontal maintenance was conducted every 3 months, and the implants have been in function and periodontally healthy for 2 years.

Conclusion: Despite initial failure of sinus augmentation to produce suitable implant sites, it is possible to rescue these sites with re-entry grafting procedures and allow successful implant placement and restoration.

Keyword: Maxilla, Complication, Implant

Background

Patients with severe periodontal disease often display severely resorbed ridges in the posterior maxilla. Implant therapy can be a challenge for those patients as available bone height is limited by the maxillary sinus. Although sinus augmentation using subantral or lateral window approaches are routinely used, complications occur that may limit bone augmentation in the sinus after any given procedure. The most common complication during sinus augmentation surgery is tearing of the Schneiderian membrane. This happens in 14–53% of surgeries. History of tobacco use and complex sinus anatomy are the most common risk factors for membrane tears. Membrane tears that develop during the surgery can be managed by placing resorbable membranes over the torn area [1–3]. Although piezoelectric surgery and surgical planning can reduce this complication [4], tears still remain a possible surgical complication and there may be incomplete bone augmentation [5].

One reason for this is that even though piezoelectric surgery can gently remove the overlying bone from the fragile Schneiderian membrane, sinus curettes still may be needed to manually lift the membrane from the interior walls of the sinus. As this procedure can tear the membrane, Dr. Muronoi and others developed an alternative procedure for lifting the Schneiderian membrane using a hemostatic nasal dilating balloon in 2003. For this

Correspondence: tboehm@westernu.edu
Western University of Health Sciences College of Dental Medicine, 309 E Second Street, Pomona, CA 91766, USA

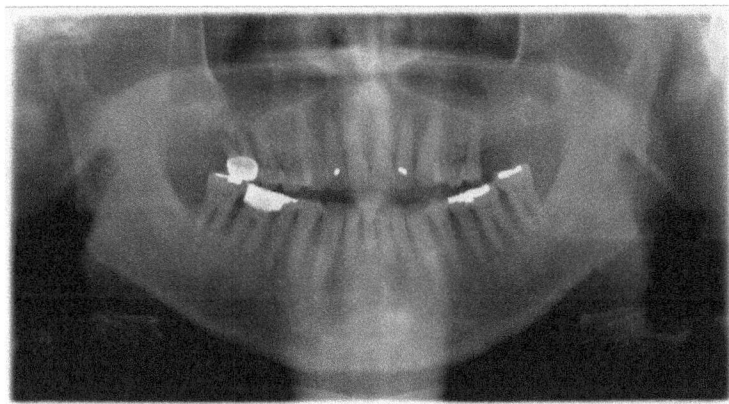

Fig. 1 Initial presentation. Panoramic radiograph taken at initial visit shows severe bone loss, supraerupted molars and furcation involvement

procedure, the surgeons created a lateral window in the posterior maxilla exposing the Schneiderian membrane, slightly elevate the membrane, insert a dilating balloon, and use hydraulic pressure to inflate the balloon, which then gently separates the membrane from the underlying bone and creates space for bone grafting materials [6]. Other clinicians refined this technique by creating successively smaller access windows and reported complications in less than 10% of cases, only minor patient discomfort and satisfactory bone formation [7–10]. Most recently, several clinicians modified the procedure by further reducing

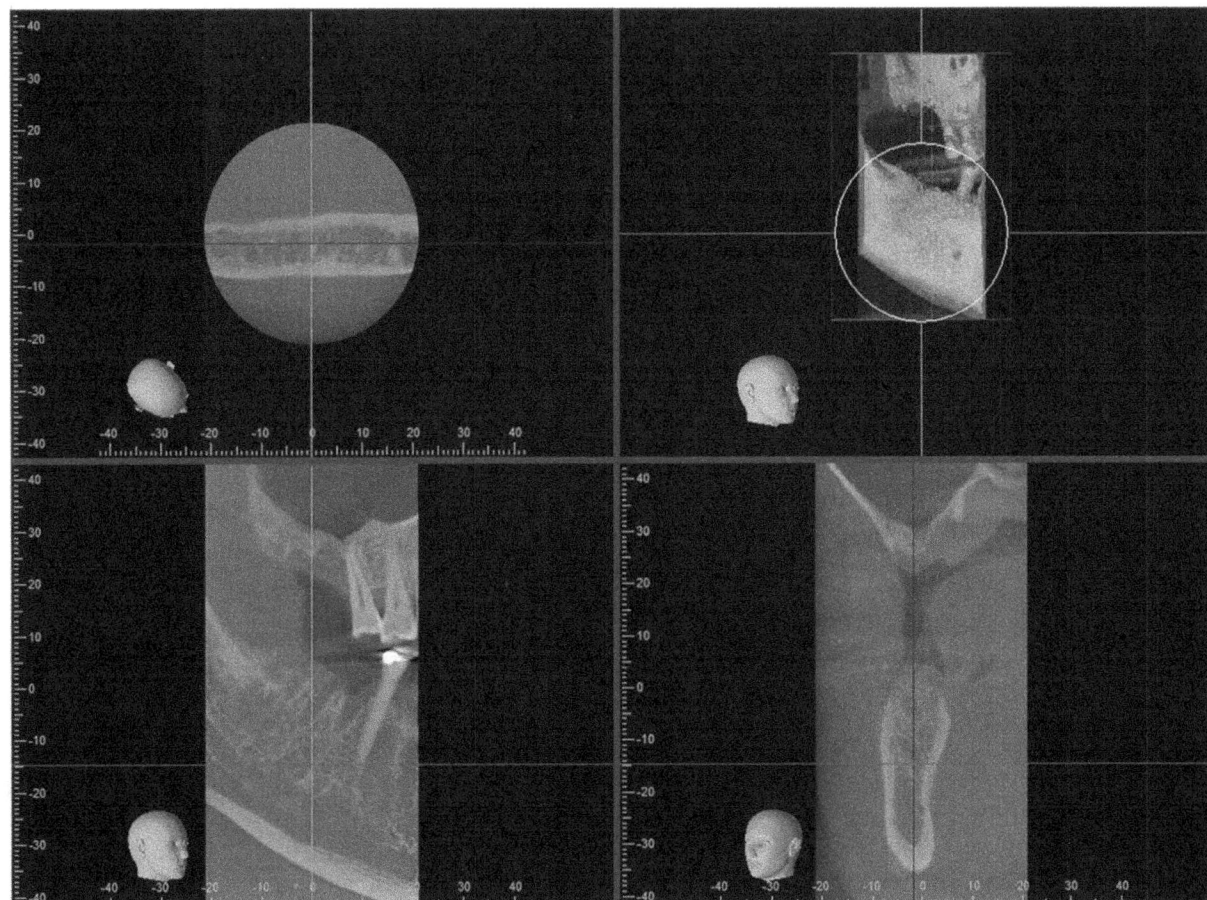

Fig. 2 Right sinus prior to first sinus grafting procedure. Cone beam CT imaging shows very little residual bone volume at implant site for the no. 3 area

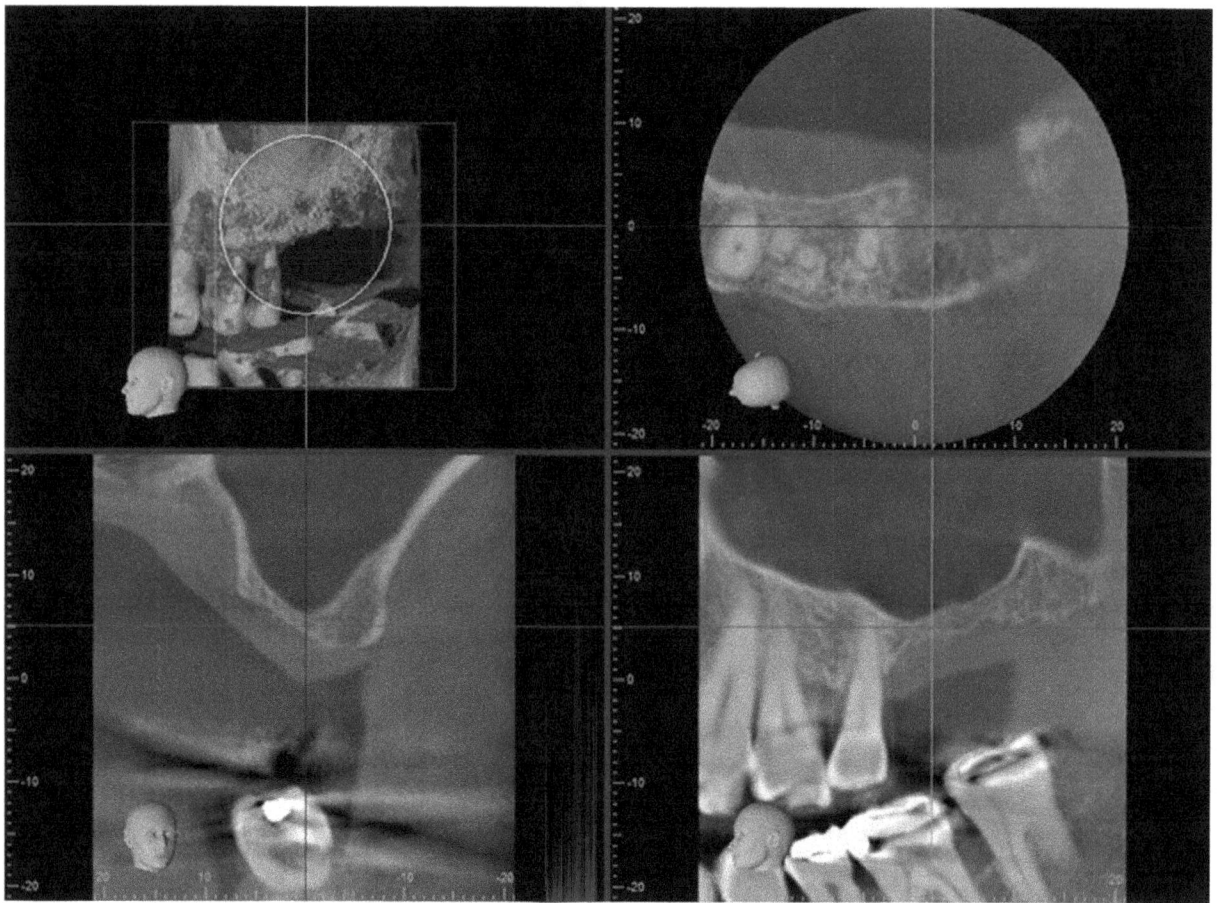

Fig. 3 Left sinus prior to first sinus grafting procedure. Cone beam CT imaging also shows very little bone volume on left side for the no. 14 area

the flap size needed for the procedure, moving the access site to the ridge crest, and limit the access window to an implant osteotomy created with osteotomes [11, 12]. Significantly for our case report, this transcrestal approach reduces the chance of post-grafting complications with patients who have sinus pathology and unusual sinus anatomy while minimizing the chance of membrane tears [13].

Membrane tears are a significant concern as they may result in postoperative complications such as an oroantral communication as reported recently. In this case, the communication was managed by inserting a fibrin sponge, but it resulted in a cyst-like concavity within grafted bone, which was subsequently managed by re-entry and grafting of the affected site prior to implant placement [14]. As seen in this case, incomplete bone formation can be managed with re-entry procedures, but incomplete bone formation often results in unusual sinus floor morphologies that make conventional sinus approaches difficult. A recent case report describes an unconventional palatal

approach for managing sinus floor anatomy complicated by previous sinus grafting [15].

There is still little data on the long-term success of these unconventional re-entry procedures after incomplete bone formation, and here, we present a case with 3-year follow-up after re-entry grafting procedures using either a palatal window or balloon-dilating device for management of previously failed sinus augmentation.

Case presentation

A 65-year-old retired Caucasian male presented to the Western University of Health Sciences Dental Center expressing an interest in implants after consulting with a private practice periodontist and a dentist from a large implant dentistry practice. He had no medical conditions or known allergies, but reported a 40-pack-year history of using tobacco and quit just before attending the Dental Center. No caries or mucosal abnormalities were found during examination other than a combined periodontal

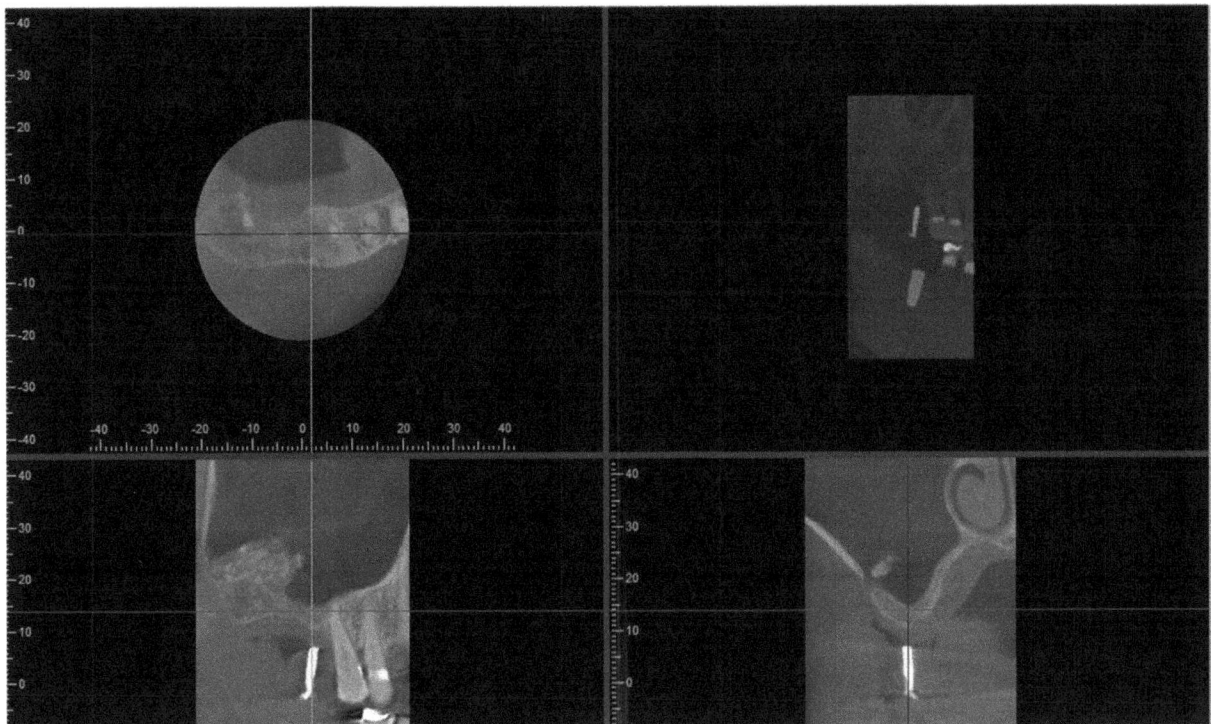

Fig. 4 Right sinus about 12 months after first grafting procedure. Cone beam CT imaging shows little suitable bone at implant site, but grafted bone displaced distal to site. Bone hydroxyapatite particles were added as radiographic marker to the graft material for the first sinus augmentation procedure and are still visible as radiopaque specks

endodontic lesion at tooth no. 3 and localized severe periodontitis at no. 31 and no. 30 with complete through-and-through furcation involvement. Tooth no. 18 protruded beyond the occlusal plane, and several areas of shallow facial abfractions were noted on mandibular incisor teeth. (See initial panoramic radiograph, Fig. 1.) For initial disease treatment, teeth no.3, no. 30, and no. 31 were gently extracted and the residual socket of no. 30 grafted with human cortical particulate allograft. While healing was uneventful and ridge width was preserved at no. 30, little bone remained at the no. 3 site (see Fig. 2). On the left side, similar low amounts of available bone prevented implant placement at the no. 14 implant site (see Fig. 3). Given the good overall health of the patient, continued tobacco abstinence, good oral mucosal health after initial therapy, and low amount of sinus anatomy complexity, we suggested lateral window sinus augmentation to the patient, and the patient accepted proposed treatment after explanation of risks, benefits, and alternatives to implant therapy.

All of the following surgeries were carried out under local anesthesia. The patient received one tablet of 0.25 mg triazolam the evening before the surgery appointment and was taking ibuprofen 600 mg every

6 h and amoxicillin 250 mg every 6 h for 1 week starting the evening before the surgery. Starting the second day after surgery, the patient was instructed to rinse twice daily with 0.5 oz. of chlorhexidine gluconate for 30 s after oral hygiene, and the patient was seen at least once 7 days after each surgical procedure for postoperative care and oral hygiene instruction.

Lateral window sinus augmentation was performed on each side during appointments spaced 3 months apart, following the technique developed by Tatum in 1974. For each site, a midcrestal mucoperiosteal incision with buccal releases was created, and the lateral Schneiderian membrane of the maxillary sinus exposed through an ovoid window osteotomy of about 15 mm diameter. Osteotomy was performed using a piezotome (Piezotome 2, Acteon North America, and Mount Laurel, NJ, USA). Thereafter, the Schneiderian membrane was reflected away from the inferior floor of the sinus cavity with a mushroom-shaped Piezotome insert (Sinus surgery kit, Acteon North America, Mount Laurel, NJ, USA) and Sinus curettes (Sinus surgery curette kit, ACE Surgical Supply, Brockton, MA, USA) until the inferior most 15 mm of the medial

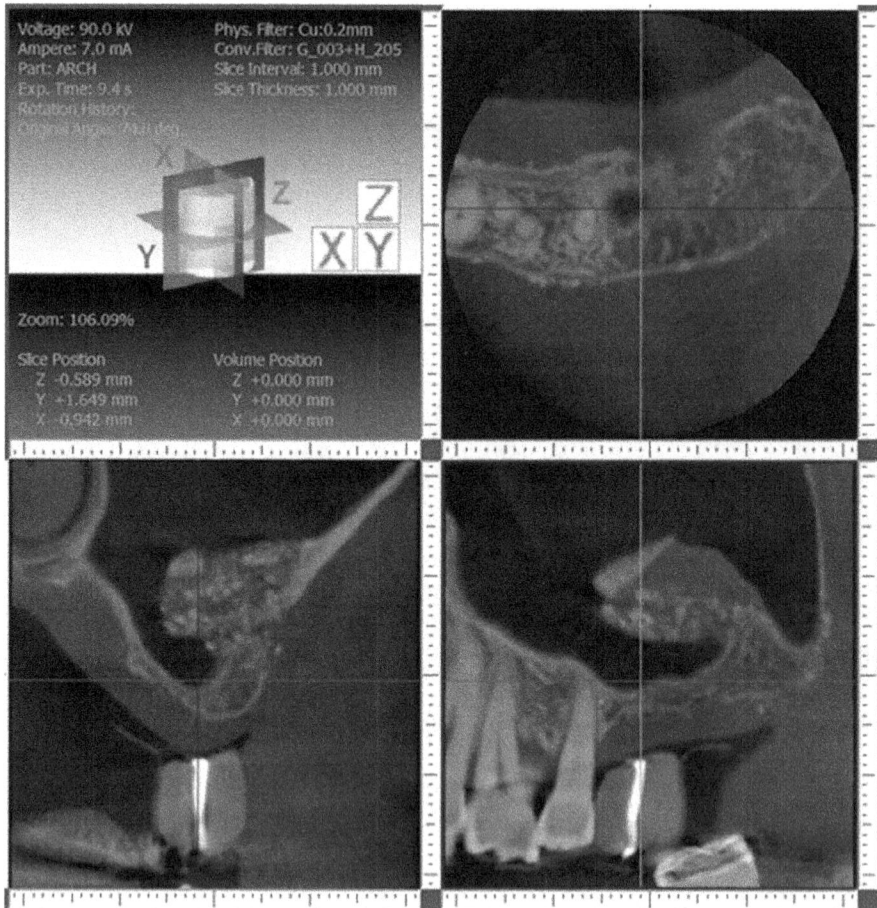

Fig. 5 Left sinus about 12 months after first grafting procedure. Cone beam CT imaging shows unusual sinus anatomy after grafting, with finger-like sinus extension at implant site, and thick-grafted bone buccal and apical to it. The infractured wall is still clearly visible, as well as the bovine bone particles used as radiographic marker

wall was felt and seen. During both surgeries, we noticed small tears of 5 mm in the mid-portion of the mobilized Schneiderian membranes and repaired those by placing a double layer of 2 cm × 2 cm × 1.5 mm thick collagen tape (RCT, cut to shape, ACE Surgical Supply, Brockton, MA, USA) over the tears, which stabilized the membrane. We then placed a 1:1:1 mixture of cancellous and cortical allograft (AlloOss, ACE Surgical Supply, Brockton, MA, USA) and bovine xenograft (NuOss, ACE Surgical Supply, Brockton, MA, USA) into the space created between the former floor of the sinus cavity and collagen tape-covered Schneiderian membrane. Buccal access windows were then covered with a resorbable collagen membrane (resorbable collagen, ConFORM, ACE Surgical, Brockton, MA, USA) as suggested by Wallace and Froum [16], and the surgical site closed with continuous sutures (PTFE 3-0, Cytoplast, Osteogenics, Lubbock, TX, USA). No complications were reported by the patient and only when questioned he reported a short-lived episode of

postnasal drip with few embedded "sand grains" after the surgery on the left side. We waited then for 10–12 months prior to further evaluation to allow complete dissolution of allograft [17] and allow complete bone formation [18].

A year later, we requested cone beam computed tomography for both posterior maxilla sites, and we found incomplete bone growth in the sinus. On the right side, bone growth had occurred only distal to the desired implant site, and there was an ovoid extension of sinus into the area planned for implant placement (Fig. 4). On the left side, a finger-like extension of sinus had developed between grafted bone and the former inferior medial wall of the sinus (Fig. 5). After explanation of findings, treatment alternatives, and risks and benefits of proposed treatments, the patient agreed on continuing with additional bone grafting.

For the right side, we decided to augment the area of insufficient bone using a balloon dilation

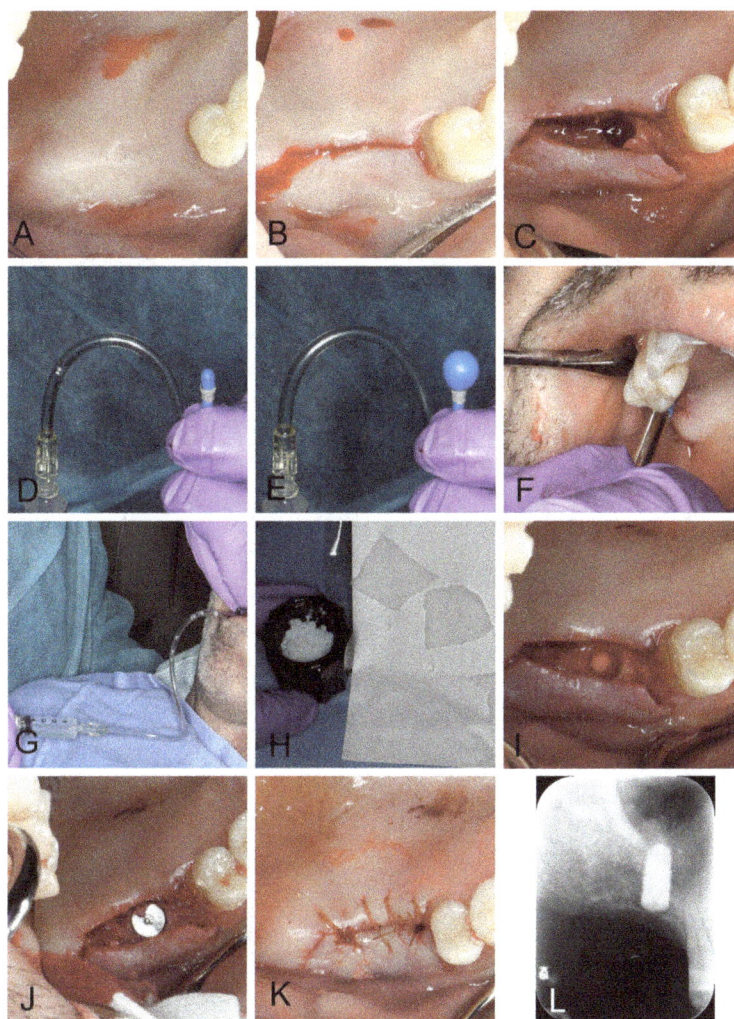

Fig. 6 Right sinus balloon dilation procedure. This photographic series shows the surgical procedure that augmented bone and allowed implant placement at the no. 3 site. **a** Preoperative view after infiltration anesthesia. **b** Full-thickness midcrestal incision. **c** Osteotomy preparation with implant drills and osteotomes. **d, e** The dilating balloon, which is inflated using saline pressure from a syringe. **f** Insertion of uninflated balloon into osteotomy. **g** Gentle inflation of balloon by 1 ml. **h** Preparation of allograft and collagen tape. **i** Collagen tape is visible at bottom of osteotomy after filling expanded Schneiderian membrane with bone graft and covering graft with collagen tape. **j** Implant placement. **k** Suturing with a continuous suture. **l** Postoperative radiograph showing implant and halo of allograft surrounding apex of implant after surgery

technique through a subantral approach since the area of the missing bone was nearly spherical and centered at the no. 3 site. We also decided to place an implant simultaneously since primary stability seemed likely with the consistent thickness of 5 mm available bone at the no. 3 site, consistent with the recommendation by Pjetursson and Lang [19]. We created sinus access in a similar fashion as developed by Tatum in the 1970s and described by Misch [20] and performed sinus augmentation with a balloon technique as described for lateral window augmentation by Muronoi et al. [6]. (See Fig. 6 for the actual procedure, Fig. 7 for a diagram.) For this

surgery, we created a mucoperiosteal flap with buccal releases for improved access (Fig. 6a, b) and created an osteotomy using osteotomy drills (Fig. 6c; Zimmer implant surgical kit, Zimmer, Carlsbad, CA, USA). Since there was sufficient ridge width and the bone was hard, we opted not to use Summer's technique [21] but used drills to take the osteotomy to its final width that was slightly undersized for a 4.7-mm implant, but wide enough to allow insertion of a balloon dilator (straight model, Osseous Technologies of America, Hamburg, NY, USA). Drilling of the osteotomy stopped short 1 mm of the sinus floor. Prior to balloon dilation, we

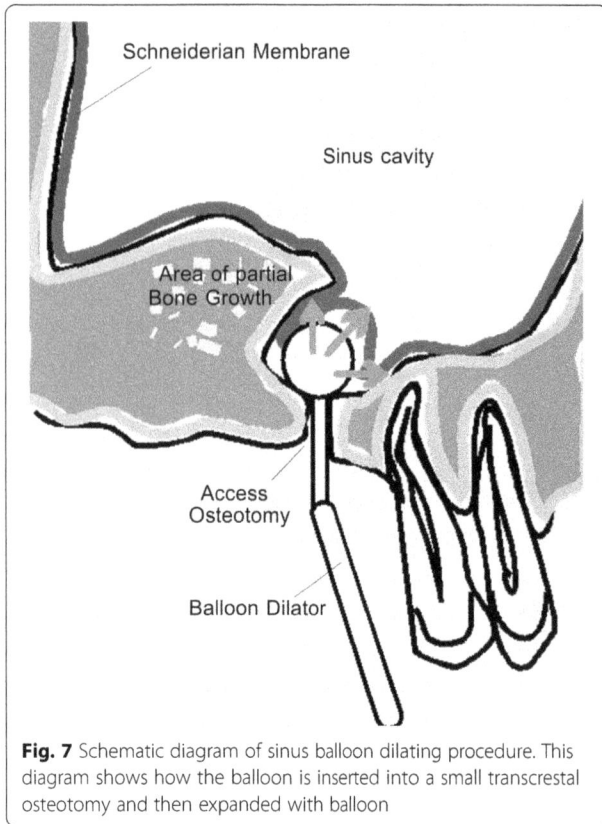

Fig. 7 Schematic diagram of sinus balloon dilating procedure. This diagram shows how the balloon is inserted into a small transcrestal osteotomy and then expanded with balloon

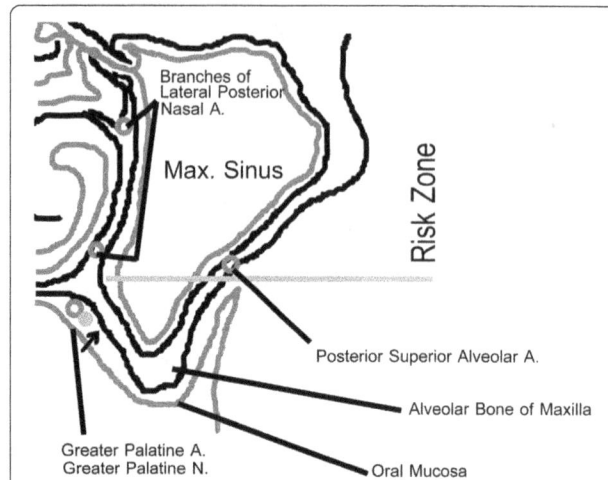

Fig. 8 Blood supply of the sinus. There are three areas in the sinus where blood vessels may be encountered during sinus augmentation procedures for implants. On the inflection point between hard palate and alveolar ridge in the posterior maxilla, the greater palatine neurovascular bundle is located embedded in soft tissue. This inflection point is matched in the internal sinus anatomy and presents a landmark that can be palpated with sinus curettes during sinus membrane elevation or seen on cone beam CT images in this patient. It is important to avoid instrumenting the area above this inflection point as branches of the lateral posterior nasal arteries may be encountered superior to this area. Injuring these blood vessels can lead to significant sinus bleeding that is difficult to stop without sinus tamponade. Often on cone beam CT images, we see a small blood vessel channel midway within the lateral wall of the sinus, which likely is the posterior superior alveolar artery and vein. This and the interior medial wall sinus inflection point can serve as anatomic landmark to delineate a risk zone superior to it and to limit sinus augmentation inferior to it

mobilized the Schneiderian membrane by gently infracturing small segments of the osteotomy floor using thin flat-ended osteotomes (ACE Surgical Supply, Brockton, MA, USA). For this, we started in the center of the osteotomy, advanced the depth of the infracture by 1 mm with a mallet and worked in a spiral fashion to the outer limits of the osteotomy floor and apical most 2 mm of the osteotomy wall. We then used a larger flat osteotome to advance the entire floor of the osteotomy by another millimeter, which resulted in a rubber-like mobility of the osteotomy floors. We verified the integrity of the membrane by gentle probing with a WHO probe and inserted the balloon dilator (Fig. 6d–g). We then slowly inflated the balloon dilator with 1 ml of saline, verified integrity of the membrane again, placed two sheets of 1 cm × 1 cm × 1.5 resorbable collagen tape, followed by 0.5 ml allograft and a 4.7 × 10 mm rootform implant (Fig. 6h–j; Tapered Screw-Vent TSVWB10, Zimmer, Carlsbad, CA, USA), which achieved good primary stability in excess of 30 Ncm. We placed a cover screw, replaced the flap, and sutured it with a continuous chromic gut 4-0 suture (Fig. 6k). Postoperative radiographs verified implant placement and showed

good confinement of graft material around the implant (Fig. 6l). Healing was uneventful with only mild short-lived postoperative pain for a few days, and implant uncovery 12 months later revealed a firmly embedded implant.

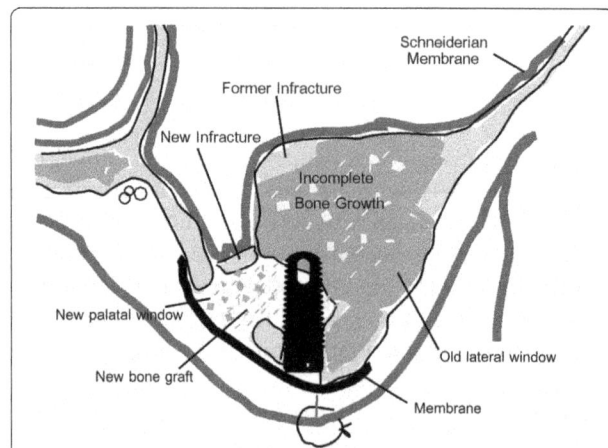

Fig. 9 Schematic diagram of palatal approach sinus augmentation. The diagram shows the location of the lateral window, avoiding the thick grafted bone on the buccal, and the greater palatal neurovascular bundle

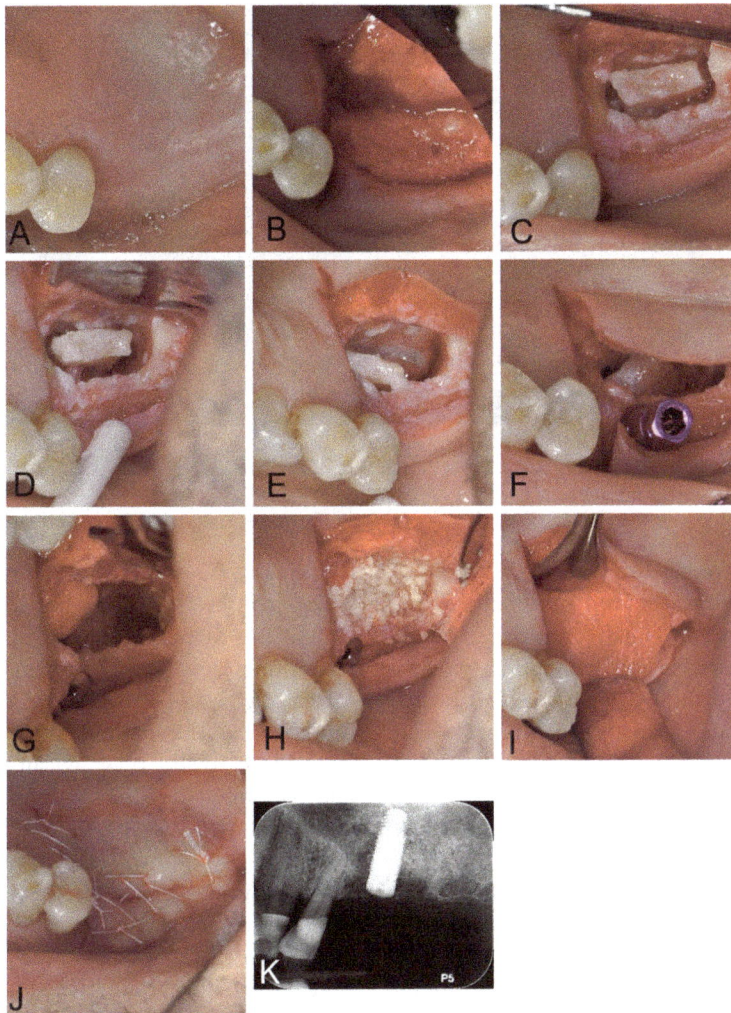

Fig. 10 Palatal approach lateral window sinus augmentation. This photographic series shows the surgical procedure that augmented bone and allowed implant placement at the no. 14 site. **a** Preoperative view prior to infiltration anesthesia. **b** Full-thickness midcrestal incision with palatal release and flap elevation. This was aided by a small bony ridge that separated the alveolar crest from the soft tissue area containing the greater palatine neurovascular bundle. **c** Sinus window created with piezosurgery. **d–f** With gentle piezocision and water pressure, the finger-like membrane is slowly mobilized and collapsed towards the remainder of the sinus cavity. The overlying bone serves to form a new floor covering the base of the finger-like cavity. **f** Conventional implant placement using osteotomy drills. **g** Any exposed sinus membrane is covered with collagen tape. **h** Particulate mineralized allograft is placed into the newly created space. **i** A resorbable collagen membrane is placed over the access window. **j** Palatal tissue is sutured over implant and grafted site with mattress sutures. **k** Postoperative radiograph taken immediately after surgery shows cloud of particulate grafted bone around implant, suggesting good bone graft containment

For the left side, we decided to access the sinus using a lateral window as the area of deficient bone was much larger in size and more complex in shape. We also decided to approach this area from the palate, as the defect was closer to the palate and required much less bone removal as a buccal approach. Most importantly, we were already familiar with the anatomical structures on the lower medial wall of the sinus in the access area as we visualized this area during the first graft surgery and CT scans showed no signs of larger intraosseous vasculature in the area. Given this specific case, and knowledge of the vascular anatomy of the maxillary sinus in the surgical area (Fig. 8, based on CT scans of this patient and Bailey et al.'s work [22]), we felt that our approach would not invade the zone of risk for bleeding complications. We performed the surgery similar to a conventional lateral window sinus augmentation surgery using piezosurgery and a buccal approach, except from the palatal side of the alveolar ridge and staying clear of the greater palatine neurovascular bundle (Fig. 9). Here, we created a

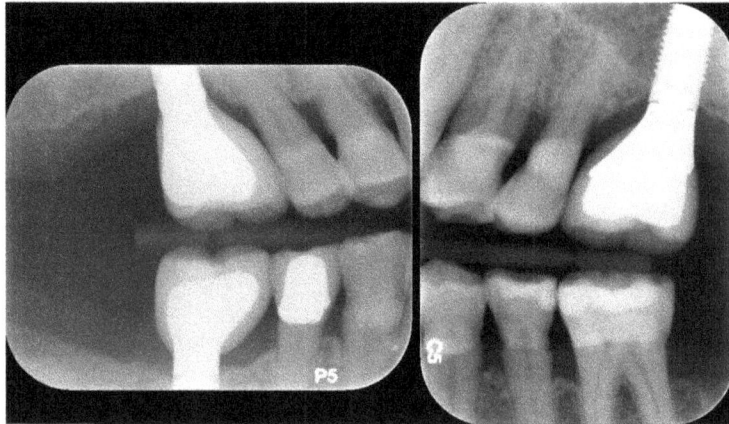

Fig. 11 Implant restoration. Implants were restored by dental students supervised by prosthodontists at the Dental Center

mucoperiosteal flap with vertical release at no. 13 (Fig. 10a, b). Using a piezotome and piezosurgery inserts (Piezotome 2, Acteon North America, Mount Laurel, NJ, USA), we created a rectangular window over the bony defect, avoiding any vascular structures (Fig. 10c). Using piezosurgery inserts and hydraulic pressure (IntraLift Kit, Acteon North America, Mount Laurel, NJ, USA), we carefully removed the Schneiderian membrane from the finger-like defect (Fig. 10d–f). We then placed a root-form 4.7 mm × 10 mm implant (Fig. 10f; Tapered Screw Vent TSWB10, Zimmer, Carlsbad, CA, USA) according to standard protocol and achieved good primary stability in excess of 30 Ncm. We placed a strip of resorbable collagen tape over any exposed Schneiderian membrane, grafted the site with 1.2 ml cortical particulate allograft (LifeNet Health, Virginia Beach, WA, USA) and placed a resorbable collagen membrane (ConFORM, ACE Surgical Supply, Brockton, MA, USA) over the palatal access window (Fig. 10g–i). We then covered the implant and graft with the palatal flap and sutured it with PTFE 3-0 (Cytoplast, Osteogenics Biomedical, Lubbock, TX, USA) continuous and horizontal mattress sutures (Fig. 10j). A postoperative radiograph showed good containment of the graft material (Fig. 10k).

Healing was uneventful with little discomfort reported by the patient during the first week, and implant uncovery revealed an implant firmly embedded in bone after 12 months. A third implant was placed at the no. 30 site and supraerupted no. 18 extracted as planned. Restoration of the implants was uneventfully performed by senior dental students supervised by various prosthodontists (Fig. 11). Periodontal maintenance was regularly performed, and 3 years after implant placement, there is no significant bone loss (Fig. 12), and probing depth remains at 2 to 4 mm with no bleeding on probing.

Conclusions

We conclude that incomplete bone formation after sinus augmentation can be managed successfully through a variety of re-entry procedures and that successful long-

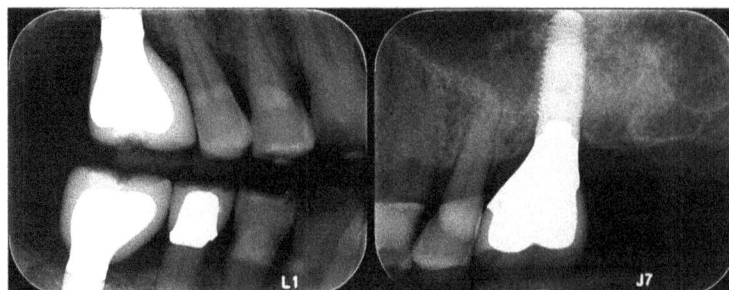

Fig. 12 Radiographic bone levels three years after placement. Bone levels remain unchanged during long-term follow-up

term implant placement and restoration is possible in a compliant patient of good overall health.

Acknowledgements
I would like to thank the former dental students Dr. Lily Hoang and Dr. Shirley Hsieh and their prosthodontic supervisors Dr. James Ywom, Dr. Steven Sanders, and Dr. Alessandro Urdaneta for providing this patient's continued restorative and preventive care after the surgeries and the dental assistants of the Western University of Health Sciences Dental Center, Mrs. Cindy Morton and Mrs. Melody Palomar for the surgical assistance. I also would like to thank Dr. Bruno Correa de Azevedo for the radiology reports and the sinus balloon dilator he obtained as a sample from Osseous Technologies of America.

Funding
This work was supported by Western University of Health Sciences through no specific grant mechanism.

Authors' contributions
The manuscript was solely created by Dr. Boehm.

Competing interests
Tobias K. Boehm declares that he has no competing interests.

References
1. Hernandez-Alfaro F, Torradeflot MM, Marti C. Prevalence and management of Schneiderian membrane perforations during sinus-lift procedures. Clin Oral Implants Res. 2008;19(1):91–8.
2. Wallace SS, Mazor Z, Froum SJ, Cho SC, Tarnow DP. Schneiderian membrane perforation rate during sinus elevation using piezosurgery: clinical results of 100 consecutive cases. Int J Periodontics Restorative Dent. 2007;27(5):413–9.
3. Testori T, Wallace SS, Del Fabbro M, Taschieri S, Trisi P, Capelli M, et al. Repair of large sinus membrane perforations using stabilized collagen barrier membranes: surgical techniques with histologic and radiographic evidence of success. Int J Periodontics Restorative Dent. 2008;28(1):9–17.
4. Toscano NJ, Holtzclaw D, Rosen PS. The effect of piezoelectric use on open sinus lift perforation: a retrospective evaluation of 56 consecutively treated cases from private practices. J Periodontol. 2010;81(1):167–71.
5. Lee KS, Kwon YH, Herr Y, Shin SI, Lee JY, Chung JH. Incomplete bone formation after sinus augmentation: a case report on radiological findings by computerized tomography at follow-up. J Periodontal Implant Sci. 2010;40(6):283–8.
6. Muronoi M, Xu H, Shimizu Y, Ooya K. Simplified procedure for augmentation of the sinus floor using a haemostatic nasal balloon. Br J Oral Maxillofac Surg. 2003;41(2):120–1.
7. Soltan M, Smiler DG. Antral membrane balloon elevation. J Oral Implantol. 2005;31(2):85–90.
8. Kfir E, Kfir V, Mijiritsky E, Rafaeloff R, Kaluski E. Minimally invasive antral membrane balloon elevation followed by maxillary bone augmentation and implant fixation. J Oral Implantol. 2006;32(1):26–33.
9. Hu X, Lin Y, Metzmacher AR, Zhang Y. Sinus membrane lift using a water balloon followed by bone grafting and implant placement: a 28-case report. Int J Prosthodont. 2009;22(3):243–7.
10. Kfir E, Goldstein M, Yerushalmi I, Rafaelov R, Mazor Z, Kfir V, et al. Minimally invasive antral membrane balloon elevation—results of a multicenter registry. Clin Implant Dent Relat Res. 2009;11 Suppl 1:e83–91.
11. Mazor Z, Kfir E, Lorean A, Mijiritsky E, Horowitz RA. Flapless approach to maxillary sinus augmentation using minimally invasive antral membrane balloon elevation. Implant Dent. 2011;20(6):434–8.
12. Penarrocha-Diago M, Galan-Gil S, Carrillo-Garcia C, Penarrocha-Diago D, Penarrocha-Diago M. Transcrestal sinus lift and implant placement using the sinus balloon technique. Med Oral Patol Oral Cir Bucal. 2012;17(1):e122–8.
13. Kfir E, Goldstein M, Abramovitz I, Kfir V, Mazor Z, Kaluski E. The effects of sinus membrane pathology on bone augmentation and procedural outcome using minimal invasive antral membrane balloon elevation. J Oral Implantol. 2014;40(3):285–93.
14. Crivellaro VR, Zielak JC, Deliberador TM, de Oliveira ND, Santos FR, Storrer CL. Pneumatization within a maxillary sinus graft: a case report. Int J Implant Dent. 2016;2(1):3.
15. Sarmiento HL, Othman B, Norton MR, Fiorellini JP. A palatal approach for a sinus augmentation procedure. Int J Periodontics Restorative Dent. 2016;36(1):111–5.
16. Wallace SS, Froum SJ. Effect of maxillary sinus augmentation on the survival of endosseous dental implants. A systematic review. Ann Periodontol. 2003;8(1):328–43.
17. Soardi CM, Suarez-Lopez del Amo F, Galindo-Moreno P, Catena A, Zaffe D, Wang HL. Reliability of cone beam computed tomography in determining mineralized tissue in augmented sinuses. Int J Oral Maxillofac Implants. 2016;31(2):352–8.
18. Hanisch O, Lozada JL, Holmes RE, Calhoun CJ, Kan JY, Spiekermann H. Maxillary sinus augmentation prior to placement of endosseous implants: a histomorphometric analysis. Int J Oral Maxillofac Implants. 1999;14(3):329–36.
19. Pjetursson BE, Lang NP. Sinus floor elevation utilizing the transalveolar approach. Periodontol 2000. 2014;66(1):59–71.
20. Misch CE. Maxillary sinus augmentation for endosteal implants: organized alternative treatment plans. Int J Oral Implantol. 1987;4(2):49–58.
21. Summers RB. A new concept in maxillary implant surgery: the osteotome technique. Compendium. 1994;15(2):152. 4-6, 8 passim; quiz 62.
22. Bailey BJ, Johnson JT, Newlands SD. Head and neck surgery—otolaryngology. Philadelphia: Lippincott Williams & Wilkins; 2006.

6

Spectrophotometric determination of platelet counts in platelet-rich plasma

Yutaka Kitamura[1], Masashi Suzuki[1], Tsuneyuki Tsukioka[1], Kazushige Isobe[1], Tetsuhiro Tsujino[1], Taisuke Watanabe[1], Takao Watanabe[1], Hajime Okudera[1], Koh Nakata[2], Takaaki Tanaka[3] and Tomoyuki Kawase[4*]

Abstract

Background: Platelet-rich plasma (PRP) is widely used in regenerative dentistry and other medical fields. However, its effectiveness has often been questioned. For better evaluation, the quality of individual PRP preparations should be assured prior to use. We proposed a spectrophotometric method for determination of platelet counts and validated its applicability using two types of PRP preparations.

Methods: Blood samples were obtained from healthy male volunteers and pure PRP (P-PRP) and leukocytes-rich PRP (L-PRP) were prepared using the double-spin method. In serial dilutions, platelet counts in P-PRP and L-PRP were determined using an automated hematology analyzer and a compact spectrophotometer. For validation, P-PRP and L-PRP independently prepared by three well-trained operators were used for comparison of the calculated and measured platelet counts.

Results: In the two types of PRP samples evaluated, platelet counts were almost equal and greater amount of both white blood cells (WBCs) and red blood cells (RBCs) were included in L-PRP preparations. The calibration curve obtained from serially diluted P-PRP showed a strong correlation ($R^2 = 0.995$), whereas that of L-PRP was relatively weaker ($R^2 = 0.975$). In validation testing, the scatter plot of the calculated platelet counts versus the measured values showed a strong correlation in P-PRP ($R^2 = 0.671$), whereas that of L-PRP showed a much weaker correlation ($R^2 = 0.0605$).

Conclusions: This method can precisely determine platelet counts in PRP preparations when the inclusion of WBCs or RBCs is minimized. Therefore, we recommend that clinicians use this method for quality assurance of individual PRP preparations.

Keywords: Platelet, Count, Spectrophotometry, Leukocytes, Red blood cells, Quality assurance

Background

Almost two decades have passed since platelet concentrates, such as platelet-rich plasma (PRP), were first introduced to the field of regenerative medicine by Marx et al. [1]. To date, PRP has been modified to create different variations and has increasingly been used in various fields of regenerative therapy around the world. However, negative data obtained from clinical applications of PRP have often been reported, leading to controversy regarding the predictability of PRP therapy [2].

Especially in cases of skeletal regeneration, the efficacy of PRP has been controversial [3–9].

One possible major reason behind this debate is the lack of large controlled clinical trials [2] or randomized clinical trials. Because there is no consensus regarding the indications and contraindications for PRP therapy, it is theoretically difficult to design appropriate experiments. In addition, there are no generally accepted guidelines on how to evaluate the condition of application sites. The second major reason, which has frequently been used as a possible explanation (actually, an "excuse") for unexpected clinical results in many clinical case reports, is individual difference. This is highly conceivable, but not convincingly supported by scientific evidence in individual cases. The third major reason is

* Correspondence: kawase@dent.niigata-u.ac.jp
[4]Division of Oral Bioengineering, Institute of Medicine and Dentistry, Niigata University, Niigata, Japan
Full list of author information is available at the end of the article

the lack of consensus regarding PRP preparation protocols [2]. Recent advances in the development of various automated preparation devices and kits are expected to reduce not only the labor of the operator but also technique-dependent variation of PRP quality. However, it should be noted that these devices cannot standardize PRP quality. In other words, it is not guaranteed that the quality of individual PRP preparations depends specifically on individual preparation devices. In fact, it is well-known that PRP and its derivatives prepared using the same devices do not necessarily induce similar clinical results.

In Japan, a new regulatory framework for PRP therapy was established in 2014. However, no evaluation indexes for PRP quality, except for aseptic handling to ensure sterility, are indicated in the regulations. In our recent review article [10], we highlighted the necessity of PRP quality indexes. The primary index is platelet counts. Specifically, it is best to check platelet counts prior to use. To assess PRP quality in clotted PRP derivatives, such as platelet-rich fibrin (PRF), we recently developed a direct counting method for platelets contained in fibrin clots [11]. However, only a few clinicians possess automated hematology analyzers (AHAs) or similar electronic devices that can be used to determine platelet counts accurately without bias or technical error.

In this study, we focused on the possibility of spectrophotometric determination and validated the applicability of the proposed method on platelet counts in PRP preparations. This idea was based on bacterial cell counting [12] and a similar challenge was reported in 1992 [13]. However, this optical method has not been further modified for PRP as a grafting material for regenerative therapy in accordance with the policy of quality assurance. Based on the count of white blood cells (WBCs) and red blood cells (RBCs) included in PRP preparations, we categorized PRP preparations into two types as follows: pure PRP (P-PRP) and leukocyte-rich PRP (L-PRP) [14–16]. As not only platelets but also WBCs are concentrated in L-PRP, we hypothesized that the inclusion of WBCs at higher levels could markedly interfere with this spectrophotometric determination. As predicted, we validated the applicability of our proposed method by precisely determining platelet counts in P-PRP, but not L-PRP.

Methods
Preparation of P-PRP and L-PRP
Blood samples were collected from 11 non-smoking healthy male volunteers aged 33 to 69 years. The study design and consent forms for all the procedures were approved by the ethics committee for human participants at the Niigata University School of Medicine (Niigata, Japan) in accordance with the Helsinki Declaration of 1964 as revised in 2013.

Peripheral blood (~ 9 mL) was collected into plastic vacuum plain blood collection tubes (Neotube; NIPRO, Osaka, Japan) containing 1 mL of the A-formulation of acid-citrate-dextrose (ACD-A; Terumo, Tokyo, Japan). The whole-blood samples were stored using a rotating agitator at ambient temperature and were used within 36 h. The whole-blood samples were centrifuged at $533 \times g$ for 10 min (first low-speed spin). For P-PRP preparation, the upper plasma fraction, which was approximately 2 mm beyond the interface between the plasma and RBC fractions, was transferred into 2-mL sample tubes for the second high-speed spin ($2656 \times g$, 5 min). For L-PRP preparation, the upper plasma fraction was transferred along with a buffy coat and the surface of the RBC fraction for the second spin. Prior to the second spin, 0.5 µg/mL prostaglandin E_1 (PGE_1) (Wako Pure Chemicals, Osaka, Japan) was added to each sample to prevent platelet aggregation. After centrifugation, 50–70% of the supernatant (PPP) was removed, and platelets (and other blood cells, if any) were resuspended in the remaining PPP fraction.

The numbers of platelets and other blood cells in the whole-blood samples and PRP preparations were determined using an AHA (pocH 100iV, Sysmex, Kobe, Japan).

Spectrophotometric determination of platelet counts and calibration curves
P-PRP and L-PRP preparations were serially diluted with the corresponding amount of PPP. The series of P-PRP and L-PRP dilutions were first subjected to measurement using the AHA and subsequently subjected to measurement with a compact scanning probe microscope (SPM; PiCOSCOPE, Ushio Inc., Tokyo, Japan) (Fig. 1). The SPM can be operated by remote control through a specific application installed on smart devices,

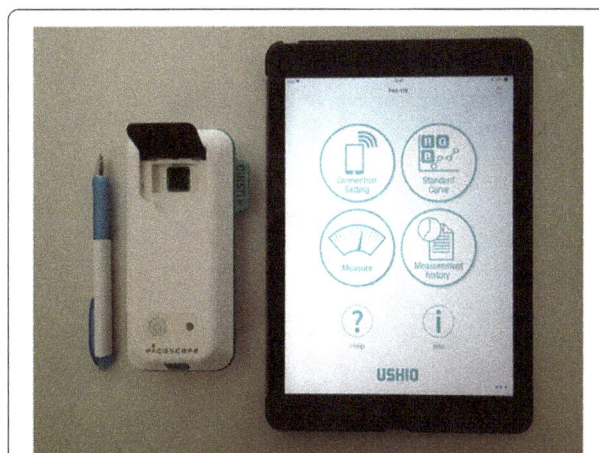

Fig. 1 A compact SPM with its remote controller installed on an iPad Air. iPhones and other Android devices can be used instead of the iPad Air

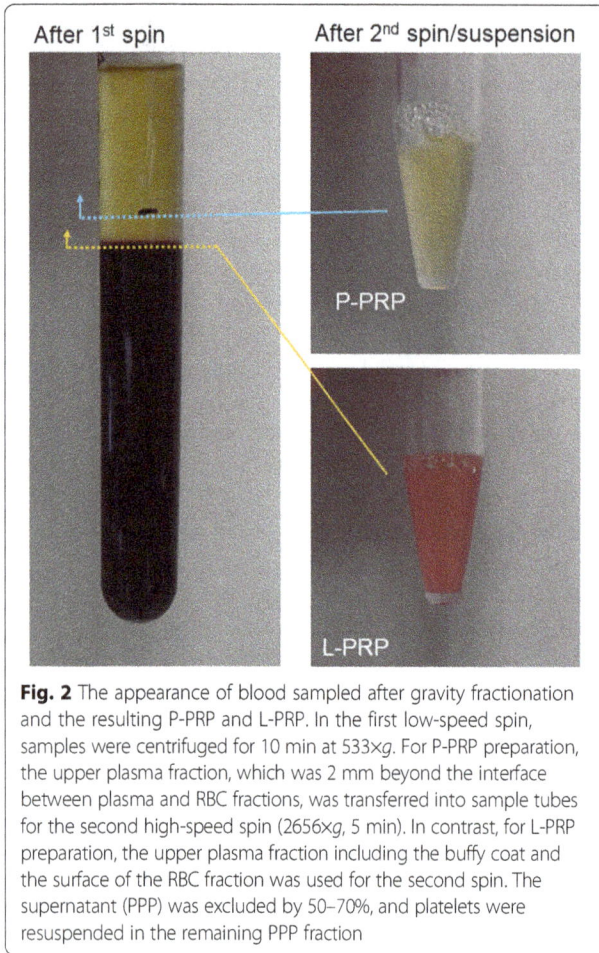

Fig. 2 The appearance of blood sampled after gravity fractionation and the resulting P-PRP and L-PRP. In the first low-speed spin, samples were centrifuged for 10 min at 533×*g*. For P-PRP preparation, the upper plasma fraction, which was 2 mm beyond the interface between plasma and RBC fractions, was transferred into sample tubes for the second high-speed spin (2656×*g*, 5 min). In contrast, for L-PRP preparation, the upper plasma fraction including the buffy coat and the surface of the RBC fraction was used for the second spin. The supernatant (PPP) was excluded by 50–70%, and platelets were resuspended in the remaining PPP fraction

including the iPad Air (Apple, Cupertino, CA, USA). PRP samples were transferred into 0.2 mL highly transparent PCR tubes (Nippon Genetics Co., Ltd., Tokyo, Japan) and were measured at 615 nm (range of wavelength 570–660 nm).

Using the data obtained with both the AHA and SPM, scattered plots were created to examine correlations and obtain formulas to calculate platelet counts.

Validation testing

P-PRP and L-PRP preparations were independently prepared from the 11 donors by three well-trained operators. Platelet counts were first determined using the AHA and aliquots of the PRP preparations were measured using the SPM. Platelet counts were calculated with the appropriate formulas and were compared with the measured platelet counts.

Statistical analysis

The data are expressed as mean ± standard deviation (SD). For two-group comparisons, statistical analyses were conducted to compare the mean values using the Student's *t* test (SigmaPlot 12.5; Systat Software, Inc., San Jose, CA, USA). *P* values of < 0.05 were considered statistically significant. The strength of a linear association between measured platelet counts and absorbance values was evaluated using the Pearson correlation coefficient (*R*). Based on these data, we obtained formulas for calculating platelet counts using absorbance values. Additionally, possible correlations between platelets and RBCs or WBCs and those between measured and calculated platelet counts were also evaluated using the Pearson correlation coefficient.

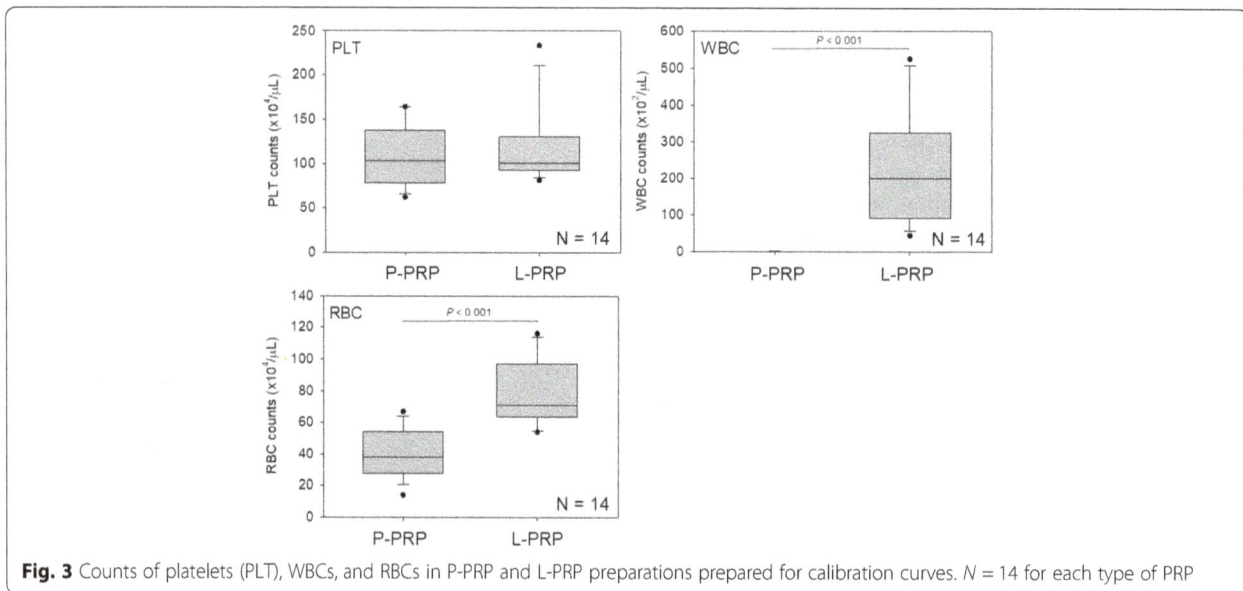

Fig. 3 Counts of platelets (PLT), WBCs, and RBCs in P-PRP and L-PRP preparations prepared for calibration curves. *N* = 14 for each type of PRP

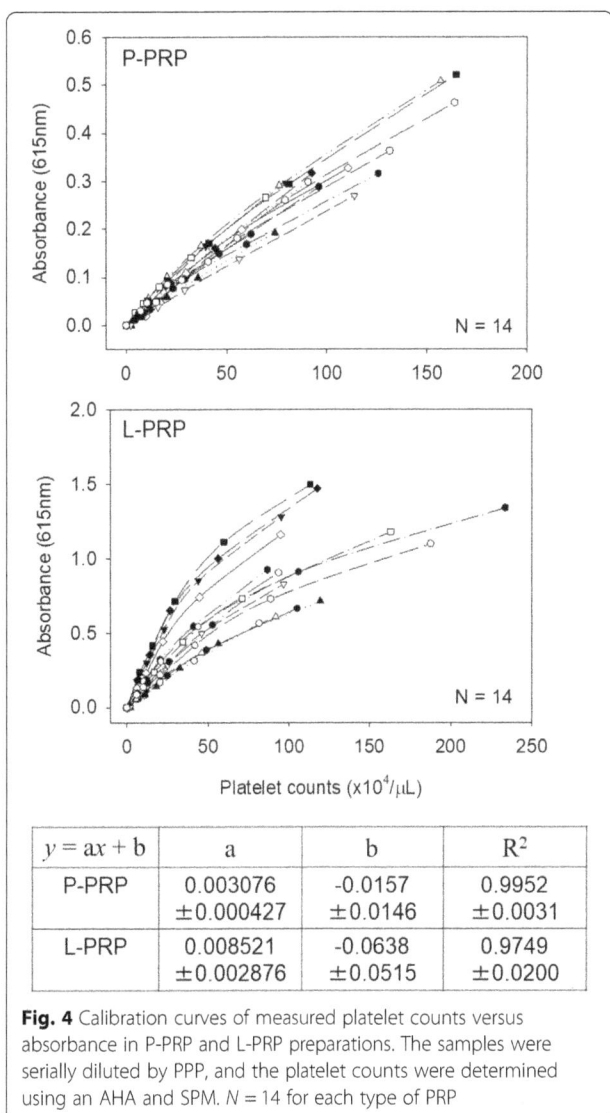

$y = ax + b$	a	b	R^2
P-PRP	0.003076 ±0.000427	-0.0157 ±0.0146	0.9952 ±0.0031
L-PRP	0.008521 ±0.002876	-0.0638 ±0.0515	0.9749 ±0.0200

Fig. 4 Calibration curves of measured platelet counts versus absorbance in P-PRP and L-PRP preparations. The samples were serially diluted by PPP, and the platelet counts were determined using an AHA and SPM. $N = 14$ for each type of PRP

Results

The appearance of the blood-collection tube after the first low-speed spin and representative P-PRP and L-PRP preparations after the second high-speed spin and subsequent re-suspension are shown in Fig. 2. Although low-speed spinning did not result in the formation of a clear buffy coat in the interface between the plasma and RBC fractions, the buffy coat corresponding to the plasma was not included in the second spin for P-PRP preparation. Therefore, the resulting P-PRP was light yellow in color, not reddish. In contrast, for the L-PRP preparation, the buffy coat and the surface of the RBC fraction just below the interface were included in the second spin. The inclusion of significant amounts of RBC turned the L-PRP red. The strength of this color was variable depending on the operators' pipetting skills; however, L-PRP preparations were more or less reddish when the maximum amount of platelets was recovered.

To characterize both the P-PRP and L-PRP preparations used for the calibration curves, blood cells were counted using an AHA (Fig. 3). For platelet counts, there was no significant difference between the two types of PRP. For WBC and RBC counts, in contrast, L-PRP contained significantly more WBCs and RBCs than P-PRP.

The samples were serially diluted, and platelets in individual dilutions were counted using the AHA. In parallel, the absorbance of each sample was measured with the SPM. The resulting calibration curves for P-PRP and L-PRP are shown in Fig. 4. Compared with P-PRP, the calibration curves for L-PRP varied with the samples and appeared generally inappropriate for linear regression. The calibration curve for P-PRP was expressed as "$y = 0.00308x - 0.0157$," while that of L-PRP was "$y = 0.00852x - 0.638$." The SD values for both the slope and intercept values were much higher in L-PRP. In addition, the R^2 value (coefficient of determination) for the linear regression of P-PRP was 0.995, while that of L-PRP was a little lower than that of P-PRP, 0.975, with almost 6.5-times higher SD values.

For validation of these calibration curves, P-PRP and L-PRP preparations prepared by three independent operators were employed. Blood cell counts are shown in Fig. 5. As observed in the calibration curves for the samples, significant differences were found in WBC and RBC counts, but not in platelet counts, between the P-PRP and L-PRP preparations. Correlations between platelet counts and WBC or RBC counts are shown in Fig. 6. Unexpectedly, strong positive correlations were observed only between platelet and RBC counts, but not between platelet and WBC counts, in both types of PRP preparations.

Measured versus calculated platelet counts are plotted in Fig. 7. In P-PRP preparations, the ratio of calculated platelet counts to the measured values was 108.6 ± 22.0%, whereas in L-PRP preparations, the ratio was 110.4 ± 64.0%. The discrepancy of SD values was reflected more clearly in the difference of R^2 values (0.671 vs. 0.0605).

Discussion

Since determination of bacterial cell number is a fundamental procedure in the field of microbiology, several methods have been developed and widely employed depending on the purpose of cell counting. SPM is one of the common methods used to estimate bacterial load [12]. The advantage of SPM is speed and convenience without additional preparation steps. On the other hand, the limitations are the inability to distinguish live bacteria from dead bacteria and a relatively narrow range of detection (10^8–10^{10} bacteria/mL) [12].

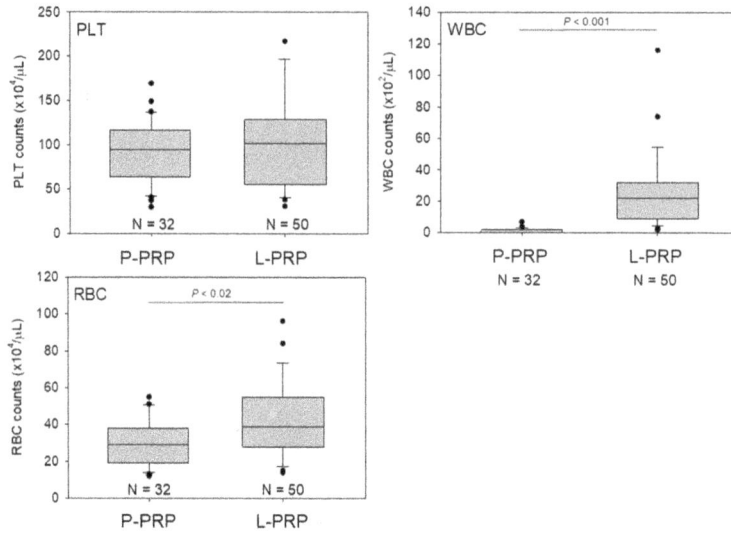

Fig. 5 Counts of platelets (PLT), WBCs, and RBCs in P-PRP and L-PRP preparations prepared for validation testing. $N = 32$ and 50 for P-PRP and L-PRP, respectively

A wide range of detection is not required for platelet counting in PRP preparations unlike in bacterial cell counting. However, it is more difficult to recognize platelets in PRP preparations compared to bacteria because WBCs and RBCs can more or less be included, especially when the buffy coat is included in the second spin. Lee and Tarassenko were probably inspired by the bacterial cell count and first reported the optical determination method for platelet counts [13]. However, the shortcomings of this method are that the range of RBC counts ($0–3 \times 10^4/\mu L$) is set below the RBC range ($30–40 \times 10^4/\mu L$ in average) of P-PRP and that WBCs were not taken into consideration.

To solve this problem, in this study, we separated PRP preparations into two types (i.e., P-PRP and L-PRP) for evaluation and successfully validated the spectrophotometric method in P-PRP preparations. In contrast, the accuracy of this method was lower than expected in L-PRP preparations, which is reflected in the difference in the coefficient values (Fig. 4). The striking difference

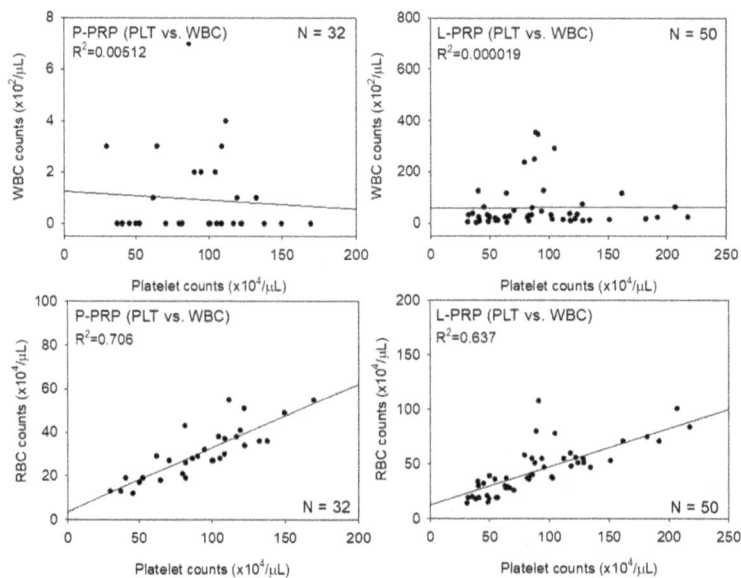

Fig. 6 Scatter plots representing possible correlations between platelet (PLT) and WBC counts and between platelet and RBC counts in P-PRP and L-PRP preparations. Note: strong positive correlations were observed between platelets and RBC in both PRP types. $N = 32$ and 50 for P-PRP and L-PRP, respectively

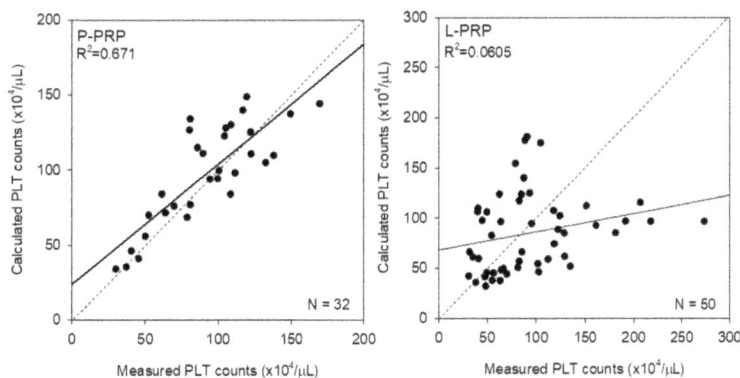

Fig. 7 Scatter plots representing correlations between measured and calculated platelet counts in P-PRP and L-PRP preparations. Note: a strong correlation was observed only in P-PRP. $N = 32$ and 50 for P-PRP and L-PRP, respectively

between P-PRP and L-PRP could be attributed to the inclusion of WBCs rather than RBCs in L-PRP as RBCs were also included in P-PRP with higher platelet counts. We speculate that WBCs were the primary factor responsible for lowering the performance and that they can disrupt light transparency more effectively than can RBCs; this is because WBCs are spherical, nucleated, and larger than disk-shaped RBCs and because the absorbance of hemoglobin contained in RBCs decreases beyond 600 nm [17] (cf., 615 nm, the peak wavelength used here). Besides counts, the size distribution of WBCs depends on individual donors. Hence, the ratios of large WBCs (e.g., neutrophils) to small WBCs (e.g., lymphocytes) widely vary across individuals, especially when they suffer from certain types of diseases, such as cancers, cardiovascular diseases, and pulmonary diseases [18–21].

Another limitation is the color of plasma. In terms of color, blood samples obtained from the donors participating in this study were light yellow and could be evaluated as "normal." However, we have sometimes encountered colored plasma samples in clinical practice. For example, when blood triglyceride levels are high, the plasma turns milky white or turbid [22–24]. Hemolytic plasma looks reddish, while icteric plasma appears yellow. When the degree of color change is not severe and when the transparency is maintained, the data may be compensated by the absorbance of PPP. However, in this case, we recommend the use of an AHA for accurate determination of the platelet counts.

We should discuss briefly how clinicians can perform quality assurance for individual PRP preparations. As described elsewhere [10, 25], PRP quality is evaluated mainly based on two major points: sterility and efficacy. Recent advances in PCR technology enable clinicians to quickly assess the contamination of targeted bacteria and mycoplasmas [26] in clinical settings. However, clinicians may require a well-trained operator for this kind

of sterility testing. The current regulatory framework for PRP therapy in Japan requires clinicians to prepare PRP on a clean bench [10]. Therefore, as long as blood samples are handled aseptically, the resulting PRP preparations are evaluated as sterile.

As for efficacy, regardless of the assay system, several hours or days are required to complete efficacy testing. Even if it takes only several hours, unfortunately, this delay is not beneficial to many patients and is not suitable for on-site preparation and immediate use in autologous PRP therapy. The only exception is platelet counting, which takes only a few minutes with the use of an AHA. However, it is a problem that the conventional form of this device is $10,000 or higher and requires installation space (500×500 mm at least). In contrast, the compact SPM used in this study costs only $800 and can be stored in a drawer. Therefore, despite several limitations, this compact SPM would be useful for fundamental quality assurance as well as for the examination of possible correlations between platelet counts and clinical outcomes.

Consistent with the clinical significance of platelet counting, several studies have reported that the platelet concentration is the most reliable criterion for the regenerative ability of PRP [27, 28] because platelets increase the number of anabolic signaling molecules. Conversely, as WBCs increase the number of catabolic signaling molecules, the quality of PRP can, perhaps, be considerably altered depending on the levels of WBCs included in PRP [29]. Despite functioning to clean wounds and prevent infection, WBCs, particularly phagocytic leukocytes, have been reported to produce matrix metalloproteinases (MMPs), oxygen and nitrogen reactive species (free radicals), and proinflammatory cytokines, which could adversely affect the stem cell behavior and, consequently, tissue regeneration [27, 30, 31]. This finding is evidenced by the fact that L-PRP induces inferior effects on the bone and cartilage regeneration compared with P-PRP [32, 33], indicating that P-PRP is, perhaps, more suitable than L-PRP in the field of regenerative dentistry. Hence, although working only in P-PRP, our spectrophotometric method would be of great use in assuring the quality of individual PRP preparations in the dental setting.

Conclusions

In normal blood samples composed of light yellow plasma, spectrophotometric determination of platelet counts would be useful for quality assurance of individual PRP preparations. For accurate determination, however, operators should handle samples with care to minimize the inclusion of WBCs and RBCs in PRP preparations.

Abbreviations
ACD: Acid-citrate-dextrose solution; AHA: Automated hematology analyzer; L-PRP: Leukocyte-rich PRP; PGE_1: Prostaglandin E_1; PPP: Platelet-poor plasma; PRF: Platelet-rich fibrin; PRP: Platelet-rich plasma; P-PRP: Pure-PRP; RBC: Red blood cell; SD: Standard deviation; SPM: Spectrophotometer; WBC: Leukocyte

Authors' contributions
YK, MS, TyTo, and TK conceived and designed the study, performed the experiments and data analysis, and wrote the manuscript. KI, TaTn, TsW, TkW, and HO designed and performed the experiments, data analysis, and intepretation. KN and TaTn conceived the study and participated in discussion of the results and manuscript preparation. All authors read and approved the final version of the manuscript.

Competing interests
Yutaka Kitamura, Masashi Suzuki, Tsuneyuki Tsukioka, Kazushige Isobe, Tetsuhiro Tsujino, Taisuke Watanabe, Takao Watanabe, Hajime Okudera, Koh Nakata, Takaaki Tanaka, and Tomoyuki Kawase declare that they have no competing interests.

Author details
[1]Tokyo Plastic Dental Society, Kita-ku, Tokyo, Japan. [2]Bioscience Medical Research Center, Niigata University Medical and Dental Hospital, Niigata, Japan. [3]Department of Materials Science and Technology, Niigata University, Niigata, Japan. [4]Division of Oral Bioengineering, Institute of Medicine and Dentistry, Niigata University, Niigata, Japan.

References
1. Marx RE, Carlson ER, Eichstaedt RM, Schimmele SR, Strauss JE, Georgeff KR. Platelet-rich plasma: Growth factor enhancement for bone grafts. Oral Surg Oral Med Oral Pathol Oral Radiol Endod. 1998;85:638–46.
2. Etulain J. Platelets in wound healing and regenerative medicine. Platelets. 2018:1–13.
3. Hou X, Yuan J, Aisaiti A, Liu Y, Zhao J. The effect of platelet-rich plasma on clinical outcomes of the surgical treatment of periodontal intrabony defects: a systematic review and meta-analysis. BMC Oral Health. 2016;16:71.
4. Pocaterra A, Caruso S, Bernardi S, Scagnoli L, Continenza MA, Gatto R. Effectiveness of platelet-rich plasma as an adjunctive material to bone graft: a systematic review and meta-analysis of randomized controlled clinical trials. Int J Oral Maxillofac Surg. 2016;45:1027–34.
5. Oryan A, Alidadi S, Moshiri A. Platelet-rich plasma for bone healing and regeneration. Expert Opin Biol Ther. 2016;16:213–32.
6. Rosello-Camps A, Monje A, Lin GH, Khoshkam V, Chavez-Gatty M, Wang HL,

Gargallo-Albiol J, Hernandez-Alfaro F. Platelet-rich plasma for periodontal regeneration in the treatment of intrabony defects: a meta-analysis on prospective clinical trials. Oral Surg Oral Med Oral Pathol Oral Radiol. 2015; 120:562–74.
7. Jovani-Sancho MD, Sheth CC, Marques-Mateo M, Puche-Torres M. Platelet-rich plasma: a study of the variables that may influence its effect on bone regeneration. Clin Implant Dent Relat Res. 2016;18:1051–64.
8. De Pascale MR, Sommese L, Casamassimi A, Napoli C. Platelet derivatives in regenerative medicine: an update. Transfus Med Rev. 2015;29:52–61.
9. Del Fabbro M, Corbella S, Taschieri S, Francetti L, Weinstein R. Autologous platelet concentrate for post-extraction socket healing: a systematic review. Eur J Oral Implantol. 2014;7:333–44.
10. Kawase T, Okuda K. Comprehensive quality control of the regenerative therapy using platelet concentrates: the current situation and prospects in Japan. Biomed Res Int. 2018; in press
11. Kitamura Y, Watanabe T, Nakamura M, Isobe K, Kawabata H, Uematsu K, Okuda K, Nakata K, Tanaka T, Kawase T. Platelet counts in insoluble platelet-rich fibrin clots: a direct method for accurate determination. Front Bioeng Biotechnol. 2018;6:4.
12. Hazan R, Que YA, Maura D, Rahme LG. A method for high throughput determination of viable bacteria cell counts in 96-well plates. BMC Microbiol. 2012;12:259.
13. Lee VS, Tarassenko L. An optical method for the determination of platelet count in platelet samples contaminated with red blood cells. J Biochem Biophys Methods. 1992;24:215–23.
14. Davis VL, Abukabda AB, Radio NM, Witt-Enderby PA, Clafshenkel WP, Cairone JV, Rutkowski JL. Platelet-rich preparations to improve healing. Part I: workable options for every size practice. J Oral Implantol. 2014;40:500–10.
15. Kossev P, Sokolov T. Platelet-rich plasma (PRP) in orthopedics and traumatology—review. In: Metodiev K, editor. Immunopathology and immunomodulation: IntechOpen limited; 2015. p. 173–95.
16. Parrish WR, Roides B, Hwang J, Mafilios M, Story B, Bhattacharyya S. Normal platelet function in platelet concentrates requires non-platelet cells: a comparative in vitro evaluation of leucocyte-rich (type 1a) and leucocyte-poor (type 3b) platelet concentrates. BMJ Open Sport Exerc Med. 2016;2: e000071.
17. Zijlstra WG, Buursma A. Spectrophotometry of hemoglobin: absorption spectra of bovine oxyhemoglobin, deoxyhemoglobin, carboxyhemoglobin, and methemoglobin. Comp Biochem Physiol B: Biochem Mol Biol. 1997;118:743–9.
18. Afari ME, Bhat T. Neutrophil to lymphocyte ratio (NLR) and cardiovascular diseases: an update. Expert Rev Cardiovasc Ther. 2016;14:573–7.
19. Faria SS, Fernandes PC, Silva MJB, Lima VC, Fontes W, Freitas-Junior R, Eterovic AK, Forget P. The neutrophil-to-lymphocyte ratio: a narrative review. Ecancermedicalscience. 2016;10:702.
20. Gao Y, Wang W-J, Zhi Q, Shen M, Jiang M, Bian X, Gong F-R, Zhou C, Lian L, Wu M-Y, Feng J, Tao M, Li W. Neutrophil/lymphocyte ratio is a more sensitive systemic inflammatory response biomarker than platelet/ lymphocyte ratio in the prognosis evaluation of unresectable pancreatic cancer. Oncotarget. 2017;8:88835–44.
21. Paliogiannis P, Fois AG, Sotgia S, Mangoni AA, Zinellu E, Pirina P, Negri S, Carru C, Zinellu A. Neutrophil to lymphocyte ratio and clinical outcomes in COPD: recent evidence and future perspectives. Eur Respir Rev. 2018;27
22. Vassallo RR, Stearns FM. Lipemic plasma: a renaissance. Transfusion. 2011;51: 1136–9.
23. Guder WG, da Fonseca-Wollheim F, Heil W, Schmitt YM, Töpfer G, Wisser H, Zawta B. The Haemolytic, Icteric and Lipemic Sample Recommendations Regarding their Recognition and Prevention of Clinically Relevant Interferences. Recommendations of the Working Group on Preanalytical Variables of the German Society for Clinical Chemistry and the German Society for Laboratory Medicine. LaboratoriumsMedizin / Journal of Laboratory Medicine. 2009;24:357–64.
24. Simundic AM, Nikolac N, Ivankovic V, Ferenec-Ruzic D, Magdic B, Kvaternik M, Topic E. Comparison of visual vs. automated detection of lipemic, icteric and hemolyzed specimens: can we rely on a human eye? Clin Chem Lab Med. 2009;47:1361–5.
25. Kawase T, Watanabe T, Okuda K. Platelet-rich plasma and its derived platelet concentrates: what dentists involved in cell-based regenerative therapy should know. Nihon Shishubyou Gakkai Kaishi. 2017;59:68–76. (in Japanese)
26. Tokuno O, Hayakawa A, Yanai T, Mori T, Ohnuma K, Tani A, Minami H, Sugimoto T. Sterility testing of stem cell products by broad-range bacterial 16S ribosomal DNA polymerase chain reaction. Lab Med. 2015;46:34–41.

27. Davis VL, Abukabda AB, Radio NM, Witt-Enderby PA, Clafshenkel WP, Cairone JV, Rutkowski JL. Platelet-rich preparations to improve healing. Part II: platelet activation and enrichment, leukocyte inclusion, and other selection criteria. J Oral Implantol. 2014;40:511–21.

28. Sundman EA, Cole BJ, Fortier LA. Growth factor and catabolic cytokine concentrations are influenced by the cellular composition of platelet-rich plasma. Am J Sports Med. 2011;39:2135–40.

29. Kobayashi Y, Saita Y, Nishio H, Ikeda H, Takazawa Y, Nagao M, Takaku T, Komatsu N, Kaneko K. Leukocyte concentration and composition in platelet-rich plasma (PRP) influences the growth factor and protease concentrations. J Orthop Sci. 2016;21:683–9.

30. Anitua E, Zalduendo MM, Prado R, Alkhraisat MH, Orive G. Morphogen and proinflammatory cytokine release kinetics from PRGF-Endoret fibrin scaffolds: evaluation of the effect of leukocyte inclusion. J Biomed Mater Res A. 2015;103:1011–20.

31. Kizil C, Kyritsis N, Brand M. Effects of inflammation on stem cells: together they strive? EMBO Rep. 2015;16:416–26.

32. Xu Z, Yin W, Zhang Y, Qi X, Chen Y, Xie X, Zhang C. Comparative evaluation of leukocyte- and platelet-rich plasma and pure platelet-rich plasma for cartilage regeneration. Sci Rep. 2017;7:43301.

33. Yin W, Qi X, Zhang Y, Sheng J, Xu Z, Tao S, Xie X, Li X, Zhang C. Advantages of pure platelet-rich plasma compared with leukocyte- and platelet-rich plasma in promoting repair of bone defects. J Transl Med. 2016;14:73.

7

Prospective multicenter non-randomized controlled study on intraosseous stability and healing period for dental implants in the posterior region

Shinya Homma[1]* , Yasushi Makabe[1], Takuya Sakai[2], Kenzou Morinaga[2], Satoru Yokoue[3], Hirofumi Kido[2] and Yasutomo Yajima[1]

Abstract

Background: A current implant body surface was treated with "rough processing" by sandblasting and acid etching for the purposes of obtaining more reliable osseointegration and shortening the treatment period. Various reports have examined the healing period with the use of these implant bodies, but a consensus opinion has not yet been obtained. The purpose of this study is to evaluate the relationship between insertion torque (IT) and implant stability quotient (ISQ) at implant treatment using the current rough-surfaced implant. We evaluated the implant treatment sites with ISQ values, IT values, and voxel values.

Methods: Participants in this study comprised 26 patients (10 males, 16 females; mean age, 55.5 years) who received posterior region dental implants at Tokyo Dental College Hospital or Fukuoka Dental College Hospital. For all participants, pretreatment computed tomography and determination of bone quality from voxel values were performed. Thirty-two implant bodies were inserted into the posterior region, and insertion torque was measured. ISQ was also measured at 0, 2, 4, 6, 8, and 12 weeks postoperatively.

Results: Eight implant bodies in the maxilla and 24 in the mandible were inserted. All ISQ values increased, exceeding 60 by 6 weeks postoperatively. For insertion torque < 30 N cm, ISQ increased significantly after 8 weeks. For ≥ 30 N cm, the ratio at which high ISQ values appeared increased significantly after 6 weeks. Compared with the treatment area with insertion torque < 40 N cm, the treatment area ≥ 40 N cm showed a significantly higher voxel value.

Conclusions: No significant relationship was found between the insertion torque value and the ISQ value. Also, it was suggested that the ISQ value was considered to be an important indicator for observing the treatment state of the implant.

Keywords: Osseointegration, Intraosseous stability, Insertion torque, Resonance frequency analysis, Voxel value, CBCT

Background

Dental implant treatments have improved in both convenience and predictability with refinements in implant bodies and treatment procedures as compared to about 50 years ago when clinical applications were started. Currently, an implant body surface is treated with "rough processing" by sandblasting and acid etching for the purposes of obtaining more reliable osseointegration and shortening treatment period. Despite previous reports about the healing period when implant bodies treated in this the procedure, a common consensus has yet to be obtained [1–3].

With implant treatment, the healing period refers to the period until an inserted implant body acquires osseointegration and can be loaded with occlusal force [4, 5]. In order to shave off the healing period, various method in which occlusal force was immediately or early loaded on the inserted implant body have been reported.

* Correspondence: honmas@tdc.ac.jp
[1]Department of Oral and Maxillofacial Implantology, Tokyo Dental College, 2-9-18 Misaki-cho, Chiyoda-ku, Tokyo 101-0061, Japan
Full list of author information is available at the end of the article

However, theories on the therapeutic effect of immediate loading or early loading of implant treatment were not unified [6, 7]. "Quantity and quality of bone in treatment area," "primary stability after implant insertion," and "intraosseous stability during the healing period" are regional factors related to the acquisition and maintenance of osseointegration [8–10].

Usually, bone quantity and bone quality are evaluated by morphometry of computed tomography (CT) images and analysis of voxel values, and primary stability is evaluated as insertion torque (IT). Intraosseous stability of the implant during the healing period is estimated from X-ray images, the Periotest, or a resonance frequency analysis device [11–15]. The estimation procedure with a non-contact-type resonance frequency analysis device has been recognized as a non-invasive and reproducible procedure [16].

Intraosseous stability of an implant that is measured with a non-contact-type resonance frequency analysis device is evaluated as ISQ value. Insertion torque (IT) value and ISQ value are important indicators of implant treatment. However, the relationship between IT and ISQ is unclear. Some articles have reported positive correlations between IT and ISQ [15, 17], but others have found no correlation [18–20].

The purpose of this study is to evaluate the relationship between IT and ISQ at implant treatment using the current rough surfaced implant. We evaluated the implant treatment sites with implant stability quotient (ISQ) values, IT values, and voxel values. We assumed that there is relevance between the insertion torque value and the ISQ value.

Methods

Research design and study participants

This prospective study was conducted jointly by Tokyo Dental College (Tokyo, Japan) and Fukuoka Dental College (Fukuoka, Japan) from January to December 2015. All study protocols were conducted in accordance with the Declaration of Helsinki [21] and were approved by the ethics committees of Tokyo Dental College (approval #416) and Fukuoka Dental College (approval #213).

Participants comprised patients at Tokyo Dental College Hospital or Fukuoka Dental College Hospital who were ≥ 20 years old, desired implant treatment in the posterior region, and consented to the details of the study protocols. The participants of this study were selected without randomization.

In this study, implant treatment was performed on 33 tooth extracted sites. The reasons for tooth extraction were periodontal diseases (14), caries (12), root fractures (7), and teeth had already been extracted (8). Tooth extraction was carried out with normal technique without socket preservation method. All participants were followed up for more than 4 months after tooth extraction and X-ray examined with multi-slice CT (MSCT) or cone beam CT (CBCT). Consequently, it was confirmed that sufficient bone mass exists to insert the implant body without bone augmentation in all treatment site. CT imaging equipment was different for each facility.

Exclusion criteria were untreated systemic disease, diabetes, cardiovascular disease, osteoporosis, mental disorder, alcohol- or drug dependence, or smoking habit; failure to follow treatment directions; presence of severe periodontal disease, shedding disorder, trismus, malocclusion, or bruxism in the oral cavity; or failure of implant treatment.

Materials and treatment procedure

The implant body used in this study was the Genesio® Plus implant with Aanchor surface (GC, Tokyo Japan). The implant body had been processed to create a rough surface by sandblasting and acid etching (Fig. 1). The implant body for the treatment of each participant was selected from two diameters (3.8 or 4.4 mm) and three lengths (8.0, 10.0, or 12.0 mm). The treatment area and the implant size used in this study are shown in Table 1.

Implant treatment was performed in accordance with the procedure recommended by the manufacturer, without bone augmentation. A healing abutment was connected to the implant bodies after insertion (implant insertion in one stage method). A total of 17 dentists (treatment experience, 5–35 years; average, 11.5 years) performed all implant treatments in this study. All dentists who performed the implant treatment in this study were specialist certified by Japan Society of Oral Implantology and had experience of more than 5 years implant treatment.

Evaluation of treatment

IT, ISQ, and voxel value were measured in this study. IT was measured immediately after the implant insertion using a torque wrench (GC, Tokyo, Japan).

ISQ was measured throughout the experimental period. To measure ISQ, a Smartpeg Type 21 (Osstell AB, Gothenburg, Sweden) was connected at 5 N cm to the implant body, measured using an Osstell ISQ™ (Osstell AB) three times from the buccal side. Average values were used for the evaluations. ISQ was measured immediately (0 week), and 4, 6, and 12 weeks after surgery in all cases, and also at 2 and 8 weeks after surgery where possible.

In the following cases, the implant body was excluded from the evaluation.

- If motion and/or rotation was observed in the implant body.

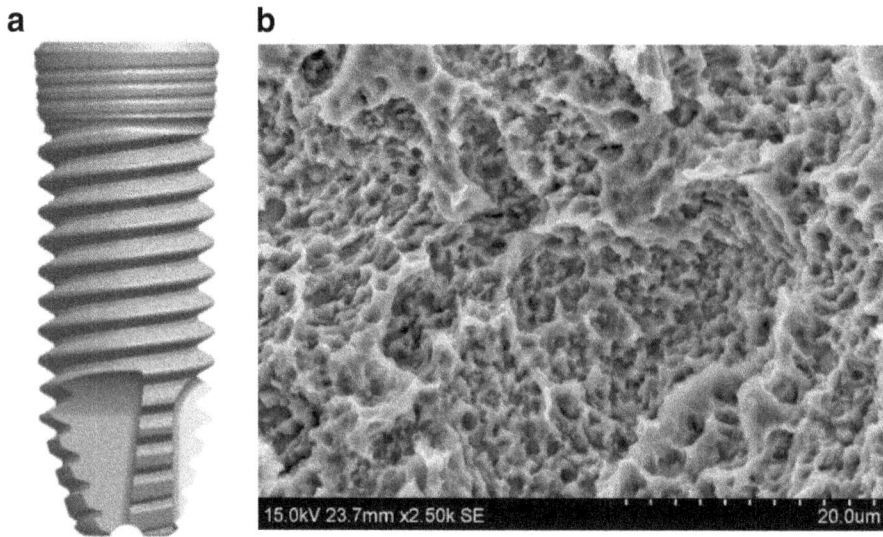

Fig. 1 Genesio® Plus implant with Aanchor surface. Scheme of the dental implant body for the Genesio® Plus implants with Aanchor surface used. **a** Overview picture of Genesio® Plus implants with Aanchor surface. **b** Image from scanning electron microscopy. Both pictures were provided by GC Corporation. To obtain osseointegration from an early stage, the dental implant body was treated with sandblasting and acid etching from the neck to apex

- If the bone surrounding the implant body showed absorption.
- If inflammation was observed in tissue surrounding the implant.
- If a mandatory ISQ measurement was not performed.

In this study, we performed X-ray image diagnosis using a multi-slice CT (MSCT) or a cone beam CT (CBCT) to confirm the healing of the bone form and volume after the tooth extraction. CT imaging equipment was different for each facility (two models of CBCT and one model of MSCT). It was difficult to make the same evaluation on voxel values obtained from different equipment. The X-ray examination performed in different two models of CBCT at 18 treatment sites and 8 treatment sites. Seven treatment sites were X-ray examined in MSCT. Therefore, bone quality was investigated at 18 treatment areas (8 in the maxilla, 10 in the mandible) on the CBCT performed under standardized conditions, as shown below.

The CBCT was performed using a 3DX Multi-Image Micro CT FPD 8 system (J. MORITA MFG., Kyoto, Japan) (tube voltage, 80 kV; imaging area, 80 × 80 mm), and voxel values were measured with coDiagnostix™ 9.7 (dental wings, Montreal, Canada). The voxel values were calculated based on CT images for bone quality diagnosis. Voxel values were measured three times at 12 locations covering the mesial, distal, buccal, and lingual sides of each of the neck, middle, and apex parts of the implant treatment area, then average voxel values for each part and for the whole treatment area were calculated (Fig. 2).

Statistical analysis

All numerical data obtained in this research were statistically analyzed with one-way analysis of variance and multiple comparison tests by Bonferroni et al. [22]. Fisher's exact test and the corresponding t test were used for statistical analysis of insertion torque values and the relationship between ISQ and insertion torque, respectively [23].

Results

Study overview

A total of 33 implant bodies (8 in the maxilla, 25 in the mandible) were inserted into the 27 participants (11 men, 16 women), with the average age of 54.6 ± 12.2 years (range, 32–78 years). The average IT value was 32.7 ± 9.2 N cm (32.5 ± 11.6 N cm in the maxilla, 32.8 ± 8.5 N cm in the mandible). The diameter of the implant body was 4.4 mm in 20 (60.6%) and 3.8 mm in 13 (39.4%), and the length of the implant body was 8.0 mm in 6 (18.2%), 10.0 mm in 19 (57.6%), and 12.0 mm in 8 (24.2%) (Table 1).

The measurement results of IT and ISQ are shown in Table 2. Due to the identification of mobility at 4 weeks postoperatively, No. 19 implant body (diameter, 4.4 mm; length, 12.0 mm) that had been inserted at the first molar position in the right mandible of a 32-year-old male patient was excluded from the evaluation. As a result, this study evaluated the 32 implant bodies (8 in the maxilla, 24 in the mandible) inserted into 26 participants. The survival rate of the implant bodies at the end of this study was 97% (maxilla, 100%; mandible, 96%).

Table 1 Treatment area and size of implant body

Number of implants	Treatment area (FDI)	Size of implant (mm)	
		Length	Diameter
1	14	10	3.8
2	14	10	3.8
3	14	10	3.8
4	16	8	3.8
5	16	10	4.4
6	16	8	4.4
7	16	8	4.4
8	17	10	4.4
9	36	10	3.8
10	36	10	4.4
11	36	8	3.8
12	36	10	3.8
13	36	12	4.4
14	36	10	4.4
15	36	10	4.4
16	36	12	3.8
17	36	10	4.4
18	36	12	4.4
19	36	12	4.4
20	37	10	4.4
21	37	12	4.4
22	37	12	4.4
23	46	10	4.4
24	46	10	4.4
25	46	10	3.8
26	46	8	3.8
27	46	12	4.4
28	46	10	3.8
29	46	12	4.4
30	47	10	3.8
31	47	8	3.8
32	47	10	4.4
33	47	10	4.4

The diameter of the implant body was selected to have a bone of 1 mm width or more in the around inserted implant body. The length of implant body was selected to leave 2 mm or more from the maxillary sinus or the mandibular canal

Evaluation of ISQ and IT

The average ISQ values of all tested implant bodies increased through this study; moreover, all tested implant bodies indicated 60 or more ISQ value 6 weeks after the implant insertion. A significant difference was observed at 0 and ≥ 6 weeks ($P < 0.01$) (Fig. 3). No significant difference of average ISQ was found on the maxilla and mandible.

The inserted implant bodies were classified by IT value as the low IT group (< 30 N cm), the medium IT group (30–40 N cm), and the high IT group (≥ 40 N cm). Nine specimens were classified as the low IT group (3 in the maxilla, 6 in the mandible), 12 as the medium IT group (1 in the maxilla, 11 in the mandible), and 11 as the high IT group (4 in the maxilla, 7 in the mandible) (Fig. 4). There was no difference between the maxilla and the mandible in the average value of the IT (maxilla 32.5 ± 11.6 N cm, mandible 32.9 ± 8.7 N cm).

Average ISQ tended to increase during the healing period in all IT groups (Fig. 5). Average ISQ of the low IT group was 59.81 at 0 week, increasing significantly after ≥ 8 weeks ($P < 0.01$). The average ISQ values of the medium and high IT groups at 0 week were 73.25 and 68.85, respectively. The average ISQ increased in a time-dependent manner at each group.

Total average ISQ in this study was 73.3 ± 9.6; therefore, an expedient reference value was defined as the ISQ 73, then the percentage of specimens showing ISQ ≥ 73 was determined (Fig. 6). ISQ ≥ 73 was observed from 8 to 12 weeks in the low IT group and from 4 to 6 weeks in the medium and high IT groups. Significant differences in the incidence of ISQ ≥ 73 was recognized at the medium and high IT groups (corresponding t test, $P < 0.05$).

Relationship between IT and voxel value

In this study, conditions and environments for CT imaging in each facility were different. Bone quality was investigated at 18 treatment areas (8 in the maxilla, 10 in the mandible) on CBCT performed under standardized conditions, as shown below. CBCT was performed using a 3DX Multi-Image Micro CT FPD 8 system (J. MORITA MFG., Kyoto, Japan) (tube voltage, 80 kV; imaging area, 80×80 mm), and voxel values were measured with coDiagnostix™ 9.7 (dental wings, Montreal, Canada).

There was no difference of average voxel value between the maxilla and the mandible (Fig. 7). In comparison between average voxel values and IT groups, the low and medium IT groups showed no significant differences, but the high IT group showed voxel values $\geq 40\%$ higher than the other groups (Fig. 8). A significant difference was observed between the low/medium IT groups and the high IT group ($P < 0.05$). A significant difference was observed between the low/medium IT groups and the high IT group ($P < 0.05$). Also, voxel values at each part of the implant (neck, middle apex) were compared with IT < 40 and ≥ 40. The results suggested that the neck and apex parts in the ≥ 40 IT group showed significantly higher voxel values than the middle and apex parts of the < 40 IT group ($P < 0.05$) (Fig. 9).

Discussion

According to the previous literature, the obtaining osseointegration is integral to the intraosseous stability of

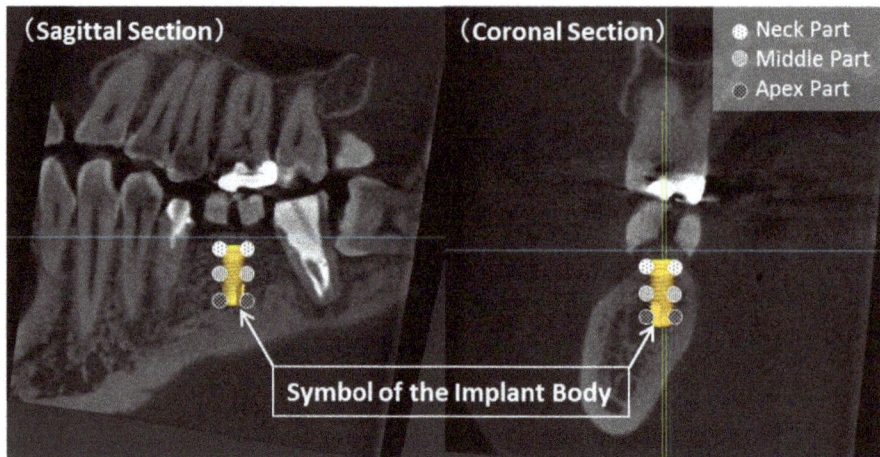

Fig. 2 The measurement of the voxel values. A case of bone quality diagnosis before treatment. Width and height of the bone were measured to select the proper size of the implant body. The selected implant body was simulated on the bone images as a symbol, and then the voxel value was calculated as described in the "Methods" section

the implant body during the healing period [24]; moreover, the importance of postoperative assessment of the intraosseous stability of the implant has also been reported [10]. Intraosseous stability of the implant body is evaluated immediately after the implant insertion and during the healing period after surgery.

The primary stability is necessary for implant treatment, and the absence of primary stability may result in treatment failure [25, 26]. Primary stability was evaluated with insertion torque immediately after the implant insertion.

This study had a short implementation period, and it was difficult to recruit a large number of participants. Therefore, participants had a bias in age and gender, and the treated area was also biased. We referred previous publication to review the effect of participant's age and gender at insertion torque value. According to the above literature reviewing, the participant's age and gender did not affect insertion torque value [27–29]. However, it was thought that there was a possibility that the number of participants influenced the result.

In this study, primary stability was evaluated with insertion torque value measured by manual torque wrench immediately after implant insertion. Manual torque wrench is the medical instrument used for implant treatment frequently. A recent study about insertion torque that compared electronically controlled torque wrench with manual torque wrench states that the measurement results of both instruments were similar [30]. Manual torque wrench is classified into three styles (coil, toggle, and beam style). In this study, beam style manual torque wrench was used. It was reported that beam style torque wrench present most precise result compared with other two kinds of torque wrenches [31]. As described above, the measurement procedure of insertion torque value in this study is thought to be acceptable.

The insertion torque value in this study showed broader (10 to 50 N cm) than the previous publication (Table 2) [22, 32], and the cause of reasons for the difference are as follows: Primary stability may be affected by the bone quantity and bone quality in the treatment area, the micro- and macro-level design of the implant body, and the accuracy of the surgical technique [18, 25]. In this study, the 17 dentists performed implant treatment. The deviation of each insertion torque value was thought by the surgical technique of each dentist. In clinical situation, the insertion torque value is considered to indicate various values.

The insertion torque value in this study showed no significant difference between each treatment area. Therefore, all of the implant bodies were considered as one population and that population was classified into three groups by insertion torque value and analyzed. In a recent literature, Anitua et al. reported that the insertion torque values were 59.29 ± 7.27 N cm at type I bone, 56.51 ± 1.62 N cm at type II bone, 46.40 ± 1.60 N cm at type III bone, 34.84 ± 2.38 N cm at type IV bone, and 5 N cm at type V bone [29]. Since the average value of insertion torque in this study was 32.7 ± 9.2 N cm, it was inferred that this study evaluated implant treatment for relatively soft bone quality.

The intraosseous stability of the healing period was evaluated by mobility measurement and/or resonance frequency analysis. A resonance frequency analysis has been reported as a non-invasive procedure that is useful for evaluating osseointegration [13, 33]. The results of the resonance frequency analysis were represented in the present study as the ISQ.

An ISQ is reportedly affected by the condition of the bone surrounding the implant, such as the range of contact between implant body and bone [33–35]. Other

Table 2 Result of IT and ISQ

Number of implants	Insertion torque value (N cm)	Implant stability quotient value					
		0 week	2 weeks	4 weeks	6 weeks	8 weeks	12 weeks
1	25	33.0	75.0	77.0	78.3	79.7	77.0
2	40	68.0	70.3	70.0	72.0	75.7	75.3
3	40	78.3	77.0	78.0	78.7	80.0	80.0
4	35	74.0	43.0	61.0	73.0	75.7	80.0
5	45	85.3	85.7	84.0	83.3	84.0	83.0
6	25	65.0	68.0	68.3	70.0	72.0	71.0
7	40	82.3	84.0	82.0	84.0	81.0	81.0
8	10	51.3	52.1	46.7	59.3	66.3	68.7
9	35	78.7	80.0	80.0	80.0	81.3	80.0
10	35	86.3	84.0	83.0	84.0	85.0	85.0
11	40	78.0	75.7	76.3	78.7	79.7	80.0
12	40	80.0	80.0	79.3	81.0	81.0	84.3
13	35	71.0	73.0	77.3	80.0	77.0	82.0
14	45	70.0	72.0	76.0	80.0	81.0	82.3
15	30	73.3	73.0	65.0	68.7	73.3	75.0
16	25	75.3	75.0	72.0	73.0	75.3	77.7
17	35	68.7	76.0	72.7	76.3	79.0	81.3
18	30	75.0	80.0	80.3	81.7	82.7	81.3
19	30	50.7	–	–	–	–	–
20	30	73.7	61.3	67.7	73.7	57.7	57.0
21	45	69.3	66.7	57.3	75.0	76.3	77.7
22	20	73.3	75.7	76.7	77.0	80.7	82.0
23	50	71.7	69.7	73.3	76.0	77.3	79.7
24	30	76.0	80.0	80.0	82.0	81.3	81.0
25	20	64.0	47.7	71.0	69.3	68.0	77.0
26	20	65.0	70.0	75.0	77.0	79.0	80.0
27	35	65.7	60.3	61.3	69.7	68.0	68.0
28	40	22.3	57.0	68.7	75.0	75.0	80.0
29	35	69.7	73.7	76.7	74.7	74.7	81.0
30	20	58.0	46.0	65.7	70.0	70.0	75.3
31	35	67.0	78.0	69.3	78.7	80.0	82.3
32	20	53.3	63.3	61.0	64.7	68.7	70.0
33	40	52.0	52.7	66.0	75.7	78.0	79.3

The primary stability of no.19 implant was evaluated as good. ISQ of this implant was measured immediately after surgery. No.19 implant had mobility at 2 weeks after surgery and did not improve even at 4 weeks after surgery. Therefore, this implant was excluded from the evaluation

studies have suggested that ISQ immediately after implant insertion should be about 60 [24, 36], with ISQ subsequently decreasing over weeks 0–4 and increasing over weeks 4–8 after surgery [13, 24, 34]. ISQ values 57–70 may indicate that intraosseous stability of the implant body is constant [34, 37].

Increases or decreases of ISQ values are explained as follows: The inserted dental implant body is supported by mechanical interdigitating force after surgery, but this interdigitating force will be reduced time-dependently by

the effects of osteoclasts activation at the initial stage of the bone remodeling process, then osseointegration will be completed by an increasing contact area between the bone and dental implant body at the bone regeneration step [38]. The period switch from ISQ decreasing to increasing was considered as the most unstable but important period during the healing period [24].

The average ISQ in this study was 68.0 ± 13.7 after surgery then increased to 71.8 ± 8.3 at 4 weeks and 78.0 ± 5.7 at 12 weeks after surgery; all inserted implants

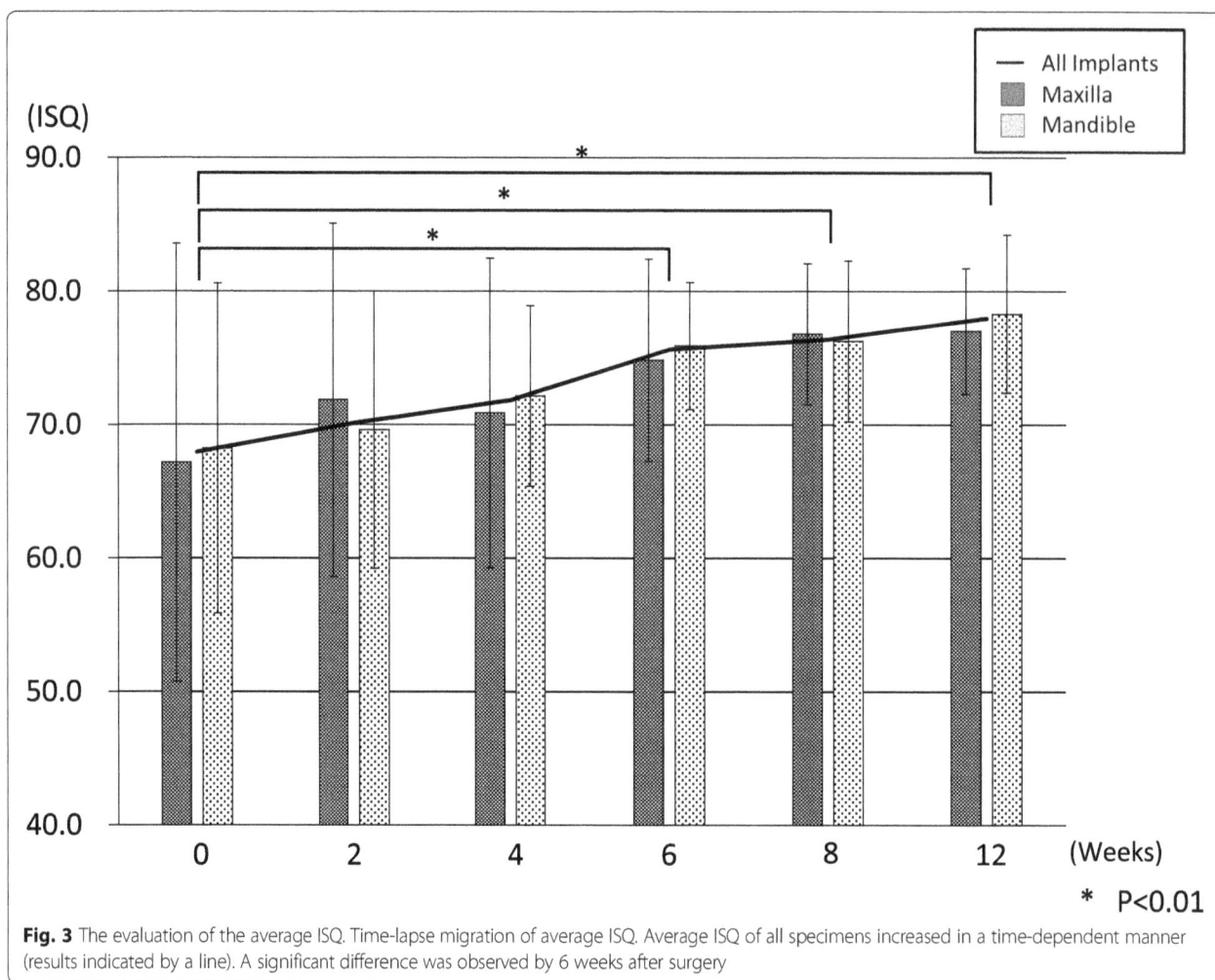

Fig. 3 The evaluation of the average ISQ. Time-lapse migration of average ISQ. Average ISQ of all specimens increased in a time-dependent manner (results indicated by a line). A significant difference was observed by 6 weeks after surgery

showed ISQ > 60 after 6 weeks (Fig. 3). In addition, the average ISQ decreasing was not observed during the experimental period. According to the publication about the relationship with ISQ value and intraosseous stability of the implant body inserted in the soft bone quality by Held et al., the ISQ value was not decreasing and tended to increase [39]. As per we evaluated implant treatment at the soft bone in this study, migration of the ISQ value in this study showed similarity with the abovementioned document.

The relationship between IT and ISQ remains unclear. Some articles have reported positive correlations between IT and ISQ [15, 17], but others have found no correlation [18–20].

While no significant relationship was found between IT and ISQ in this study, the migration pattern of ISQ differed between the low IT group and medium/high IT group. ISQ in the low IT group was initially low, increasing over time. A significant difference was observed between 0 and ≥ 8 weeks (Fig. 5). The ISQ did not change significantly during the experimental period in

the medium or high IT groups, but the percentage of high ISQ (≥ 73) specimens was significantly higher at 4 to 6 weeks compared to other time periods in both groups (Figs. 5 and 6). The results in this study suggest that if the implant insertion has been performed with low insertion torque, progress of peri-implant bone maturation (transfer from mechanical interdigitation to osseointegration) slowly stabilizing at 8 weeks after surgery, or if the insertion torque value was moderate or higher, peri-implant bone will maturate following a safe healing period and show stabilization at 6 weeks after surgery.

In this study, we could not find a significant relationship between insertion torque value and ISQ value. However, insertion torque value is an important indicator for predicting the progress of implant treatment, and ISQ value is considered to be an important indicator for observing the treatment state of the implant. Currently, the insertion torque value is used as the major decision index for the determination of the loading period on the implant body. Lozano-Carrascal et al. explained that if

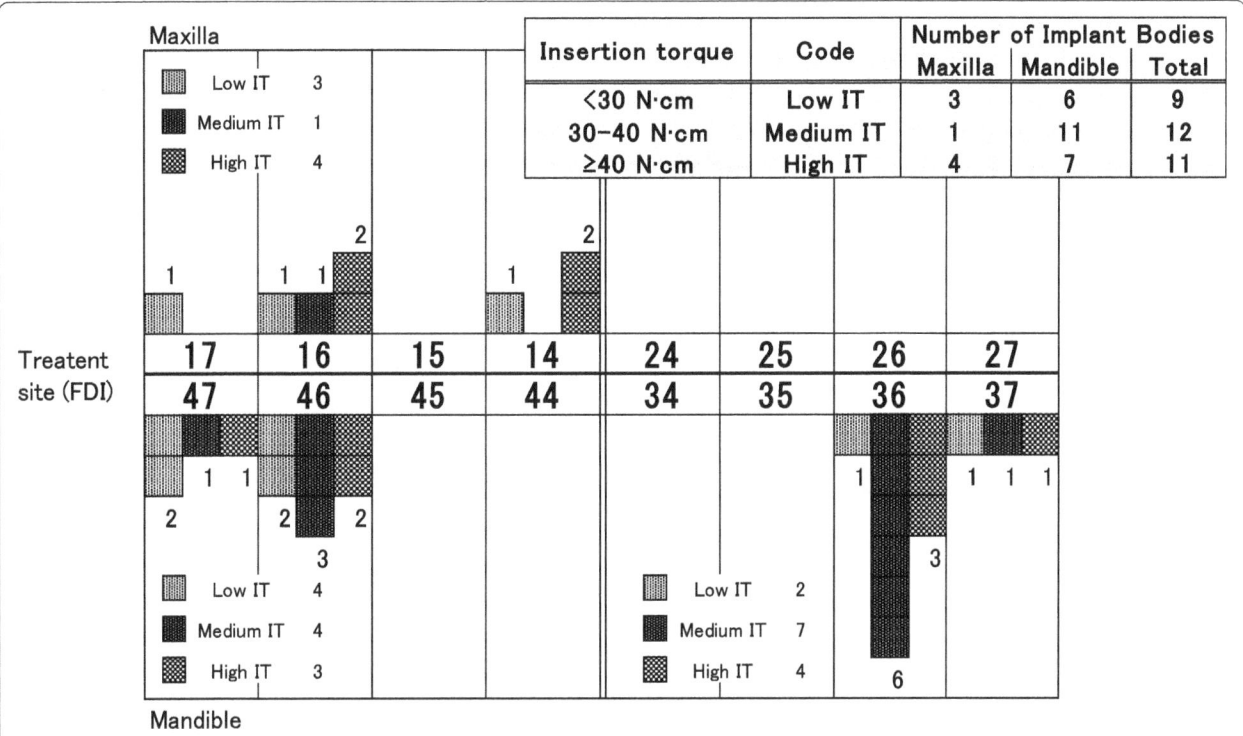

Fig. 4 The classification of the insertion torque. All specimens classified into three groups according to insertion torque. Criteria for the classification are shown in the figure and in the "Methods" section

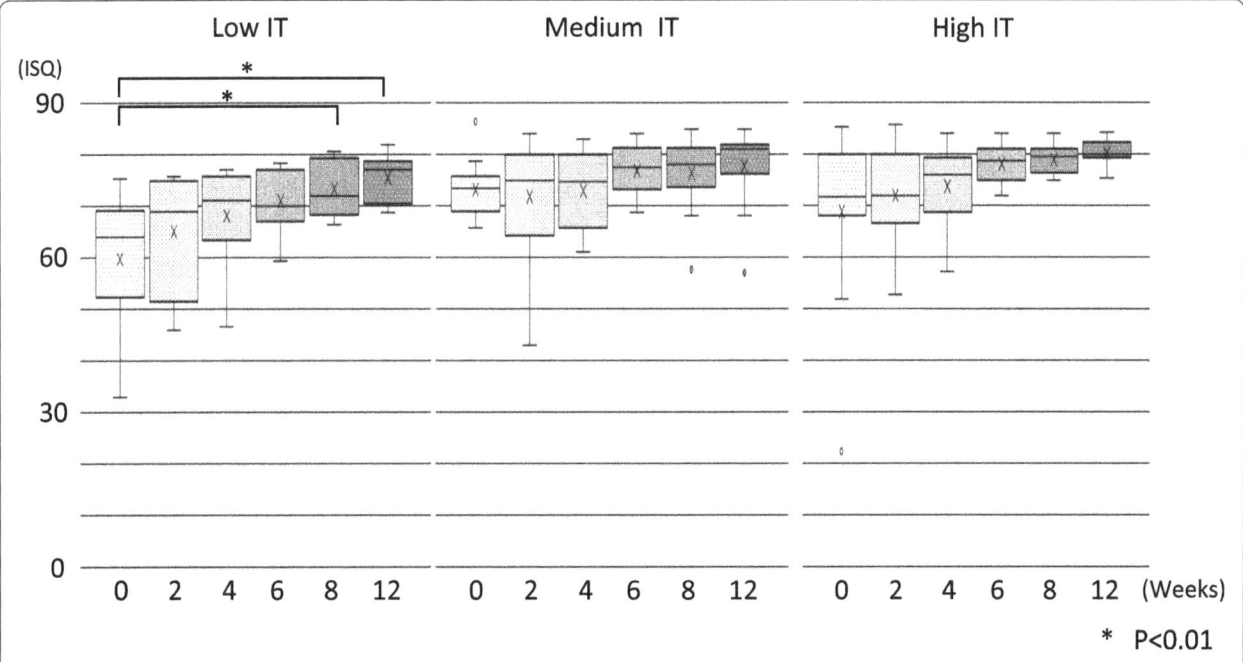

Fig. 5 The comparison of ISQ values by the insertion torque. Time-lapse migration of ISQ values was compared with IT groups. Each IT group displayed similar migration. A significant difference in The ISQ was found in the low IT group after 8 weeks

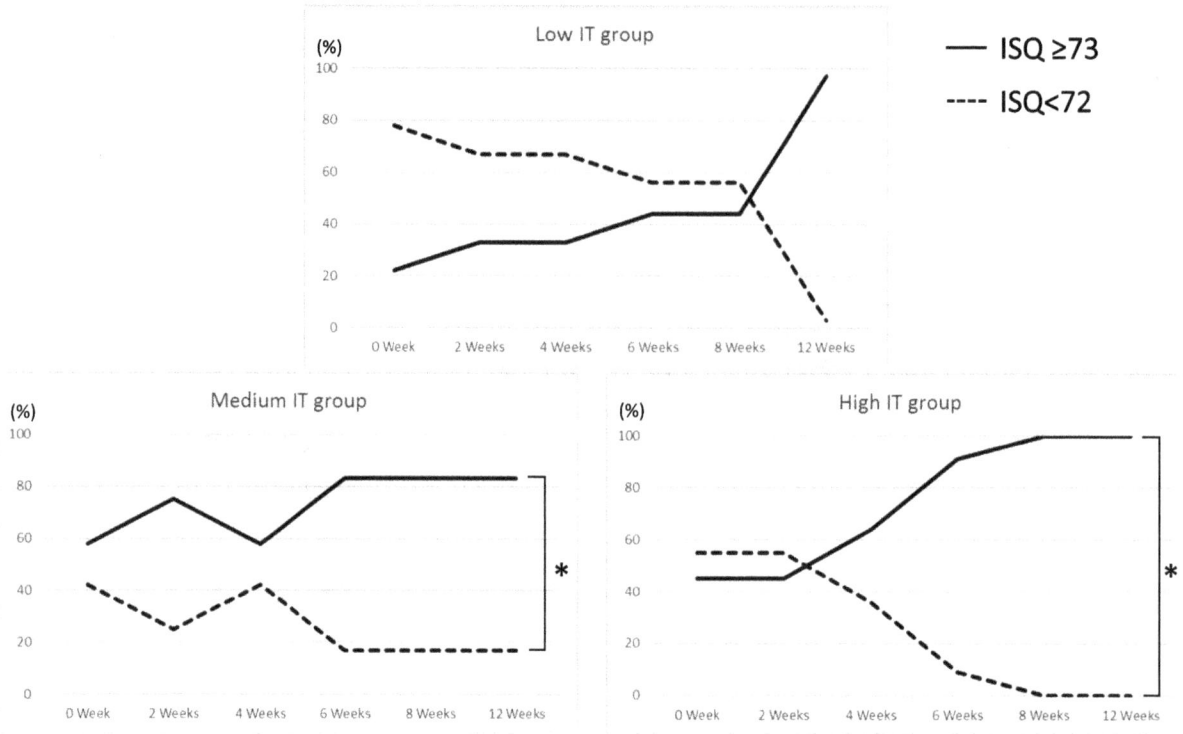

Fig. 6 The relationship between ISQ and insertion torque. Percentage of specimens showing ISQ ≥ 73 compared with groups by week. In all groups, a period of rapidly increasing percentages was observed (8–12 weeks in the low IT group, 4–6 weeks in the medium and high IT groups). In the medium and high IT Group, a statistically significant difference was observed between ISQ ≥ 73 and ISQ < 72 (P < 0.05)

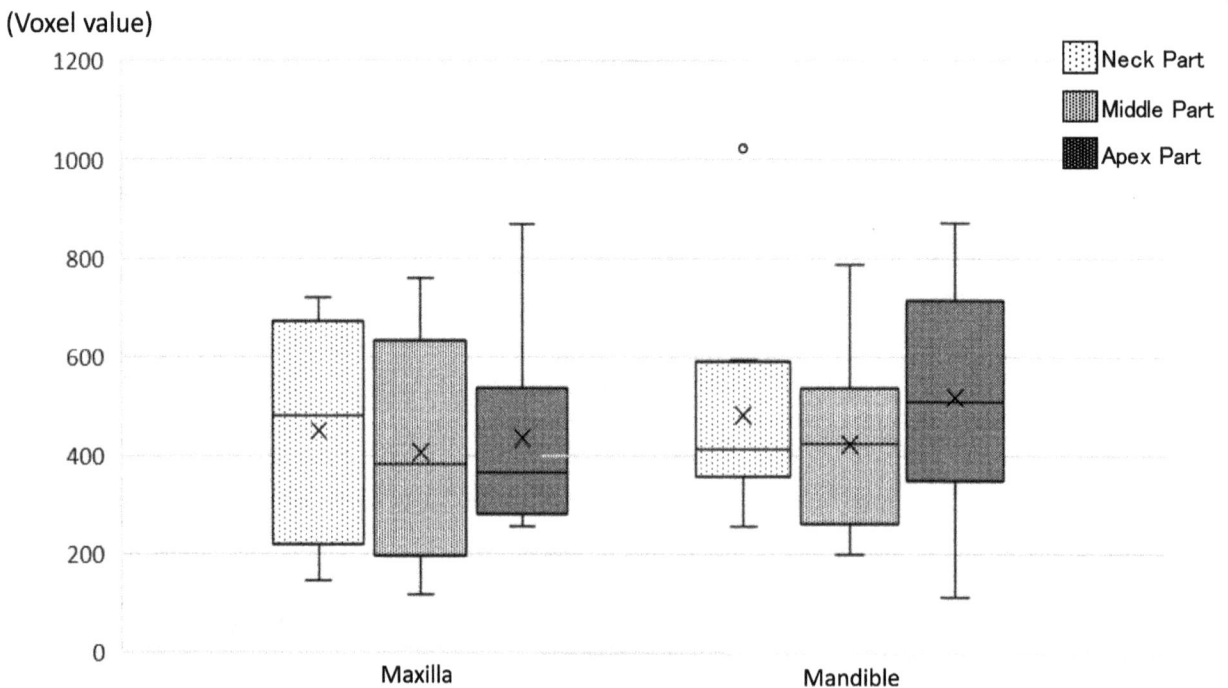

Fig. 7 The average voxel value between the maxilla and mandible. There was no difference between the maxilla (430.9 ± 211.6) and the mandible (475.6 ± 211.5) in the average voxel value. Also, no difference was found in each part

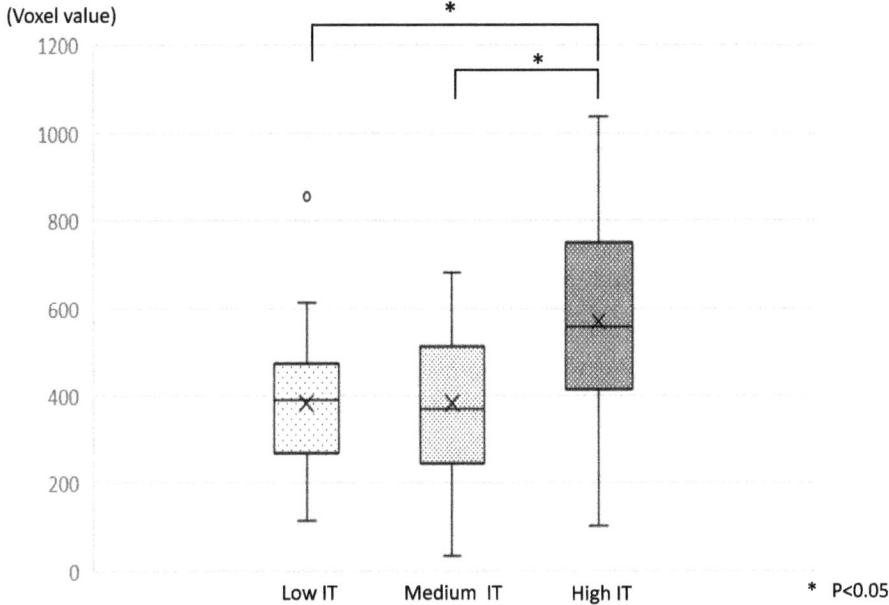

Fig. 8 The relationship between average voxel value and insertion torque (averaged over the entire treatment area). The comparison of average voxel value among IT groups. Average voxel value was 384.0 ± 154.6 in the low IT group, 387.7 ± 147.7 in the medium IT group, and 619.2 ± 200.4 in the high IT group

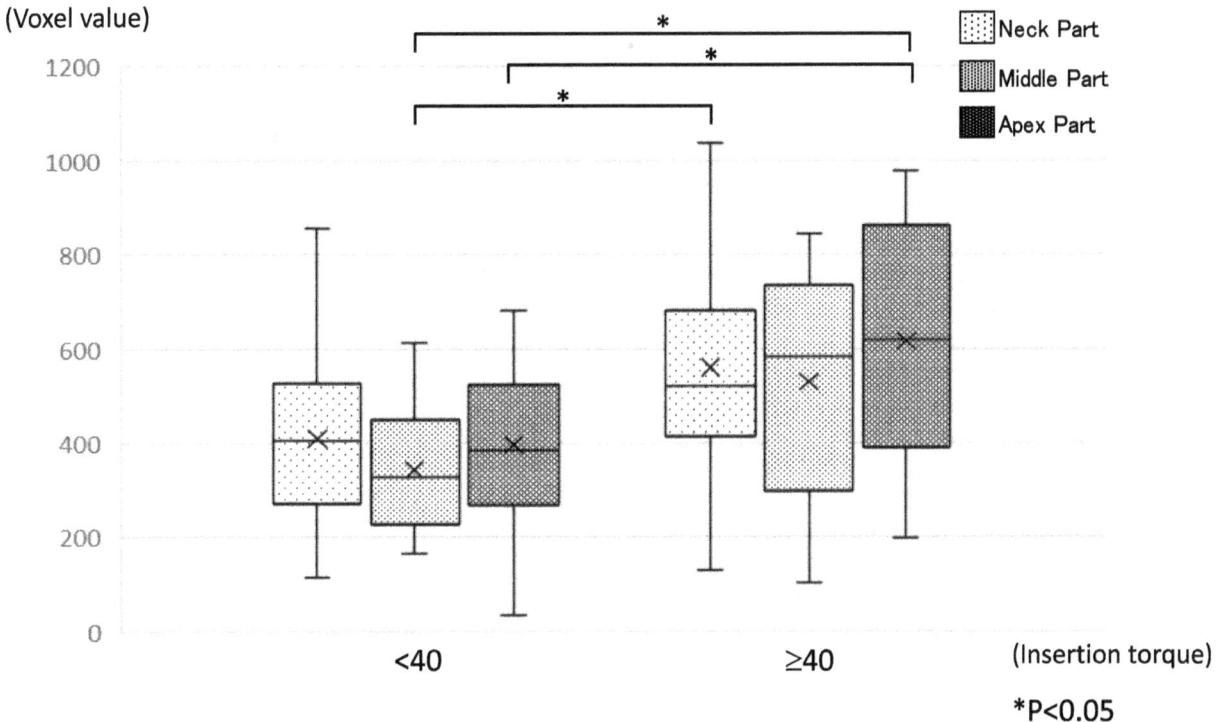

Fig. 9 The comparison of two groups at average voxel values for each part. The comparison of voxel values by insertion torque. All specimens were classified into two groups by insertion torque < 40 and ≥ 40. The < 40 group represents a combination of the low and medium IT groups

the insertion torque value shows between 32 to 50 N cm, the implant treatment with immediate loading protocol is able to apply [40]. Also, Anitua et al. applied immediate loading protocol when the insertion torque value was 40 to 65 N cm (the average insertion torque value is 55 ± 3.48 N cm) [29]. As described above, the insertion torque value used as a decision index of the loading period of the implant is yet undefined. Therefore, the loading period of the implant should not be determined immediately after insertion but should be determined after careful follow-up observation. When deciding to load period, the ISQ value will be an important decision index.

A bone quality of the treated area may affect primary stability as described above, preoperative analysis of bone quality is important for clarifying the primary stability of dental implants. This study analyzed bone quality using voxel values obtained using Digital Imaging and Communications in Medicine (DICOM) data from CBCT. According to the result of that analysis, it was suggested that insertion torque is high when inserting the implant body used in this study into the bone with high voxel value (Fig. 7). Moreover, in this study, the ISQ values of implant bodies showing insertion torque of 30 or more N cm were stabilized at a high value (ISQ was 73 or more) in 6 weeks after insertion (Figs. 5 and 6). These results may suggest that if the implant body used in this study is inserted into the bone of sufficient quality, high IT then intraosseous stability during the healing period can be expected, and osseointegration may be completed by 6 weeks after surgery. In addition, in order to judge the completion of osseointegration, an evaluation of intraosseous stability in the healing process after insertion of the implant body is necessary. There was a possibility that the implant body used in this study could be treated with the early loading method [1, 2]. In order to make this result more reliable evidence, it seems necessary to conduct a randomized controlled study on more participants.

As accurate CT attenuation was not measured due to the lower spatial resolution of CBCT compared with MSCT, a CBCT was recognized as unsuitable for evaluating bone quality. However, several groups have recently reported the potential use of CBCT systems as an apparatus for estimating bone quality. Isoda et al. described a high correlation between voxel values obtained by CBCT and IT of the implant [41]. Moreover, Nomura et al. reported a high correlation between density values from the CBCT and MSCT systems [42].

According to the measurement of the average voxel values in this study, a significant difference was seen between the high IT group and the low/medium IT group,

but no significant difference was found between the low and medium IT groups (Fig. 7). Specimens showing IT ≥ 40 N cm were thought to have a good bone quality, and voxel values at each part of the implant (neck, middle apex) were compared between groups with IT < 40 (combined low and medium IT groups) and ≥ 40 (high IT group) (Fig. 8). The results suggested that the neck and apex parts in the high IT group showed significantly higher voxel values than the middle and apex parts of the low/medium IT group.

Using a MSCT system for preoperative diagnosis of bone quality, classified as five stages according to CT attenuation, and detailed diagnosis was performed for the whole treatment area [43]. In this study, no significant difference was found when bone quality was compared between the three different IT groups, but when comparisons were made between two groups (low/medium vs high), significant differences were observed between groups and also between measurement sites (Figs. 6 and 7). Diagnosis of bone quality using CBCT does not seem as detailed as results from MSCT, but the diagnosis of whether bone quality is sufficient appears feasible.

CBCT systems offer many advantages over MSCT systems, including low exposure doses, high resolution, reduction of metal artifacts, ease of installation, and utility as a diagnostic tool in implant treatment [41, 42]. Due to the expanded utility of CBCT systems for dental implant diagnosis, the establishment of techniques for diagnosing bone quality by CBCT is necessary.

Conclusions

The purpose of this study was to evaluate the relationship between the insertion torque value and the ISQ value at the implant treatment using the current rough-surfaced implant. As a result, no significant relationship was found between the insertion torque value and the ISQ value. Also, it was suggested that the ISQ value was considered to be an important indicator for observing the treatment state of the implant. In addition, it was considered that there is a possibility that the early loading protocol can be applied to the implant body used in this study.

Abbreviations
CBCT: Cone beam CT; CT: Computed tomography; DICOM: Digital Imaging and Communications in Medicine; ISQ: Implant stability quotient; IT: Insertion torque; MSCT: Multi-slice CT

Authors' contributions
SH, YM, TS, KM, SY, HK, and YY contributed to the data collection and evaluation. SH contributed to the statistical analysis, manuscript writing, and creation of figures. All authors approved the contents of this manuscript.

Competing interests

Shinya Homma, Yasushi Makabe, Takuya Sakai, Kenzou Morinaga, Satoru Yokoue, Hirofumi Kido, and Yasutomo Yajima declare that they have no competing interests.

Author details

[1]Department of Oral and Maxillofacial Implantology, Tokyo Dental College, 2-9-18 Misaki-cho, Chiyoda-ku, Tokyo 101-0061, Japan. [2]Section of Oral Implantology, Department of Oral Rehabilitation, Fukuoka Dental College, 2-15-1 Tamura, Sawara-ku, Fukuoka-City, Fukuoka 814-0175, Japan. [3]Center for Oral Diseases, Fukuoka Dental College, 3-2-1 Hakataekimae, Hakata-ku, Fukuoka City, Fukuoka 812-0011, Japan.

References

1. Aparicio C, Rangert B, Sennerby L. Immediate/early loading of dental implants. A report from the Sociedad Española de Implantes World Congress consensus meeting in Barcelona, Spain 2002. Implant Dent Relat Res. 2003;5:57–60.
2. Cochran DL, Moeton D, Weber HP. Consensus statements and recommended clinical procedures regarding loading protocols for endosseous dental implants. Int J Oral Maxillofac Implants. 2004;19(Suppl):109–13.
3. Proceedings of the 4th International Team for Implantology (ITI) Consensus Conference, August 2008, Stuttgart, Germany. Int J Oral Maxillofac Implants. 2009;24 Suppl:7–278.
4. Brånemark PI, Hansson BO, Adell R, Breinr U, Lindström J, Hallén O, Ohman A. Osseointegrated implants in the treatment of the edentulous jaw. Experience from a 10-year period. Scand J Plast Reconstr Surg. 1977; 16(Suppl):1–132.
5. Buser D, Nydegger T, Hirt HP, Cochran DL, Nolte LP. Removal torque values of titanium implants in the maxilla of miniature pigs. Int J Oral Maxillofac Implants. 1998;13(5):611–9.
6. Sennerby L, Gottlow J. Clinical outcomes of immediate/early loading of dental implants. A literature review of recent controlled prospective clinical studies. Aust Dent J. 2008;53(Suppl 1):S82–8. https://doi.org/10.1111/j.1834-7819.2008.00045.x.
7. Henry PJ, Liddelow GJ. Immediate loading of dental implants. Aust Dent J. 2008;53(Suppl 1):S69–81. https://doi.org/10.1111/j.1834-7819.2008.00044.x.
8. Parsa A, Ibrahim N, Hassan B, van der Stelt P, Wismeijer D. Bone quality evaluation at dental implant site using multislice CT, micro-CT, and cone beam CT. Clin Oral Implants Res. 2015;26(1):e1–7. https://doi.org/10.1111/clr.12315. Epub 2013 Dec 11
9. Fuh LJ, Huang HL, Chen CS, Fu KL, Shen YW, Tu MG, Shen WC, Hsu JT. Variations in bone density at dental implant sites in different regions of the jawbone. J Oral Rehabil. 2010;37(5):346–51. https://doi.org/10.1111/j.1365-2842.2010.02061.x. Epub 2010 Jan 25
10. Chang WJ, Lee SY, Wu CC, Lin CT, Abiko Y, Yamamichi N, Huang HM. A newly designed resonance frequency analysis device for dental implant stability detection. Dent Mater J. 2007;26(5):665–71.
11. Lindh C, Petersson A, Robin M. Assessment of the trabecular pattern before endosseous implant treatment: diagnostic outcome of periapical radiography in the mandible. Oral Surg Oral Med Oral Pathol Oral Radiol Endod. 1996;82(3):335–43.
12. Schulte W, Lukas D. The Periotest method. Int Dent J. 1992;42(6):433–40.
13. Meredith N, Book K, Friberg B, Jemt T, Sennerby L. Resonance frequency measurements of implant stability in vivo. A cross-sectional and longitudinal study of resonance frequency measurements on implants in the edentulous and partially dentate maxilla. Clin Oral Implants Res. 1997;8(3):226–33.
14. Meredith N. Assessment of implant stability as a prognostic determinant. Int J Prosthodont. 1998;11(5):491–501.
15. Friberg B, Sennerby L, Meredith N, Lekholm U. A comparison between cutting torque and resonance frequency measurements of maxillary implants. A 20-month clinical study. Int J Oral Maxillofac Surg. 1999; 28(4):297–303.
16. Ostman PO, Hellman M, Wendelhag I, Sennerby L. Resonance frequency analysis measurements of implants at placement surgery. Int J Prosthodont. 2006;19(1):77–83. discussion 84
17. Ohta K, Takechi M, Minami M, Shigeishi H, Hiraoka M, Nishimura M, Kamata N. Influence of factors related to implant stability detected by wireless resonance frequency analysis device. J Oral Rehabil. 2010;37(2):131–7. https://doi.org/10.1111/j.1365-2842.2009.02032.x. Epub 2009 Nov 30
18. Sakoh J, Wahlmann U, Stender E, Nat R, Al-Nawas B, Wagner W. Primary stability of a conical implant and a hybrid, cylindric screw-type implant in vitro. Int J Oral Maxillofac Implants. 2006;21(4):560–6.
19. Degidi M, Daprile G, Piattelli A. RFA values of implants placed in sinus grafted and nongrafted sites after 6 and 12 months. Clin Implant Dent Relat Res. 2009;11(3): 178–82. https://doi.org/10.1111/j.1708-8208.2008.00113.x. Epub 2008 Sep 9
20. Levin BP. The correlation between immediate implant insertion torque and implant stability quotient. Int J Periodontics Restorative Dent. 2016;36(6): 833–40. https://doi.org/10.11607/prd.2865.
21. World Medical Association. World Medical Association Declaration of Helsinki: ethical principles for medical research involving human subjects. JAMA. 2013;310(20):2191–4.
22. Wadhwa B, Jain V, Bhutia O, Bhalla AS, Pruthi G. Flapless versus open flap techniques of implant placement: a 15-month follow-up study. Indian J Dent Res. 2015;26(4):372–7. https://doi.org/10.4103/0970-9290.167629.
23. Alvira-González J, Díaz-Campos E, Sánchez-Garcés MA, Gay-Escoda C. Survival of immediately versus delayed loaded short implants: a prospective case series study. Med Oral Patol Oral Cir Bucal. 2015;20(4):e480–8.
24. Boronat López A, Balaguer Martínez J, Lamas Pelayo J, Carrillo García C, Peñarrocha DM. Resonance frequency analysis of dental implant stability during the healing period. Med Oral Patol Oral Cir Bucal. 2008;13(4):E244–7.
25. Gapski R, Wang HL, Mascarenhas P, Lang NP. Critical review of immediate implant loading. Clin Oral Implants Res. 2003;14(5):515–27.
26. Esposito M, Hirsch JM, Lekholm U, Thomsen P. Biological factors contributing to failures of osseointegrated oral implants. (II). Etiopathogenesis. Eur J Oral Sci. 1998;106(3):721–64.
27. Maluf PS, Ching AW, Angeletti P, Bretos JL, Ferreira LM. Insertion torque of dental implants after microvascular fibular grafting. Br J Oral Maxillofac Surg. 2015;53(7): 647–9. https://doi.org/10.1016/j.bjoms.2015.03.016. Epub 2015 Jun 17
28. Tsukioka T, Sasaki Y, Kaneda T, Buch K, Sakai O. Assessment of relationships between implant insertion torque and cortical shape of the mandible using panoramic radiography: preliminary study. Int J Oral Maxillofac Implants. 2014;29(3):622–6. https://doi.org/10.11607/jomi.3451.
29. Anitua E, Alkhraisat MH, Piñas L, Orive G. Efficacy of biologically guided implant area preparation to obtain adequate primary implant stability. Ann Anat. 2015; 199:9–15. https://doi.org/10.1016/j.aanat.2014.02.005. Epub 2014 Mar 12
30. Nevins M, Nevins M, De Angelis N, Ghaffari S, Bassir H, Kim DM. Comparative clinical and histologic assessments of dental implants delivered with a manual torque limiting wrench versus with an electronically controlled torque limiting device. Int J Periodontics Restorative Dent. 2015;35(6):819–23. https://doi.org/10.11607/prd.2585.
31. Neugebauer J, Petermöller S, Scheer M, Happe A, Faber FJ, Zoeller JE. Comparison of design and torque measurements of various manual wrenches. Int J Oral Maxillofac Implants. 2015;30(3):526–33. https://doi.org/10.11607/jomi.3733.
32. González-García R, Monje F, Moreno-García C. Predictability of the resonance frequency analysis in the survival of dental implants placed in the anterior non-atrophied edentulous mandible. Med Oral Patol Oral Cir Bucal. 2011;16(5):e664–9.
33. Barewal RM, Oates TW, Meredith N, Cochran DL. Resonance frequency measurement of implant stability in vivo on implants with a sandblasted and acid-etched surface. Int J Oral Maxillofac Implants. 2003;18(5):641–51.
34. Nedir R, Bischof M, Szmukler-Moncler S, Bernard JP, Samson J. Predicting osseointegration by means of implant primary stability. Clin Oral Implants Res. 2004;15(5):520–8.
35. Ito Y, Sato D, Yoneda S, Ito D, Kondo H, Kasugai S. Relevance of resonance frequency analysis to evaluate dental implant stability: simulation and histomorphometrical animal experiments. Clin Oral Implants Res. 2008;19(1): 9–14. Epub 2007 Nov 6
36. Boronat-López A, Peñarrocha-Diago M, Martínez-Cortissoz O, Mínguez-Martínez I. Resonance frequency analysis after the placement of 133 dental implants. Med Oral Patol Oral Cir Bucal. 2006;11(3):E272–6.
37. Rowan M, Lee D, Pi-Anfruns J, Shiffler P, Aghaloo T, Moy PK. Mechanical versus biological stability of immediate and delayed implant placement using resonance frequency analysis. J Oral Maxillofac Surg. 2015;73(2):253–7. https://doi.org/10.1016/j.joms.2014.09.024. Epub 2014 Oct 13

38. Brånemark R, Ohrnell LO, Skalak R, Carlsson L, Brånemark PI. Biomechanical characterization of osseointegration: an experimental in vivo investigation in the beagle dog. J Orthop Res. 1998;16(1):61–9.

39. Held U, Rohner D, Rothamel D. Early loading of hydrophilic titanium implants inserted in low-mineralized (D3 and D4) bone: one year results of a prospective clinical trial. Head Face Med. 2013;9:37. https://doi.org/10.1186/1746-160X-9-37.

40. Lozano-Carrascal N, Salomó-Coll O, Gilabert-Cerdà M, Farré-Pagés N, Gargallo-Albiol J, Hernández-Alfaro F. Effect of implant macro-design on primary stability: a prospective clinical study. Med Oral Patol Oral Cir Bucal. 2016;21(2):e214–21.

41. Isoda K, Ayukawa Y, Tsukiyama Y, Sogo M, Matsushita Y, Koyano K. Relationship between the bone density estimated by cone-beam computed tomography and the primary stability of dental implants. Clin Oral Implants Res. 2012;23(7):832–6. https://doi.org/10.1111/j.1600-0501.2011.02203.x. Epub 2011 May 5

42. Nomura Y, Watanabe H, Honda E, Kurabayashi T. Reliability of voxel values from cone-beam computed tomography for dental use in evaluating bone mineral density. Clin Oral Implants Res. 2010;21(5):558–62. https://doi.org/10.1111/j.1600-0501.2009.01896.x.

43. Misch CE, editor. Dental implant prosthetics. 1st ed. Philadelphia: Elsevier Health Sciences; 2004.

8

Implant therapy for a patient with osteogenesis imperfecta type I

Shamit S. Prabhu[1,4]* ⓘ, Kevin Fortier[2], Michael C. May[3] and Uday N. Reebye[4]

Abstract

Bone fragility and skeletal irregularities are the characteristic features of osteogenesis imperfecta (OI). Many patients with OI have weakened maxillary and mandibular bone, leading to poor oral hygiene and subsequent loss of teeth. Improvements in implant therapy have allowed for OI patients to achieve dental restoration. However, there is limited available literature on implant therapy for patients with OI. The greatest challenge in the restoration process for OI patients in an outpatient setting is ensuring primary stability and osseointegration. Improvements in synthetic grafts improve successful implant placement and prevent predisposing patients to unnecessary procedures. This report details the successful restoration process of an OI type I patient's maxillary arch in addition to a review of the currently available literature.

Keywords: Osteogenesis imperfecta type I, Implant therapy, Brittle bone disease

Introduction

Osteogenesis imperfecta (OI), colloquially known as "brittle bone disease," is a broad term for a group of congenital disorders affecting the connective tissue resulting in a susceptibility to fractures. In 1979, Sillence et al. conducted an epidemiological and genetic study of OI patients [1]. These patients were grouped according to four distinct syndromes: (1) dominantly inherited OI with blue sclerae, (2) lethal perinatal OI with radiographically crumpled femora and beaded ribs, (3) progressively deforming OI with normal sclerae, or (4) dominantly inherited OI with normal sclerae [1]. These groupings would later become the clinical features in identifying OI types I–IV. Since then, additional types of OI have been classified based on allelic heterogeneity, histological variance, radiological features, and clinical manifestations (Table 1).

In studies conducted in Europe and the US, the birth prevalence of OI was estimated to be 0.3–0.7 per 10,000 births [2, 3]. Incidence in males and females is roughly equal. The pathophysiology for OI type I is characterized by mutations in the genes for proα1 chains on *COL1A1* on chromosome 17 or for proα2 chains on *COL1A2* on chromosome 7 [4]. The prominence of type I collagen in the extracellular matrix of bones and skin results in patients with OI having qualitative or quantitative defects. In OI type I, individuals have quantitative defects in their normal type I collagen in that the collagen is functionally normal but produced in smaller quantities. Individuals with qualitative defects produce structurally defective type I collagen resulting in moderate deformations as seen in OI type IV, to severe deformation as seen in OI type III, and can even be lethal in OI type II [5].

Clinically, patients with OI type I present with an increased risk of bone fractures due to fragile bone, osteoporosis, blue sclerae, short stature, joint hypermobility, and susceptibility to conductive hearing loss progressing from adolescence to adulthood [6]. OI type I can be further categorized based on the presence, Ia, or absence, Ib, of dentinogenesis imperfecta (DI) [7]. Patients with DI will have opalescent teeth due to abnormal dentin exposure through the translucent enamel with a variable blue-gray or yellow-brown hue. Radiographical features of dentinogenesis imperfecta include deposition of dentin resulting in a marked reduction of the pulp chamber and root canals, short roots with constricted

---
* Correspondence: shamitprabhu@gmail.com
[1]Wake Forest School of Medicine, Winston-Salem, USA
[4]Triangle Implant Center, 5318 NC Highway 55, Suite 106, Durham, NC 27713, USA
Full list of author information is available at the end of the article

Table 1 Osteogenesis imperfecta classifications

Type	Inheritance	Gene	Locus	Clinical features	OMIM
I [1, 4]	AD	COL1A1 or COL1A2	17q21.33 or 7q21.3	Variable bone fragility, moderate bone deformity, blue sclerae, possible dentinogenesis imperfecta	166,200
II [1, 26]	AD	COL1A1 or COL1A2	17q21.33 or 7q21.3	Perinatally lethal	166,210
III [1, 27]	AD	COL1A1 or COL1A2	17q21.33 or 7q21.3	Severe bone fragility, progressively deforming, normal sclerae, dentinogenesis imperfecta, cardiovascular complications, spinal curvature, kyphoscoliosis	259,420
IV [1]	AD	COL1A1 or COL1A2	17q21.33 or 7q21.3	Moderate bone fragility, moderate deformity, normal sclerae, short stature, possible dentinogenesis imperfecta, kyphoscoliosis	166,220
V [28, 29]	AD	IFITM5	11p15.5	Moderate to severe bone fragility, radial head dislocation, normal to blue sclerae, normal dentin	610,967
VI [30]	AR	SERPINF1	17p13.3	Moderately to severe deformity, fish-scale pattern of lamellae, excessive osteoid, normal dentin	613,982
VII [31]	AR	CRTAP	3p22.3	Severe bone fragility, progressively deforming, normal sclerae, severe rhizomelia and coxa vera, normal dentin	610,682
VIII [32]	AR	LEPRE1	1p34.2	Severe bone fragility, normal sclerae, bulbous metaphyses, round face, short barrel-shaped chest	610,915
IX [33]	AR	PPIB	15q22.31	Severe bone deformity, gray sclerae	259,440
X [34]	AR	SERPINH1	11q13.5	Multiple bone deformities and fractures, osteopenia, dentinogenesis imperfecta, blue sclerae	613,848
XI [35]	AR	FKBP10	17q21.2	Mild to severe bone deformity, normal to gray sclerae	610,968
XII [36]	AR	SP7	12q13.13	Mild bone deformity, normal dentin, normal hearing, normal sclerae	613,849
XIII [37]	AR	BMP1	8p21.3	Severe growth deficiency, severe bone deformity, normal dentin, light blue sclerae	614,856
XIV [38]	AR	TMEM38B	9q31.2	Variable bone deformity, variable osteopenia, normal dentin, normal sclerae, normal hearing	615,066
XV [39, 40]	AR	WNT1	12q13.12	Severe bone deformity, short stature, early and recurrent fractures, normal dentin, possible blue sclerae, normal hearing	615,220
XVI [41]	AR	CREB3L1	11p11.2	Severe bone deformity, beaded ribs, callus formation, cardiac irregularities	616,229
XVII [42]	AR	SPARC	5q33.1	Progressive severe bone fragility, kyphoscoliosis, mild joint hyperlaxity, short stature	616,507

AD autosomal dominant, *AR* autosomal recessive, *OMIM* Online Mendelian Inheritance in Man

corono-radicular junctions, and bulbous crowns [8, 9]. Improper dentin formation predisposes patients to an increased risk of dental fractures and increased wear on teeth, subsequently requiring corrective dental procedures [10]. Navigating treatment options for patients with OI type I pose many challenges for dental professionals. In particular, successful dental implant treatment is difficult to achieve due to requiring strong, dense bone for acceptance of the implant. To avoid implant failure, patients must maintain routine oral care in addition to closely monitoring bone healing around the implant site. Implant treatment is even more challenging if the patient is prescribed bisphosphonates. These drugs are often administered to reduce osteoclast activity to limit bone resorption, subsequently improve bone microarchitecture, and bone density and correct vertebral size and shape

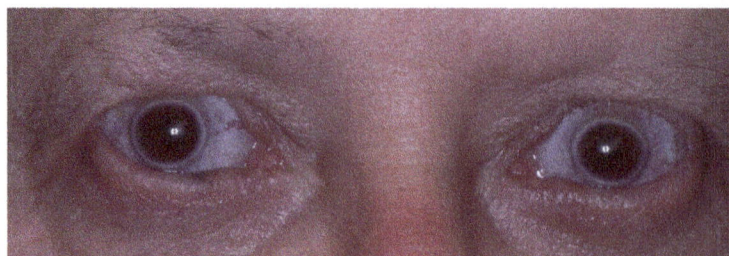

Fig. 1 Characteristic blue sclerae

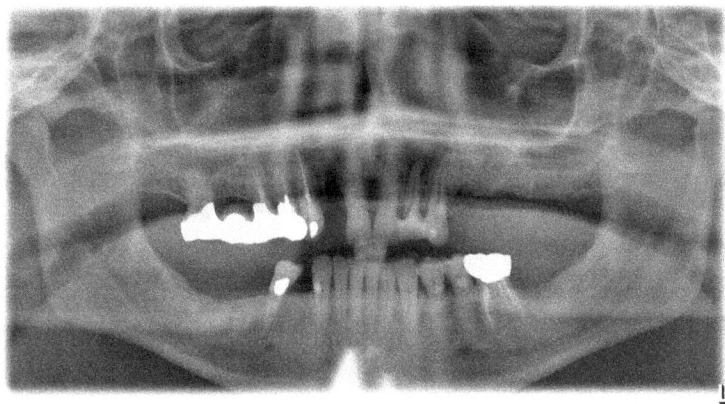

Fig. 2 Pre-operative panoramic radiograph

[11–13]. One randomized, double-blind, placebo-controlled trial on the effectiveness of Risedronate in children with OI showed a significant reduction in the risk of fractures [13]. While bisphosphonate treatment may assist in the prevention of long bone fractures, it can be a detriment in the oral restoration process.

In this report, we focus on the 3-year dental implant therapy and restorative process of a 53-year-old male patient diagnosed with OI type I.

Case presentation
Evaluation
A 53-year-old male diagnosed with OI type I was referred to our clinic for extraction of the remaining maxillary teeth and evaluation for full arch immediate load hybrid prosthesis. His clinical history included osteogenesis type 1, bipolar disorder, alopecia, and hypothyroidism. The patient presented with normal stature, measuring 170.18 cm and weighing 81.65 kg with characteristic blue sclerae of OI type I (Fig. 1). Throughout his life, he has had multiple orthopedic fractures due to his OI. At the time of surgery, he was on Lamictal, Xarelto, Synthroid, lisinopril, and hydrochlorothiazide.

Extraoral, TMJ, intraoral soft tissue, and lymph node examinations produced no abnormal findings. An examination of the dentition revealed the maxillary teeth were in poor repair with a fixed bridge extending from site number 2 to site number 5 with site number 3 serving as the pontic abutment. Sites number 8, number 9, number 10, and number 11 have periodontal involvement as well as recurrent decay. He was edentulous on the posterior left maxillary arch. His lower dentition consisted of sites number 19 through number 27 with number 28 being edentulous and number 29 having a root fracture (Fig. 2). The upper jaw had good ridge width with reproducible centric relation and centric occlusion. The patient was otherwise healthy apart from medical issues directly related to his OI.

Due to his significant gag reflex, he was unable to wear a removable prosthesis. Lengthy conversations regarding implant therapy and implant options were reviewed as well as risks with his OI. Options presented included no treatment, placement of fixtures to support a removable prosthesis, placement of fixtures to support a fixed hybrid, and placement of axial implants for fixed denture prosthesis. He elected for a fixed denture prosthesis. Our

Table 2 Chronological timeline of the implant therapy of the maxilla

Date	Site number	Implant diameter (mm)	Implant length (mm)	Immediate load	Bone graft augmentation
3/26/14	12	4.3	10	Yes	Allograft
3/26/14	14	4.3	10	Yes	None
11/10/14	10	3.5	13	Yes	Allograft
3/5/15	7	3.5	13	Yes	Allograft
4/19/16	11	4.3	11.5	Yes	None
2/22/17	3	4.3	10	Yes	Allograft
2/22/17	4	5.0	10	Yes	Allograft
2/22/17	6	4.3	13	Yes	Allograft
2/22/17	8	3.5	10	Yes	Allograft
2/22/17	9	3.5	10	Yes	Allograft

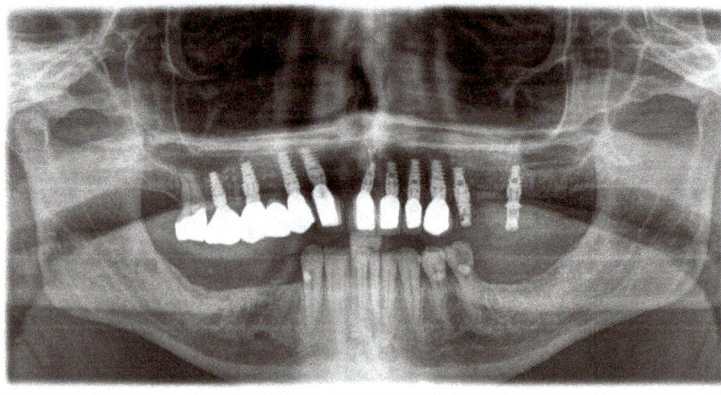

Fig. 3 Post-operative panoramic radiograph

patient was apprehensive towards having full edentulation and implant placement completed all at once and decided to have the implants placed in stages (Table 2).

Surgical technique

The patient underwent implant therapy in stages under general anesthesia with immediate load protocol. Intravenous access was obtained, and the patient was anesthetized under general anesthesia by our anesthesiologist. Carpules of 2% lidocaine with 1:100,000 epinephrine, 4% articaine hydrochloride with 1:100,000 epinephrine (Septocaine), and 0.5% bupivacaine hydrochloride with 1:200,000 epinephrine (Marcaine) were used as needed. For each site, a 15 blade was used to make a sulcular incision from the mesial to the distal aspect of the tooth. A full thickness mucoperiosteal flap was elevated with a periosteal elevator exposing the buccal alveolus. Buccal bone was removed using a surgical fissure bur to allow for osteotomes and elevators to atraumatically elevate and deliver the teeth, while preserving lingual, mesial, and distal walls. Next, a straight elevator was positioned between the alveolus and the root surface. The tooth was elevated, and

the periodontal ligament was separated from the alveolus. The tooth was extracted using a no. 150 upper universal forcep. The socket was curetted and irrigated with copious amounts of normal saline solution. A bone file and rongeur were used to smoothen the alveolus.

To deliver implants, all bony walls were checked with a perio probe to verify the depth. A series of osteotomy burs were used at 1000 RPM and 50 Ncm of torque with copious sterile normal saline irrigation. At each step, angulation was checked. Once the final osteotomy was completed, the site was checked to verify that all bony walls were stable. A NobelActive implant was torqued into position at greater than 30 Ncm followed by placement of a cover screw. In instances where grafting was necessary, the graft material was positioned to obliterate the bony defect using a periosteal elevator and curette to place in the bony voids. The gingival tissues were repositioned using an Adson Tissue Forcep. A tension-free closure was attained with a periosteal release technique. The sites were closed with interrupted 3-0 gut sutures. All procedures were accomplished without any further complications.

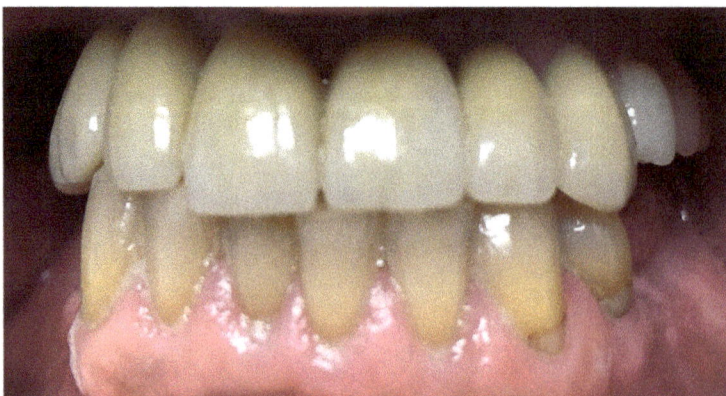

Fig. 4 Post-operative frontal view with teeth in occlusion

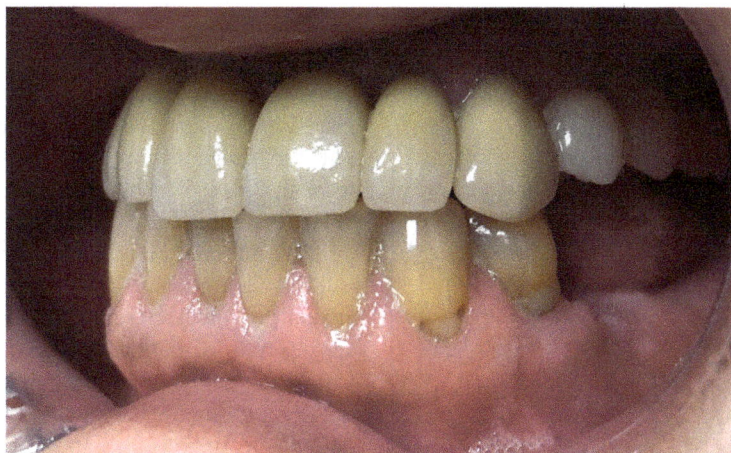

Fig. 5 Post-operative lateral view of the left maxillary arch

Prosthetic procedure

The standard immediate loading procedures were followed as the patient met the guidelines of a minimum torque value of 35 Ncm. All fixtures placed had intraoperative open tray impressions taken. Impressions were sent to the laboratory, and fabrication of a screw-retained temporary was completed. Temporaries were placed within 24 h of surgery and were torqued at 15 Ncm. Following a 6-month period of functioning in temporary prostheses, final impressions were taken via open-tray technique. He was placed in his final prostheses with no complications. Our patient settled on final prostheses consisting of a four-unit bridge cemented at sites number 3 through number 6; individual crowns placed at sites number 7, number 8, number 9, number 10, and number 11; and a screw-retained, three-unit bridge placed at sites number 12 through number 14 (Figs. 3, 4, 5, 6, and 7). The restorative dentist placed a polymethyl methacrylate (PMMA) prosthesis on the left side, and our patient will transition to his final crowns once he is financially ready.

Follow-up

Regular hygiene visits show that our OI patient has greatly improved his overall home care routine. No areas of gingival inflammation were found. Probing depths have remained 2–4 mm with no bleeding or purulent drainage at the fixtures sites. There have been no issues with implant mobility, and all healing post-operatively was uneventful.

Discussion

The vast majority of published articles regarding OI type I revolve around fractures of the long bones and treatment strategies. An extensive literature search for manuscripts detailing the implant therapy for patients diagnosed with OI produced a marginal amount of literature (Table 3). Our case posits that oral restoration is attainable without implant failure for OI type I patients. In OI type I, the collagen produced is of normal quality but in reduced quantities [14]. As a result, OI type I is considered the mildest form of OI with the majority of fractures occurring in childhood and adolescence as the

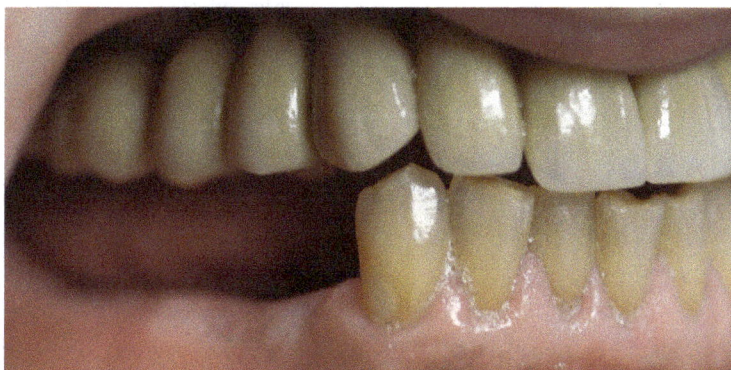

Fig. 6 Post-operative lateral view of the right maxillary arch

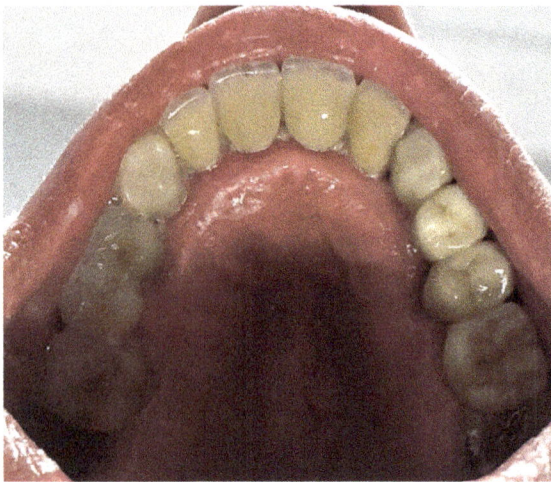

Fig. 7 Post-operative occlusal photograph of the maxilla

bones continue to grow. Since the collagen is of normal quality, successful osseointegration of implants can be attained with proper planning. To account for poor bone strength, Marx et al. proposed using implants as a "tent-pole" for bone graft to be placed around to consolidate and maintain the graft's volume [15].

The same factors that must be considered when placing implants in any patient are also pertinent to OI patients. However, extra emphasis should be placed on bone quantity and bone quality. In placing implants for our patient, we ensured that all fixtures attained a final torque value greater than 35 Ncm. Traditional endosseous implants require a bone healing period post-extraction of 3 months for the mandible and 6 months for the maxilla before the implant can be loaded [16]. Innovation in implant technology allows for immediate implant loading following extraction due to design changes that provide a stronger mechanical connection to the surrounding tissue [17]. While these innovations have made implant delivery much more time-effective, primary stability can be challenging in

patients with diminished bone quantity and quality. Bone graft augmentation can be utilized to ensure the osseointegration of the implant and has been utilized to achieve positive results in some OI cases [18–22]. However, some cases found successful osseointegration without the usage of bone grafts, including some of the implants placed in our patient [23, 24]. While we were able to successfully deliver implants using synthetic grafting material or no grafting material, other literature utilized autogenous bone from either the ascending ramus [21] or iliac crest [18–20, 22]. In determining the success rate of dental implants, there is a great deal of variability due in part to the varying degrees of bone quality and quantity in the OI subtypes, patient compliance to treatment plans and dental care, and a multitude of other factors typically involved in implant therapy. One retrospective and prospective study cites strong success rates in implant delivery for OI patients with a survival rate between 93 and 100% [25]. Our patient is now 4 years post-placement of his first implant procedure and has been functioning without any issues. The diagnosis of OI type I should not be a contraindication of implant therapy as our case, and others [18–25], have shown. This case differs from other cases in utilizing synthetic grafts to aid in stability and providing another case to illustrate the advancements in implant delivery for patients with bone abnormalities.

Conclusion

In conclusion, this case shows that implant therapy for patients with OI type I is a viable treatment option with appropriate planning, surgical skill, and routine care. Advancements in the fields of implants, prosthetics, and bone grafting will continue to make implants an increasingly practical treatment option for patients with OI. However, dental practitioners should always take great precaution in ensuring that bone quality and quantity is appropriate to ensure primary stability and successful osseointegration.

Table 3 Reported implant therapy for patients diagnosed with osteogenesis imperfecta

Reference	Age (years)	Gender	OI type	Bone graft augmentation	Number of implants	Implant location	Implant type
Friberg [23]	51	F	N/A**	No	6	Full maxilla	Regular platform TiUnite Brånemark System
Wannfors [18]	30	F	III	Yes	4	Full mandible	OsseoSpeed
Payne [19]	34	F	IV	Yes	11	Full maxilla and mandible	Brånemark Mk III Ti-Unite
Prabhu [24]	32	M	IV	No	11	Full maxilla and mandible	Brånemark titanium bone-tapped
Binger [20]	32	F	N/A**	Yes	5	Full maxilla	ITI dental standard
Lee [21]	43	F	III	Yes	2	Right posterior mandible	Paragon Screwvent internal hexed
Zola [22]	32	M	N/A**	Yes	13	Left and right posterior maxilla and left and right posterior mandible	Not specified

**OI type was not specified

Abbreviation
OI: Osteogenesis imperfecta

Acknowledgements
Not applicable

Funding
Not applicable

Authors' contributions
Primary author SSP drafted the manuscript, revised the manuscript, and assisted in the surgical implant procedures. Second author KF assisted in the revision of the manuscript and tables. Third author MCM revised the manuscript and participated in drafting the literature review. Fourth author UNR carried out all surgical procedures and coordinated the report. All authors have read and approved of this manuscript.

Competing interests
Shamit S. Prabhu, Kevin Fortier, Michael C. May, and Uday N. Reebye declare that they have no competing interests.

Author details
[1]Wake Forest School of Medicine, Winston-Salem, USA. [2]Boston University Henry M. Goldman School of Dental Medicine, Boston, USA. [3]Virginia Commonwealth University School of Dentistry, Richmond, USA. [4]Triangle Implant Center, 5318 NC Highway 55, Suite 106, Durham, NC 27713, USA.

References
1. Sillence DO, Senn A, Danks DM. Genetic heterogeneity in osteogenesis imperfecta. J Med Genet. 1979;16:101–16.
2. Orioli IM, Castilla EE, Barbosa-Neto JG. The birth prevalence rates for the skeletal dysplasias. J Med Genet. 1986;23:328–32.
3. Stevenson DA, Carey JC, Byrne JL, Srisukhumbowornchai S, Feldkamp ML. Analysis of skeletal dysplasias in the Utah population. Am J Med Genet A. 2012;158A:1046–54.
4. Byers PH. Brittle bones-fragile molecules: disorders of collagen gene structure and expression. Trends Genet. 1990;6:293–300.
5. Sillence DO, Rimoin DL, Danks DM. Clinical variability in osteogenesis imperfecta-variable expressivity or genetic heterogeneity. Birth Defects Orig Artic Ser. 1979;15:113–29.
6. Van Dijk F, Sillence D. Osteogenesis imperfecta: clinical diagnosis, nomenclature and severity assessment. Am J Med Genet A. 2014;164:1470–81.
7. Levin LS, Brady JM, Melnick M. Scanning electron microscopy of teeth in dominant osteogenesis imperfecta. Am J Med Genet. 1980;5:189–99.
8. Rios D, Vieira AL, Tenuta LM, Machado MA. Osteogenesis imperfecta and dentinogenesis imperfecta: associated disorders. Quintessence Int. 2005;36:695–701.
9. Bailleul-Forestier I, Berdal A, Vinchier F, de Ravel T, Fryns JP, Verloes A. The genetic basis of inherited anomalies of the teeth. Part 2: syndromes with significant dental development. Eur J Med Genet. 2008;51:383–408.
10. American Academy of Pediatric Dentistry. Guideline on dental management of heritable dental developmental anomalies. Pediatr Dent. 2016;38:302–7.
11. Land C, Rauch F, Montpetit K, Ruck-Gibis J, Glorieux FH. Effect of intravenous pamidronate therapy on functional abilities and level of ambulation in children with osteogenesis imperfecta. J Pediatr. 2006;148:456–60.
12. Rauch F, Munns C, Land C, Glorieux FH. Pamidronate in children and adolescents with osteogenesis imperfecta: effect of treatment discontinuation. J Clin Endocrinol Metab. 2016;91:1268–74.
13. Bishop N, Adami S, Ahmed SF, Anto'n J, Arundel P, Burren CP, Devogelaer J, et al. Risedronate in children with osteogenesis imperfecta: a randomised, double-blind, placebo-controlled trial. Lancet. 2013;382:1424–32.

14. Marini J, Forlino A, Bächinger H, Bishop N, Byers P, Paepe A, et al. Osteogenesis imperfecta. Nat Rev Dis Primers. 2017;3:17052.
15. Marx RE, Shellenberger T, Wimsatt J, Correa P. Severely resorbed mandible: predictable reconstruction with soft tissue matrix expansion (tent pole) grafts. J Oral Maxillofac Surg. 2002;60:878–88.
16. Brånemark PI. Osseointegration and its experimental background. J Prosthet Dent. 1983;50:399–410.
17. Javed F, Ahmed HB, Crespi R, Romanos GE. Role of primary stability for successful osseointegration of dental implants: factors of influence and evaluation. Interv Med Appl Sci. 2013;5:162–7.
18. Wanfors K, Johansson C, Donath K. Augmentation of the mandible via a "tent-pole" procedure and implant treatment in a patient with type III osteogenesis imperfecta: clinical and histologic consideration. Int J Oral Maxillofac Implants. 2009;24:1144–8.
19. Payne M, Postlethwaite K, Smith D, Nohl F. Implant-supported rehabilitation of an edentate patient with osteogenesis imperfecta: a case report. Int J Oral Maxillofac Implants. 2008;23:947–52.
20. Binger T, Rucker M, Spitzer WJ. Dentofacial rehabilitation by osteodistraction, augmentation and implantation despite osteogenesis imperfecta. Int J Oral Maxillofac Surg. 2006;35:559–62.
21. Lee C, Ertel S. Bone graft augmentation and dental implant treatment in a patient with osteogenesis imperfecta: review of the literature with a case report. Implant Dent. 2003;12:291–3.
22. Zola MB. Staged sinus augmentation and implant placement in a patient with osteogenesis imperfecta. J Oral Maxillofac Surg. 2000;58:443–7.
23. Friberg B. Brånemark system implants and rare disorders: a report of six cases. Int J Periodontics Restorative Dent. 2013;33:139–48.
24. Prabhu N, Stevenson A, Cameron A. The placement of osseointegrated dental implants in a patient with type IV B osteogenesis imperfecta: a 9-year follow-up. Oral Surg Oral Med Oral Pathol Oral Radiol Endod. 2007;103:349–51.
25. Jensen JL, Brox HT, Storhaug K, Ambjørnsen E, Støvne SA, Bjørnland T. Dental implants in patients with osteogenesis imperfecta: a retrospective and prospective study with review of the literature. Oral Surg. 2011;4:105–14.
26. Barnes AM, Chang W, Morello R, Cabral WA, Weis M, Eyre DR, et al. Deficiency of cartilage-associated protein in recessive lethal osteogenesis imperfecta. New Eng J Med. 2006;355:2757–64.
27. Radunovic Z, Wekre LL, Diep LM, Steine K. Cardiovascular abnormalities in adults with osteogenesis imperfecta. Am Heart J. 2011;161:523–9.
28. Glorieux FH, Rauch F, Plotkin H, Ward L, Travers R, Roughley P, et al. Type V osteogenesis imperfecta: a new form of brittle bone disease. J Bone Miner. 2000;15:1650–8.
29. Cho TJ, Lee KE, Lee SK, Song SJ, Kim KJ, Jeon D, et al. A single recurrent mutation in the 5-prime UTR of IFITM5 causes osteogenesis imperfecta type V. Am J Hum Genet. 2012;91:343–8.
30. Glorieux FH, Ward LM, Rauch F, Lalic L, Roughley PJ, Travers R. Osteogenesis imperfecta type VI: a form of brittle bone disease with a mineralization defect. J Bone Miner. 2002;17:30–8.
31. Ward LM, Rauch F, Travers R, Chabot G, Azouz EM, Lalic L, et al. Osteogenesis imperfecta type VII: an autosomal recessive form of brittle bone disease. Bone. 2002;31:12–8.
32. Cabral WA, Chang W, Barnes AM, Weis M, Scott MA, Leikin S, et al. Prolyl 3-hydroxylase 1 deficiency causes a recessive metabolic bone disorder resembling lethal/severe osteogenesis imperfecta. Nat Genet. 2007;39:359–65.
33. Van Dijk FS, Nesbitt IM, Zwikstra EH, Nikkels PGJ, Piersma SR, Fratantoni SA, et al. PPIB mutations cause severe osteogenesis imperfecta. Am J Hum Genet. 2009;85:521–7.
34. Christiansen HE, Schwarze U, Pyott SM, AlSwaid A, Al Balwi M, Alrasheed S, et al. Homozygosity for a missense mutation in SERPINH1, which encodes the collagen chaperone protein HSP47, results in severe recessive osteogenesis imperfecta. Am J Hum Genet. 2010;86:389–98.
35. Alanay Y, Avaygan H, Camacho N, Utine GE, Boduroglu K, Aktas D, et al. Mutations in the gene encoding the RER protein FKBP65 cause autosomal-recessive osteogenesis imperfecta. Am J Hum Genet. 2010;86:551–9.
36. Lapunzina P, Aglan M, Temtamy S, Caparros-Martin JA, Valencia M, Leton R, et al. Identification of a frameshift mutation in Osterix in a patient with recessive osteogenesis imperfecta. Am J Hum Genet. 2010;87:110–4.
37. Martinez-Glez V, Valencia M, Caparros-Martin JA, Aglan M, Temtamy S, Tenorio J, et al. Identification of a mutation causing deficient BMP1/mTLD proteolytic

activity in autosomal recessive osteogenesis imperfecta. Hum Mutat. 2012;33: 343–50.

38.   Shaheen R, Alazami AM, Alshammari MJ, Faqeih E, Alhashmi N, Mousa N, et al. Study of autosomal recessive osteogenesis imperfecta in Arabia reveals a novel locus defined by TMEM38B mutation. J Med Genet. 2012;49:630–5.

39.   Keupp K, Beleggia F, Kayserili H, Barnes AM, Steiner M, Semler O, et al. Mutations in WNT1 cause different forms of bone fragility. Am J Hum Genet. 2013;92:565–74.

40.   Pyott SM, Tran TT, Leistritz DF, Pepn MG, Mendelsohn NJ, Temme RT, et al. WNT1 mutations in families affected by moderately severe and progressive recessive osteogenesis imperfecta. Am J Hum Genet. 2013;92:590–7.

41.   Symoens S, Malfait F, D'hondt S, Callewaert B, Dheedene A, Steyaert W, et al. Deficiency for the ER-stress transducer OASIS causes severe recessive osteogenesis imperfecta in humans. Orphanet J Rare Dis. 2013;8:154.

42.   Mendoza-Londono R, Fahiminiya S, Majewski J, Care4Rare Canada Consortium, Tetreault M, Nadaf J, et al. Recessive osteogenesis imperfecta caused by missense mutations in SPARC. Am J Hum Genet. 2015;96:979–85.

9

Cast accuracy obtained from different impression techniques at different implant angulations (in vitro study)

Enas A. Elshenawy[1*], Ahmed M. Alam-Eldein[2] and Fadel A. Abd Elfatah[2]

Abstract

Background: Angulated implants may result in inaccurate impressions, and the impression technique may affect the accuracy of the definitive cast. This study was designed to compare the dimensional accuracy of casts obtained from three impression techniques for three definitive lower casts with implants at different angulations.

Methods: Three Osseolink implants were placed in three reference models with different angles (parallel, 15° and 30°). Impressions of each model were made with three techniques ($n = 10$ per group): indirect, unsplinted direct, and acrylic resin-splinted direct technique. Impressions were poured with type IV dental stone. Inter-implant distances were measured for casts using a coordinate measuring machine, and the deviations from the reference models (Δr) were calculated. Data were analyzed using one-way ANOVA followed by post hoc tests to detect significance between groups ($a = 0.05$).

Results: This study showed that the deviations in micrometers from the reference model were the least for acrylic resin-splinted direct technique ($\Delta r1 = 49.96$, $\Delta r2 = 50.36$) versus indirect ($\Delta r1 = 93.8$, $\Delta r2 = 90.9$) and unsplinted direct techniques (($\Delta r1 = 67.07$, $\Delta r2 = 68.66$) in 30° angulated implant situation (p value < 0.0001[*] for both $\Delta r1$ and $\Delta r2$). In 15° angulated implants, both the acrylic resin-splinted direct ($\Delta r1 = 44.64$, $\Delta r2 = 45.58$) and unsplinted direct techniques ($\Delta r1 = 47.39$, $\Delta r2 = 55.28$) were more accurate than indirect technique ($\Delta r1 = 64.8$, $\Delta r2 = 68.3$) (p value < 0.0001[*] for both $\Delta r1$ and $\Delta r2$). While in parallel condition, no difference was found between all three techniques (p value = 0.085, 0.056 for $\Delta r1$ and $\Delta r2$, respectively).

Conclusions: The impression technique affected the accuracy of definitive casts. The acrylic resin splinted direct technique produced the most accurate casts, followed by direct unsplinted and indirect techniques. Furthermore, implant angulation affected the impression accuracy. When implant angulation increased from parallel implants to 30°, the forces of deformation increased, which resulted in increased distortion.

Keywords: Direct technique, Indirect technique, Internal connection implant, Splinting procedure

Background

Precise working casts are essential to fabricate passively fitting implant prostheses. Accurate implant impressions play a significant role and serve as a starting point in the process of producing good working casts [1]. Thus, the comparative accuracy of the impression techniques becomes a significant issue in consideration of passive fit. An inaccurate impression may result in prosthesis misfit, which can lead to further problems such as mechanical and/or biological complications [2].

Impression technique, type of impression material [3], splinting or non-splinting impression copings, type of splinting material, and number and angulation of implants [4] are the factors that affect the accuracy of impression.

Two main implant impression techniques are used for transferring the intra-oral spatial relationship of the implants to the working cast. One impression technique is the direct open tray technique that uses a custom tray with windows exposing the impression copings. The other

* Correspondence: Elshenawy.enas@yahoo.com;
Enas_elshenawy@dent.tanta.edu.eg
[1]Dental Biomaterials Department, Faculty of dentistry, Tanta University, Tanta, Egypt
Full list of author information is available at the end of the article

impression technique is the indirect technique that uses closed tray [5]. With the direct technique, both splinting and non-splinting of impression copings to improve the accuracy of impressions have been advocated [6].

In the open tray technique, the impression coping is incorporated in the impression and is removed from the mouth together with the set impression [1]. In the closed tray technique, the impression copings are retained in the mouth when the set impression is removed, and then, these copings are unscrewed from the mouth and connected to the implant analogs. This coping-implant analog assembly is repositioned into its respective position within the impression [7].

To ensure maximum accuracy, some authors emphasized the importance of splinting impression copings together intraorally before making an impression and some authors sectioned the splint material leaving a thin space and then rejoining with a minimal amount of the same material to minimize polymerization shrinkage. However, inconsistent results have been obtained [8, 9].

The implant impression can be at the abutment or implant level. The implant level impression is preferred in the esthetic zones and reduces the number of treatment visits. However, it presents unique challenges to the prosthodontist and errors can be introduced in many ways due to a rotation error that occurs when implants are connected to impression copings and to dislodgement of the impression material during removal of the impression tray from the mouth [10].

The adoption of tilted implants for the rehabilitation of both edentulous mandibles and maxillae has been proposed in the recent years. In the mandible, tilting of the distal implants may prevent damage to the mandibular nerve. Implants of conventional length can be placed, allowing engagement of as much cortical bone as possible, thus increasing primary stability [11]. However, the lack of parallelism between implants may result in increased distortion of impression material during removal from the mouth that may generate an inaccurate model [12–14].

Several impression materials have been used for multiunit implant impression; the most commonly described were addition silicone and polyether impression materials. This can be correlated to their improved accuracy [7]. Polyvinylsiloxanes show the smallest dimensional changes in comparison to the other elastomeric impression materials since they do not produce a volatile by-product during polymerization [15, 16].

This study was conducted to evaluate the effect of impression techniques and implant angulations on the accuracy of impressions in parallel and angulated implants in three mandibular models simulating clinical situations.

Three null hypotheses were tested:

1. There is no significant difference in impression accuracy whether an indirect, direct unsplinted, or direct acrylic resin splinted impression techniques were used.
2. There is no significant difference in impression accuracy whether implants had a 0°, 15°, or 30° angulation to a reference line perpendicular to the cast.
3. There is no significant interaction between the impression technique and implant angulation.

Method
Master model fabrication

Three epoxy resin (Ramses medical products factory, Alex, Egypt) completely edentulous mandibular models representing a clinical situation were used as definitive casts. Each cast had three implants (OsseoLink USA LLC. 4 mm × 9 mm, internal connection type) arranged with one implant at the midline and the other two implants at the premolar regions.

Cast (1) had all the three implants parallel to each other and perpendicular to the plane of the cast.
Cast (2) had implant at the midline perpendicular to the plane of the cast and implants at the premolar regions angulated at 15° to a line drawn perpendicular to the occlusal plane.
Cast (3) had implant at the midline perpendicular to the plane of the cast and implants at the premolar regions angulated at 30° to a line drawn perpendicular to the occlusal plane.

Each definitive cast was held in a vertical milling machine (Milling & Drilling machine, RF-Sakkary, Taiwan), and a protractor was used to align the cutting bur in the proper angulation by tilting the machine table.

The implants were placed in each definitive cast with a hand wrench and were numbered as follows: the middle implant was number 1, the left premolar implant was number 2, and the right premolar implant was number 3; and this numbering was used throughout the study.

Custom tray fabrication
Preparation of stone duplicate for each model

After the impression copings were connected to the definitive models, the space for impression material was created with baseplate wax (Cavex Setup Waxes, Haarlem, Holland). Stoppers were made on the molar regions to standardize the tray position.

An impression was taken from each model, using condensation silicone (Zetaplus, Zhermack SpA, Italy). Impressions were boxed and poured with type IV dental stone (Elite® Stone, Zhermack GmbH Deutschland) in a vacuum device. The resulting three stone casts were used to fabricate the custom trays.

Preparation of the master custom tray

Self-cured acrylic resin (Acrostone cold cure special tray material, Cairo, Egypt) was used to make the master custom trays. There are two master trays for each cast: one closed tray for the indirect technique and one with three windows for the direct unsplinted and acrylic resin-splinted technique.

Preparation of replicate custom trays

Dental flask was used for fabricating replicate trays from each master tray using the master custom tray and type IV dental stone to fabricate a two-part mold to make 30 custom trays for each cast, ten closed and twenty open trays.

The trays were made of self-cured acrylic resin (Acrostone cold cure special tray material, Cairo, Egypt). The trays were perforated for added retention of the impression material. Tray handles were made and attached to the custom trays. The trays were stored at the room temperature for 24 h before impression taking.

Impression procedure

Three different groups of implant level impression techniques were made ($n = 10$ per group) for each reference cast, a total of nine subgroups.

Addition silicone impression material (Enthus PVS Impression Material, Dharma Research, USA) with medium consistency was used for all impression procedures.

The impression procedure was standardized as follows:

1. A 1.5 kg metal block exerted a standardized pressure on each tray during the polymerization.
2. The copings were secured to the implants using dedicated torque wrench calibrated at 10 Ncm.
3. Tray adhesive was painted on the trays before making impressions.
4. The impression material was mixed using an impression gun.

5. The reference models were painted with separating medium before the impression procedures to simulate oral condition.

In the indirect technique

Closed tray impression copings remained on the definitive cast after removal of the impression. These impression copings were removed one at a time from the definitive cast and attached to an implant analog. The combined impression coping analog unit was inserted into the impression by firmly pushing it into place to full depth and slightly rotating clockwise to feel for the anti-rotational resistance (Fig. 1 a, b).

In the direct unsplinted technique

The guide pins were loosened with a hex driver and removed, and the tray was separated with the impression copings locked in the impression. The guide pins were placed back into the impression copings from the top, while an implant analog was connected to the hex on the bottom, and the guide pins were tightened with the driver (Fig. 2).

In the direct acrylic resin-splinted technique

The direct impression copings were tied up with four complete loops of dental floss (REACH® Mint Waxed Floss, Johnson and Johnson Personal Products) using a forceps. Autopolymerizing acrylic resin (Acrostone cold cure special tray material, Cairo, Egypt) was applied around the impression copings using an incremental application technique till the surface of the transfer copings are fully covered with a layer about 2 mm in thickness. A silicone index (Zetaplus, Zhermack SpA, Italy) was made after the first splint for each cast to standardize the amount of acrylic resin used and used as a reference for splinting.

After 17 min, the splint was sectioned into three pieces with a diamond disk. The impression copings were then resplinted with same acrylic resin (Fig. 3 a, b). Another 17-min interval was allowed after additional splinting to reduce the effects of polymerization shrinkage.

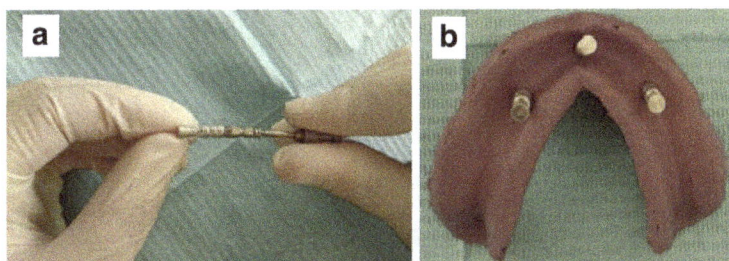

Fig. 1 a Attaching the analog to the coping using the screw driver. **b** Impression after insertion of the coping-analog till hearing the audible click

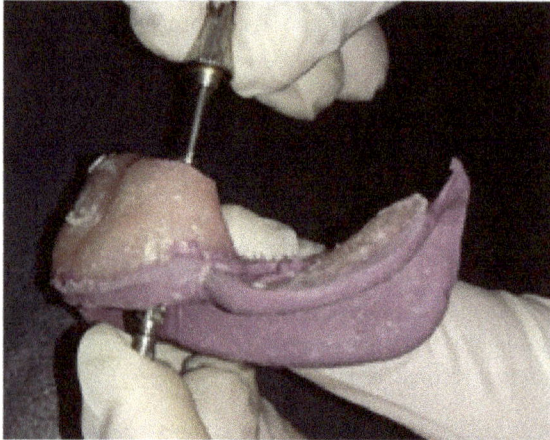

Fig. 2 Connecting the analog with the coping using the guide pin

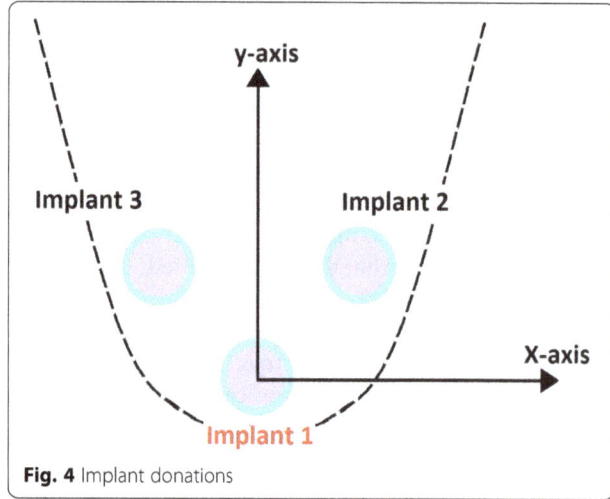

Fig. 4 Implant donations

Impressions were inspected and repeated when any inaccuracy was found.

Cast production procedure

All the impressions were poured with type IV dental stone (elite® stone, Zhermack GmbH Deutschland) using a single prefabricated mold made with laboratory silicone (Ramses medical products factory, Alex, Egypt).

After setting of stone, the casts were separated from the impressions. The three healing abutments were tightened to the implant analogs before the measuring procedures. All casts were labeled and stored at room temperature for 24 h prior to measurements.

Measurement procedure

A coordinate measuring machine (CMM) (Mitutoyo CRYSTA-Apex S544, Japan) was used to evaluate the positional accuracy of the samples with accuracy of 0.0001 mm.

The implant abutments were donated as seen in (Fig. 4).

The center of abutment 1 was considered as the reference point for all measurements. The planar surface from this point was regarded as XY. Two imaginary XZ

lines were considered between the centers of the analogs 1, 2 and 1, 3. The XZ planes were perpendicular to XY plane. Therefore, the center of analog 1 was laid on the origin (0, 0, 0). CMM measured the coordinates of each analog with respect to the reference point (Fig. 5).

The center of each implant abutments was located using a CMM probe by touching eight points on the circumference of the outer diameter of the implant abutments.

Four points on the upper surface of each implant abutment were measured to form a plane used to calculate the vertical distances between implant abutments 1 and 2, and 1 and 3 in the z-axis (Fig. 6).

The distances (in micrometers) between the implant centers with the reference point were calculated according to the following formula [9]:

The distance from the reference point $(r) = \sqrt{x^2 + y^2 + z^2}$.

Absolute error (Δr) was calculated by comparing the Euclidean distance between the analogs in the duplicated cast with the distance in the definitive cast:

Absolute error $\Delta r = \sqrt{x_{m+}^2 y_m^2 z_m^2} - \sqrt{x_{d+}^2 y_d^2 z_d^2}$

where m = master and d = duplicated.

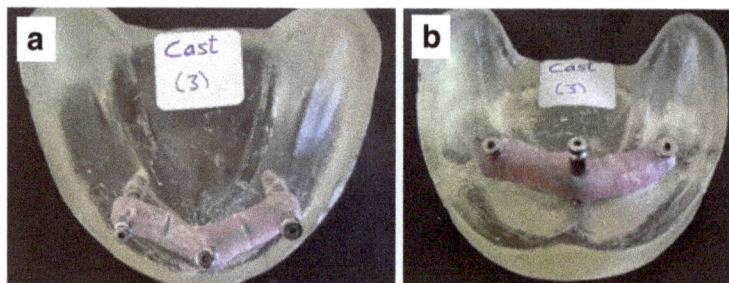

Fig. 3 a The splint sectioned into three separate pieces. **b** Resplinting with acrylic resin

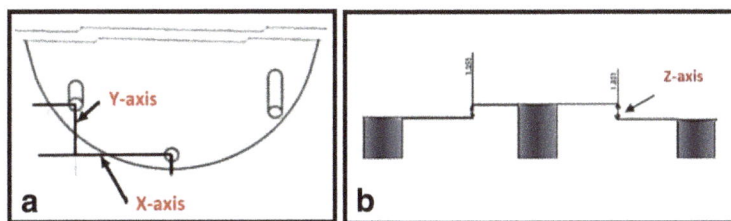

Fig. 5 a Inter-implant distances in *x*- and *y*-axes. **b** Inter-implant distance in *Z* axis

Each model has two Euclidean distances and named $\Delta r1$ (absolute error between implant abutments 1 and 2) and $\Delta r2$ (absolute error between implant abutments 1 and 3).

Statistical analysis

Mean and standard deviation were calculated for each Euclidean distance. One-way ANOVA followed by post hoc tests was performed to detect significance between groups. Statistical analysis was performed using SPSS statistics software for Windows. P values ≤ 0.05 were considered to be statistically significant in all tests.

Two-way ANOVA was used to evaluate the influence of different impression techniques and implant angulations on the accuracy of impressions at a significance level of .05 (SPSS version 20, IBM).

Results

The mean and standard deviation values of each of the two Euclidean distances measured in micrometer (μm) for the nine study groups are presented in Table 1.

Comparing between study groups
Effect of impression technique on accuracy of final impression

In cast (1):One-way ANOVA revealed no statistically significant differences in deformation between the three impression techniques ($F = 2.694$, 3.276; p value = .085, 0.056 for $\Delta r1$ and $\Delta r2$, respectively) as shown in Table 2.

In cast (2): One-way ANOVA revealed statistically significant differences in deformation between the three impression techniques ($F = 30.03$, 22.95; p value = $< .0001^*$ for $\Delta r1$ and $\Delta r2$, respectively) as shown in Table 3. Post hoc test showed that indirect technique was significantly ($p < 0.05$) less accurate than direct unsplinted and direct splinted techniques which were not significantly different from each other ($p > 0.05$) for $\Delta r1$ and $\Delta r2$.

In cast (3): One-way ANOVA revealed statistically high significant differences in deformation between the three impression techniques ($F = 85.65$, 83.56 p value = $< .0001^*$ for $\Delta r1$ and $\Delta r2$, respectively) as shown in Table 4. Post hoc test showed that indirect technique was significantly ($p < 0.05$) less accurate than direct unsplinted which was significantly ($p < 0.05$) less accurate than direct splinted techniques for $\Delta r1$ and $\Delta r2$.

Effect of implant angulation on accuracy of final impression

For (group 1) the indirect technique One-way ANOVA revealed statistically significant differences in deformation between cast 3(30°), cast 2 (15°), and cast 1(0°) groups ($F = 100.65$, 71.39; p value = $< .0001^*$ for $\Delta r1$ and $\Delta r2$, respectively). Post hoc test showed that indirect technique was significantly ($p < 0.05$) less accurate in case of 30° angulated implants in cast 3 than 15° angulated implants in cast 2, which was significantly ($p < 0.05$) less accurate than parallel implants in cast 1 for $\Delta r1$ and $\Delta r2$.

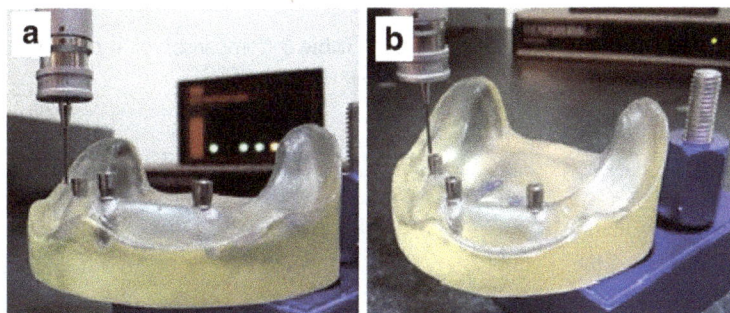

Fig. 6 a Measuring the outer diameter. **b** Measuring the upper surface

Table 1 Mean and standard deviation values of each of the two Euclidean distances measured in micrometer (μm) for the study groups

Groups	Subgroups	Mean ± SD	
		Δr1	Δr2
Group 1: Indirect technique n = 10 per subgroup	Subgroup A: cast 1	48.11 ± 8.2	54.08 ± 7.2
	Subgroup B: cast 2	64.8 ± 8.2	68.3 ± 8.6
	Subgroup C: cast 3	93.8 ± 4.83	90.9 ± 4.2
Group 2: Direct unsplinted technique n = 10 per subgroup	Subgroup A: cast 1	41.4 ± 9	50.7 ± 13.3
	Subgroup B: cast 2	47.39 ± 5.51	55.28 ± 7.3
	Subgroup C: cast 3	67.07 ± 5.7	68.66 ± 4.7
Group 3: Direct splinted technique n = 10 per subgroup	Subgroup A: cast 1	40.3 ± 6.7	42.8 ± 8.5
	Subgroup B: cast 2	44.64 ± 4.63	45.58 ± 3.4
	Subgroup C: cast 3	49.96 ± 10.6	50.36 ± 10.3

Δr1 the absolute error between implant abutments 1 and 2, Δr2 the absolute error between implant abutments 1 and 3

For (group 2) direct unsplinted technique One-way ANOVA revealed statistically significant differences in deformation between cast 3 (30°), cast 2 (15°), and cast 1 (0°) groups ($F = 36.2$, 9.33 p value = $< 0.0001^*$, 0.0008^* for Δr1 and Δr2, respectively). Post hoc test showed that the distortion values of the duplicate casts obtained from cast 3 (30°) was significantly higher than distortion values for cast 1 (0°) and cast 2 (15°) ($p < 0.05$), which were not significantly different from each other ($p > 0.05$) for Δr1 and Δr2.

For (group 3) direct splinted technique One-way ANOVA revealed no statistically significant differences in deformation (Δr1 or Δr2) between cast 3 (30°), cast 2(15°), and cast 1(0°) groups ($F = 3.14$, 2.18; p value = .059, .132 for Δr1 and Δr2, respectively).

Interaction between variables

A two-way ANOVA was performed to study the effect of impression technique and implant angulation on the accuracy of duplicate casts. The data obtained in this study reveals significant interaction between impression technique and implant angulation ($p = < .0001^*$) in the two Euclidean distances and that both variables affect the implant impression accuracy as shown in Tables 5 and 6.

Discussion

An impression that precisely records the 3-dimensional positions of implants is essential to achieve a passively fitting prosthesis [1, 17]. Therefore, comparative accuracy of impression techniques becomes an important issue in consideration of passive fit [8].

In this study, epoxy resin models were used as reference models because they have appropriate elastic modulus for a bone analog material [18]. They were also found to have better stability than plaster models used in other studies [19, 20].

The models were selected to be with no undercuts because undercuts need high removal forces, which can confound the results. Therefore, removing them from the study favors the reliability of the findings [21].

In the present study, the three implants were placed in each reference model with different angulations to simulate common clinical situations that may necessitate placement of angulated implants in lower premolar region. Furthermore, unlike most of previous studies, the implants in this study were also tilted to the mesial side, which better represents clinical conditions [21].

Table 2 Comparison of impression techniques in cast 1 using one-way ANOVA

	Comparison of impression techniques in cast 1 (parallel condition)			F	p value
	Group 1 Indirect	Group 2 D.unsplinted	Group 3 D.splinted		
	Mean ± SD	Mean ± SD	Mean ± SD		
Δr1	48.11 ± 8.2	41.4 ± 9	40.3 ± 6.7	2.694	.085
Δr2	54.08 ± 7.2	50.7 ± 13.3	42.8 ± 8.5	3.276	0.056

Δr1 the absolute error between implant abutments 1 and 2, Δr2 the absolute error between implant abutments 1 and 3

Table 3 Comparison of impression techniques in cast 2 using one-way ANOVA

	Comparison of impression techniques in cast 2 (angulated 15°)			F	p value
	Group 1 Indirect	Group 2 D.unsplinted	Group 3 D.splinted		
	Mean ± SD	Mean ± SD	Mean ± SD		
Δr1	64.8 ± 8.2	47.39 ± 5.51	44.64 ± 4.63	30.0341	$< 0.0001^*$
Δr2	68.3 ± 8.6	55.28 ± 7.3	45.58 ± 3.4	22.9561	$< 0.0001^*$

Δr1 the absolute error between implant abutments 1 and 2, Δr2 the absolute error between implant abutments 1 and 3

Table 4 Comparison of impression techniques in cast 3 using one-way ANOVA

	Comparison of impression techniques in cast 3 (angulated 30°)			F	p value
	Group 1 Indirect	Group 2 D.unsplinted	Group 3 D.splinted		
	Mean ± SD	Mean ± SD	Mean ± SD		
$\Delta r1$	93.8 ± 4.83	67.07 ± 5.7	49.96 ± 10.6	85.6521	< 0.0001*
$\Delta r2$	90.9 ± 4.2	68.66 ± 4.7	50.36 ± 10.3	83.5686	< 0.0001*

$\Delta r1$ the absolute error between implant abutments 1 and 2, $\Delta r2$ the absolute error between implant abutments 1 and 3

In this study, impressions were made at implant level because it allows for the selection of the most proper abutments and is helpful in situations where angulation of the abutments is difficult to be determined intraorally [19, 22].

The impression material used for this study was polyvinylsiloxane as it exhibits accuracy and adequate rigidity [23]. Medium consistency was more advantageous than putty consistency because the implants used caused a higher level of stress to the impression copings during the impression procedure. Therefore, the use of a more elastic consistency is advantageous in evaluating the effect of splinting impression copings on impression accuracy [19]. In addition, the single-step technique allows the material to record finer details without slumping of the material in the tray, less time-consuming, and simple to perform [24].

Custom trays were utilized because elastomeric materials are more accurate if used in 2 to 3-mm uniform thickness. All the custom trays were perforated to ensure good retention with the trays [25]. Standardization of custom trays was done through modification of reference models with spacer and making stoppers and then making of the duplicate casts from the modified reference models [26].

Self-cure acrylic resin was selected as a splinting material in this study as it is easy to use and it does not require a dry environment [27]. Acrylic resin splint was sectioned and resplinted after 17 min in

Table 5 Effect of implant angulation and impression technique on impressions by two-way ANOVA for $\Delta r1$

Source of variation	DF	Mean square	F	Sig.
Angulation	2	5668.941	104.382	.000*
Imp.tech.	2	4562.156	84.003	.000*
Angulation * imp.tech.	4	860.574	15.846	.000*
Error	81	54.309		
Total	90			
Corrected total	89			

DF degree of freedom
*Significant (p < 0.05)

Table 6 Effect of implant angulation and impression technique on impressions by two-way ANOVA for $\Delta r2$

Source of variation	DF	Mean square	F	Sig.
Angulation	2	3356.616	50.873	.000*
Imp.tech.	2	4557.783	69.077	.000*
Angulation * imp.tech.	4	581.127	8.808	.000*
Error	81	65.981		
Total	90			
Corrected total	89			

DF degree of freedom
*Significant (p < 0.05)

order to minimize any discrepancies due to polymerization shrinkage. Mojon et al [28] and other studies [19, 29–31] have stated that separation and reuniting of acrylic splint when done 17 min after the setting reaction allows 80% reduction in the effects of polymerization shrinkage. A silicone index was made to standardize the dimensions of the acrylic resin splints for each specimen [19, 32].

A prefabricated mold was used for pouring all impressions to control the setting expansion and standardize the amount of dental stone used [26]. All stone casts were stored at room temperature for 24 h prior to measurements to make sure that they have reached their optimal mechanical properties [19, 26, 33].

Studies comparing the accuracy of implant impression techniques with methods such as micrometers, Vernier calipers, strain gauges, or measuring microscopes could merely carry out two-dimensional measurements [5, 34–36]. However, when the measurements are two dimensional only, relevant information is lost. Therefore, CMM was used as the measuring device in this study because it made three-dimensional evaluation of any distortion possible. When points from different implant casts have a common reference within a coordinate system, the 3D orientation of analogs can be recorded [37].

The results show that there was no significant difference in accuracy between the impression techniques used with parallel implants. The similar accuracy may be due to removal of the custom tray along the same path as the implant angulation. These results are in agreement with several studies showing no difference between the three impression techniques [19, 20, 30, 38–40].

While in the case of 15° angulated implants, direct unsplinted technique and direct acrylic resin-splinted technique exhibited more accuracy compared to indirect technique. This was in agreement with some studies that found that direct impression technique whether splinted or not is significantly more accurate than indirect technique when angulation of implants increased up to 15° [33, 39].

Furthermore, in the case of 30° angulated implants, the direct acrylic resin-splinted technique was significantly more accurate than the direct unsplinted technique, which was significantly more accurate than the indirect technique. This finding is in agreement with several studies, which reported the superiority of the splinted technique over the non-splinted technique for making an impression of angulated internal connection implants [6, 29, 31, 39, 41].

Regarding implant angulation, the results of this study found that increasing implant angulation to 15° or 30° affected the accuracy of indirect impression technique. While in the direct unsplinted technique, no difference in accuracy was found between parallel condition and 15° angulated condition. The increased displacement of impression material and the difficult removal of the impression tray in case of angulated implant were believed to be the source of error in the indirect impression technique. In the direct technique, the impression coping remains in the impression, which reduces the effect of implant angulation and the impression material deformation upon removal from mouth.

These findings agreed with Lee et al. [33] and Carr et al. [42] who found significant difference in accuracy of indirect technique with angulated implants, while no difference in accuracy of direct technique up to 10° and 15° angulations, respectively. Conrad et al. [20] found that angulation of implants up to 15° did not affect the accuracy of both indirect and direct techniques.

In this study, increasing the angulation between implants to 30° affected the accuracy of direct unsplinted technique while it did not affect the accuracy of direct splinted technique significantly. This is in agreement with Tsagkalidis et al. [39] and Martínez-Rus et al. [31]. This may be because splinting the impression copings using a rigid material prevented individual coping movement during the impression making procedure [1].

This study showed that significant interaction existed between impression technique and implant angulations and that both affected implant impression accuracy. As implant angulations increase, distortion in the experimental cast increases. This can be explained with increased material deformation upon impression removal. These results find support in some other studies [39, 43].

According to the recorded data, the null hypothesis was partially rejected because the accuracy of the impression techniques was only different in angulated implant conditions and there was an interaction between impression technique and implant angulations and that both affect impression accuracy.

Conclusions

The accuracy of definitive casts was affected by the impression technique only in angulated implant conditions where direct splinted technique provided the most accurate position transfer. In parallel implant situation, the three techniques were similar.

When implant angulation increases, the forces of deformation increase which requires an impression technique that allows precise inter-implant relationship. The indirect technique showed the highest distortion values when angulated implants were used followed by direct-unsplinted technique then direct acrylic resin-splinted technique.

Authors' contributions
EE carried out samples preparation, measurements, data collection, and drafting the manuscript. AM participated in the design of experiment and performed the statistical analysis and interpretation of data, and FA participated in conception, design, and revising manuscript critically for important intellectual content. All authors read and approved the final manuscript.

Competing interests
Enas A. Elshenawy, Ahmed M. Alam-Eldein, and Fadel A. Abd Elfatah declare that they have no competing interests.

Author details
[1]Dental Biomaterials Department, Faculty of dentistry, Tanta University, Tanta, Egypt. [2]Prosthodontic Department, Faculty of dentistry, Tanta University, Tanta, Egypt.

References
1. Lee H, So JS, Hochstedler JL, Ercoli C. The accuracy of implant impressions: a systematic review. J Prosthet Dent. 2008;100:285–91.
2. Goodacre CJ, Bernal G, Rungcharassaeng K, Kan JY. Clinical complications with implants and implant prostheses. J Prosthet Dent. 2003;90:121–32.
3. Wee AG. Comparison of impression materials for direct multi-implant impressions. J Prosthet Dent. 2000;83:323–31.
4. Ma J, Rubenstein JE. Complete arch implant impression technique. J Prosthet Dent. 2012;107:405–10.
5. Del Acqua MM, Chavez AM, Amarat AL, Compagnoni MM, Mollo FA. Comparison of impression techniques and materials for an implant-supported prosthesis. Int J Oral Maxillofac Implants. 2010;25(4):771–6.
6. Vigolo P, Fonzi F, Majzoub Z, Cordioli G. An evaluation of impression techniques for multiple internal connection implant prostheses. J Prosthet Dent. 2004;92:470–6.
7. Lee H, Ercoli C, Funkenbusch PD, Feng C. Effect of subgingival depth of implant placement on the dimensional accuracy of the implant impression: an in vitro study. J Prosthet Dent. 2008;99:107–13.
8. Al Quran FA, Rashdan BA, Zomar AA, Weiner S. Passive fit and accuracy of three dental implant impression techniques. Quintessence Int. 2012;43:119–25.
9. Kim S, Nicholls JI, Han CH, Lee KW. Displacement of implant components from impressions to definitive casts. Int J Oral Maxillofac Implants. 2006;21:747–55.
10. Daoudi MF, Setchell DJ, Searson LJ. A laboratory investigation of the accuracy of two impression techniques for single-tooth implants. Int J Prosthodont. 2001;14:152–8.
11. Aparicio C, Perales P, Rangert B. Tilted implants as an alternative to maxillary sinus grafting: a clinical, radiological, and periotest study. Clin Implant Dent Relat Res. 2001;3:39–49.
12. Assuncao WG, Filho HG, Zaniquelli O. Evaluation of transfer impressions for osseointegrated implants at various angulations. Implant Dent. 2004;13:358–66.
13. Seyedan K, Sazgara H, Kalalipour M, Alavi K. Dimensional accuracy of

polyether and poly vinyl siloxane materials for different implant impression technique. Res J Appl Sci. 2008;3:257–63.

14. Lee SJ, Cho SB. Accuracy of five implant impression technique: effect of splinting materials and methods. J Adv Prosthodont. 2011;3:177–85.

15. ISO 4823: 2015. Dentistry–elastomeric impression materials. Geneva: International Organization for Standardization; 2015. Available at https://www.iso.org/standard/60586.html. Accessed 17 Jan 2018.

16. JF MC, AWG W. Applied dental materials. 9th ed. Munksgaard: Blackwell Publishing; 2008. p. 167–72.

17. Sahin S, Cehreli MC. The significance of passive framework fit in implant prosthodontics: current status. Implant Dent. 2001;10:85–92.

18. Lee CK, Karl M, Kelly JR. Evaluation of test protocol variables for dental implant fatigue research. Dent Mater. 2009;25(11):1419–25.

19. Choi JH, Lim YJ, Yim SH, Kim CW. Evaluation of the accuracy of implant-level impression techniques for internal-connection implant prostheses in parallel and divergent models. Int J Oral Maxillofac Implants. 2007;22:761–8.

20. Conrad HJ, Pesun IJ, DeLong R, Hodges JS. Accuracy of two impression techniques with angulated implants. J Prosthet Dent. 2007;97:349–56.

21. Geramipanah F, Sahebi M, Davari M, Hajimahmoudi M, Rakhshan V. Effects of impression levels and trays on the accuracy of impressions taken from angulated implants. Clin Oral Implants Res. 2015;26(9):1098–105.

22. Sorrentino R, Gherlone EF, Calesini G, Zarone F. Effect of implant angulation, connection length, and impression material on the dimensional accuracy of implant impressions: an in vitro comparative study. Clin Implant Dent Relat Res. 2010;12(s1):63–76.

23. Moreira AH, Rodrigues NF, Pinho AC, Fonseca JC, Vilaça JL. Accuracy comparison of implant impression techniques: a systematic review. Clin Implant Dent Relat Res. 2015;17(2):751–64.

24. Prithviraj DR, Pujari M, Garg P, Shruthi DP. Accuracy of implant impression obtained from different impression materials and techniques: review. J Clin Exp Dent. 2011;3:106–11.

25. Burns J, Palmer R, Howe L, Wilson R. Accuracy of open tray implant impressions: an in vitro comparison of stock versus custom trays. J Prosthet Dent. 2003;89:250–5.

26. Vojdani M, Torabi K, Ansarifard E. Accuracy of different impression materials in parallel and nonparallel implants. Dent Res J (Isfahan). 2015;12(4):315–22.

27. Phillips KM, Nicholls JI, Ma T, Rubenstein J. The accuracy of three implant impression techniques: a three-dimensional analysis. Int J Oral Maxillofac Implants. 1994;9(5):533–40.

28. Mojon P, Oberholzer JP, Oberholzer JP, Meyer JM, Belser UC. Polymerization shrinkage of index and pattern acrylic resins. J Prosthet Dent. 1990;64:684–8.

29. Naconecy MM, Teixeira ER, Shinkai RS, Frasca LC, Cervieri A. Evaluation of the accuracy of 3 transfer techniques for implant-supported prostheses with multiple abutments. Int J Oral Maxillofac Implants. 2004;19:192–8.

30. Hazboun GB, Masri R, Romberg E, Kempler J, Driscoll CF. Effect of implant angulation and impression technique on impressions of NobelActive implants. J Prosthet Dent. 2015;113(5):425–31.

31. Martínez-Rus F, García C, Santamaría A, Özcan M, Pradíes G. Accuracy of definitive casts using 4 implant-level impression techniques in a scenario of multi-implant system with different implant angulations and subgingival alignment levels. Implant Dent. 2013;22(3):268–76.

32. Shankar YR, Sahoo S, Krishna MH, Kumar PS, Kumar TS, Narula S. Accuracy of implant impressions using various impression techniques and impression materials. J Dent Implant. 2016;6(1):29–36.

33. Lee YJ, Heo SJ, Koak JY, Kim SK. Accuracy of different impression techniques for internal-connection implants. Int J Oral Maxillofac Implants. 2009;24:823–30.

34. Cehreli MC, Akca K. Impression techniques and misfit induced strains on implant-supported superstructures: an in vitro study. Int J Periodontics Restorative Dent. 2006;26:379–85.

35. Daoudi MF, Setchell DJ, Searson LJ. An evaluation of three implant level impression techniques for single tooth implant. Eur J Prosthodont Restor Dent. 2004;12(1):9–14.

36. Mostafa TM, Elgendy MN, Kashef NA, Halim MM. Evaluation of the precision of three implant transfer impression techniques using two elastomeric impression materials. Int J Prosthodont. 2010;23:525–8.

37. Holst S, Blatz MB, Bergler M, Goellner M, Wichmann M. Influence of impression material and time on the 3-dimensional accuracy of implant impressions. Quintessence Int. 2007;38:67–73.

38. Wenz HJ, Hertrampf K. Accuracy of impressions and casts using different implant impression techniques in a multi-implant system with an internal hex connection. Int J Oral Maxillofac Implants. 2008;23:39–47.

39. Tsagkalidis G, Tortopidis D, Mpikos P, Kaisarlis G, Koidis P. Accuracy of 3 different impression techniques for internal connection angulated implants. J Prosthet Dent. 2015;114(4):517–23.

40. Chang WG, Vahidi F, Bae KH, Lim BS. Accuracy of three implant impression techniques with different impression materials and stones. Int J Prosthodont. 2012;25(1):44–7.

41. Hariharan R, Shankar C, Rajan M, Baig MR, Azhagarasan NS. Evaluation of accuracy of multiple dental implant impressions using various splinting materials. Int J Oral Maxillofac Implants. 2010;25:38–44.

42. Carr AB. Comparison of impression techniques for a five-implant mandibular model. Int J Oral Maxillofac Implants. 1991;6(4):448–55.

43. Kurtulmus-Yilmaz S, Ozan O, Ozcelik TB, Yagiz A. Digital evaluation of the accuracy of impression techniques and materials in angulated implants. J Dent. 2014;42(12):1551–9.

10

Electro-chemical deposition of nano hydroxyapatite-zinc coating on titanium metal substrate

N. A. El-Wassefy[1*], F. M. Reicha[2] and N. S. Aref[1]

Abstract

Background: Titanium is an inert metal that does not induce osteogenesis and has no antibacterial properties; it is proposed that hydroxyapatite coating can enhance its bioactivity, while zinc can contribute to antibacterial properties and improve osseointegration.

Aims: A nano-sized hydroxyapatite-zinc coating was deposited on commercially pure titanium using an electro-chemical process, in order to increase its surface roughness and enhance adhesion properties.

Methods: The hydroxyapatite-zinc coating was attained using an electro-chemical deposition in a solution composed of a naturally derived calcium carbonate, di-ammonium hydrogen phosphate, with a pure zinc metal as the anode and titanium as the cathode. The applied voltage was −2.5 for 2 h at a temperature of 85 °C. The resultant coating was characterized for its surface morphology and chemical composition using a scanning electron microscope (SEM), energy dispersive x-ray spectroscope (EDS), and Fourier transform infrared (FT-IR) spectrometer. The coated specimens were also evaluated for their surface roughness and adhesion quality.

Results: Hydroxyapatite-zinc coating had shown rosette-shaped, homogenous structure with nano-size distribution, as confirmed by SEM analysis. FT-IR and EDS proved that coatings are composed of hydroxyapatite (HA) and zinc. The surface roughness assessment revealed that the coating procedure had significantly increased average roughness (Ra) than the control, while the adhesive tape test demonstrated a high-quality adhesive coat with no laceration on tape removal.

Conclusions: The developed in vitro electro-chemical method can be employed for the deposition of an even thickness of nano HA-Zn adhered coatings on titanium substrate and increases its surface roughness significantly.

Keywords: Hydroxyapatite-zinc coating, Titanium metal, Surface roughness, Surface morphology, Coating adhesion, Electrochemical deposition

Background

Titanium metal is one of the most widely used biomedical orthopedic materials because of its decent mechanical properties [1]. However, as an inert material, it cannot induce osteogenesis and has no antibacterial properties [2]. In order to improve surface bioactivity of titanium substrates, numerous methods have been proposed to cover it with bio-ceramic coatings [1]. Various clinical studies demonstrated that the hydroxyapatite coating

of prosthesis can promote earlier osseous response which could increase the prosthesis fixation and the bonding strength [3–5].

Titanium implants are usually placed in contact with bones and gingival tissues so they are partially exposed to the oral cavity during and after implantation. This increases the hazard of bacterial infection, which is known as peri-implantitis [6, 7].

For centuries, Zinc (Zn) as one of the essential elements of tissues in the human body has a stimulating role in the metabolism of bones and has been used as bacteriostatic and bactericidal agents [8, 9]. Zinc can enhance the retention strength and osseointegration of

* Correspondence: nohahmed@mans.edu.eg
[1]Dental Biomaterials Department, Faculty of Dentistry, Mansoura University, 35516 El Gomhoria St., Mansoura, Egypt
Full list of author information is available at the end of the article

implants [10, 11], by stimulating alkaline-phosphatase activity and collagen production, thus can increase bone deposition and reduce bone resorption [12]. Zn deficiency results in skeletal changes, including retardation of skeletal growth [10] and prolonged bone recovery [13]. Moreover, Zn species are also known to possess excellent antibacterial qualities. Zinc showed inhibitory effects against several bacteria, including *Streptococcal mutans* [14–16].

The metals' antibacterial activity has been contingent on their contact surface; thus, a greater nanoparticles' surface area permits larger interfaces and increases their interactions with other particles [17].

Although HA coatings revealed an enhanced bone attachment and thus better implants integration, long-term coating stability is quite a provoking concern [18]. Numerous coating techniques like plasma spraying, sol-gel, electrophoretic deposition, electro deposition have been employed to deposit hydroxyapatite on titanium implants. Plasma spraying is the most widely used technique for coating, but it leads to decomposition of HA due to the high temperature used, and it cannot be employed for complex structures. In electrophoretic deposition, high voltage was applied to the metal surface in order to attract the dispersed particles which leads to anodic polarization of metal substrate. This might increase the corrosion risk of metal and suppress the adhesion of HA particles [19–21]. Electro-chemical deposition (ED) is a frequently used approach with increasing popularity, due to variability of coating composition, process simplicity, and its applicability for multidimensional implant surfaces [22].

The aim of the present work was to develop well-adhered and uniform hydroxyapatite-zinc coatings on titanium metal substrate, through an in vitro electro-chemical deposition method. The coating was characterized for functional chemical group, surface morphology, surface chemical analysis, surface roughness, and coat adhesive bonding by Fourier transform infrared spectrometer (FT-IR), scanning electron microscope (SEM), energy dispersive spectroscope (EDS), profilometer, and tape adhesive test respectively.

Methods

Cathode preparation

Commercially pure Ti (CpTi) grade II specimens were cut down into plates with dimensions $10 \times 10 \times 2$ mm and used as substrates (cathode material) for depositing HA and Zn. CpTi specimens were polished with successive grades of silicon carbide papers, ultra-sonicated in acetone (99.5%, EM Science), rinsed in distilled water, and then air dried at room temperature, before they were used for the electro-chemical process.

Electro-chemical deposition of HA and Zn

The electro-chemical deposition process was carried in an electrolytic solution. The Ca source of the electrolyte was prepared from dry cuttlebone (CB) (Sepia officinalis L., from the Mediterranean Sea). The CB was cut into blocks and immersed into 5% household bleach NaClO for 2 days, in order to eliminate the organic component [23], then rinsed with water and dried in an oven at 80 °C for 6 h. The starting $CaCO_3$ material of CB was made to react with nitric acid 69% (SD Fine Chem Limited, India) to form $Ca(NO_3)_2$ solution in water. After the complete evolution of CO_2, water was evaporated by heating and the resultant powder was examined by FT-IR spectrometer (Nicolet iS10, Thermo Electron Corporation, UK) which utilized the selected range of 400 to 4000 wave numbers (cm^{-1}) to confirm its chemical structure of $Ca(NO_3)_2 \cdot 4H_2O$. The other salts were purchased from Sigma Aldrich and added to form an electrolytic solution containing 0.6 M $Ca(NO_3)_2 \cdot 4H_2O$, 0.36 M $(NH_4) \cdot 2HPO_4$, 1 M $NaNO_2$, 6% H_2O_2, and NH_4OH to adjust the solution pH to 6. Pure zinc (Zn) particles (Zinc Tres Pur, Prolabo, N 29050, $N = 99.999$) were pressed in a bench press; Craver Laboratory Press (Model C 31000-823, USA) to produce a $10 \times 10 \times 2$mm plates that acted as the anode. Platinum wires were used to hang the electrodes in the solution. A thermometer was used to monitor the temperature during the process. The deposition process was carried out with a power supply unit (LT ECOS, 7972, Italy) by applying an electrode potential of ~2.5 V at 85 °C temperature stabilized by a thermostatic water bath (MLW, U4, 74010, Germany) for 2 h, during the deposition process a continuous stirring was carried out by a magnetic stirrer. The electro-chemical deposition setup is shown in the schematic diagram in Fig. 1. After the deposition, specimens were taken out from the electrolytic bath, rinsed with deionized water, and left to dry for 24 h on a clean bench. The coated CpTi specimens were then sintered at 400 °C for 2 h in an electric furnace with a heating rate of 5 °C/min and gradually cooled to room temperature inside the furnace.

Characterization of the deposited HA-Zn coating
Infrared analysis

The coating was scrapped from Ti specimen's surface and investigated for its chemical structure using FT-IR spectroscopy. The powder was investigated by double-beam dispersive IR spectrometer (Nicolet iS10, Thermo Electron Corporation, UK) which utilized the selected range of 400 to 4000 wave numbers (cm^{-1}) at 4 cm^{-1} resolution and averaging of 100 scans. Two milligrams of scrapped powder was mixed with 300 mg of KBr and pressed into a disc before the measurement.

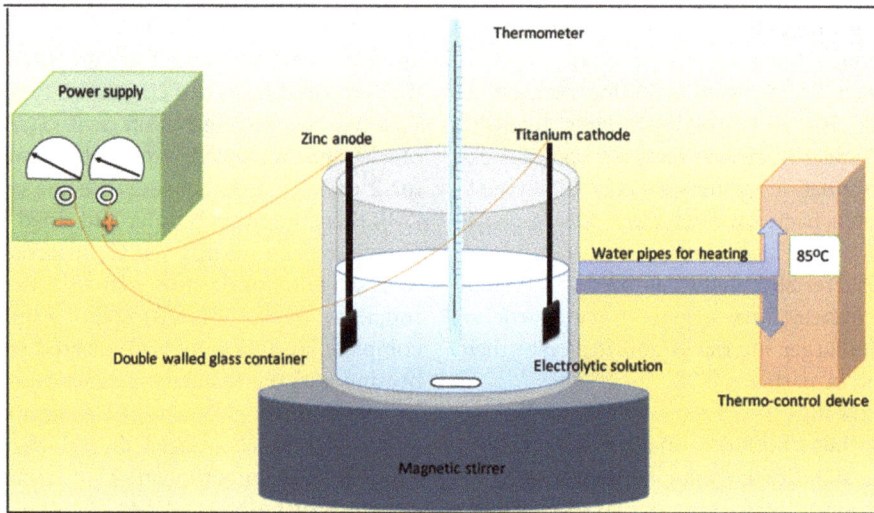

Fig. 1 Graphical presentation of the electrochemical-deposition coating process' equipment

Surface characterization of coatings

Scanning electron microscope (SEM) (JSM 6300, JEOL, Japan) and energy dispersive spectroscope (EDS) were used to examine the morphological qualities and the elemental composition of the HA-Zn deposits. The working distance was 15 mm at 20 V. Three specimens were examined for each group of the study.

Surface-mechanical testing of coatings

Roughness of coatings Specimens of control and HA-Zn coated groups were evaluated by a surface roughness profilometer tester (Surftest SJ-210, Mitutoyo Corporation, Tokyo, Japan,) according to ISO 4287-1997 [24] with a diamond tip radius of 5 μm, a scanning speed 0.5 mm/s, a

resolution of 0.01 μm, a Gaussian filter, and a cut-off length of 8 mm. Seven specimens from each group were scanned and evaluated for the average roughness parameter, each specimen was scanned five times, and the mean was calculated in μm. The roughness parameter (Ra) values were compared for statistical significance using the Student t test in SPSS software version 20 (SPSS Inc. Chicago, IL, USA).

Coating adhesion test The adhesion of coating is qualitatively assessed by the tape test. A standard test method (Tape test-ASTM D 3359-97) was used for assessing the adhesion of the HA-Zn coating on the titanium substrate. In this method, a part of a pressure-sensitive adhesive tape (masking tape, M&G pen AJD97355) is

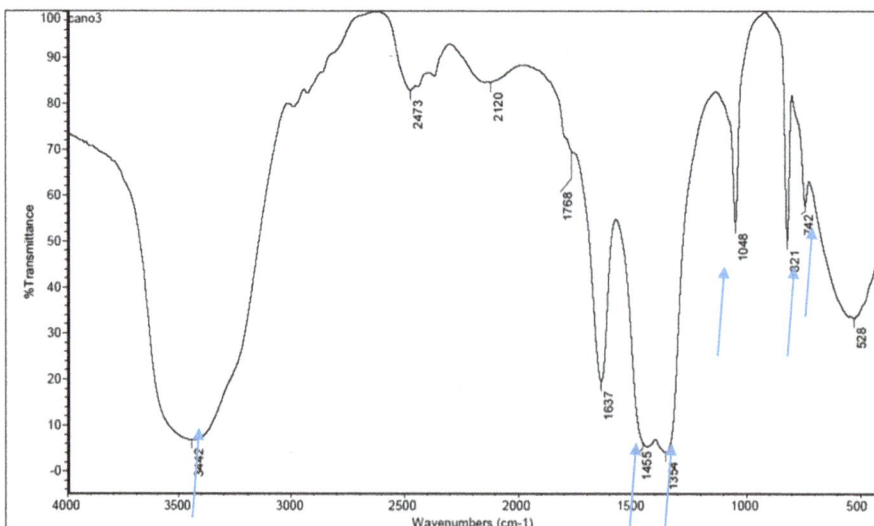

Fig. 2 IR spectra of $Ca(NO_3)_2 \cdot 4 H_2O$ powder prepared from a natural source (CB)

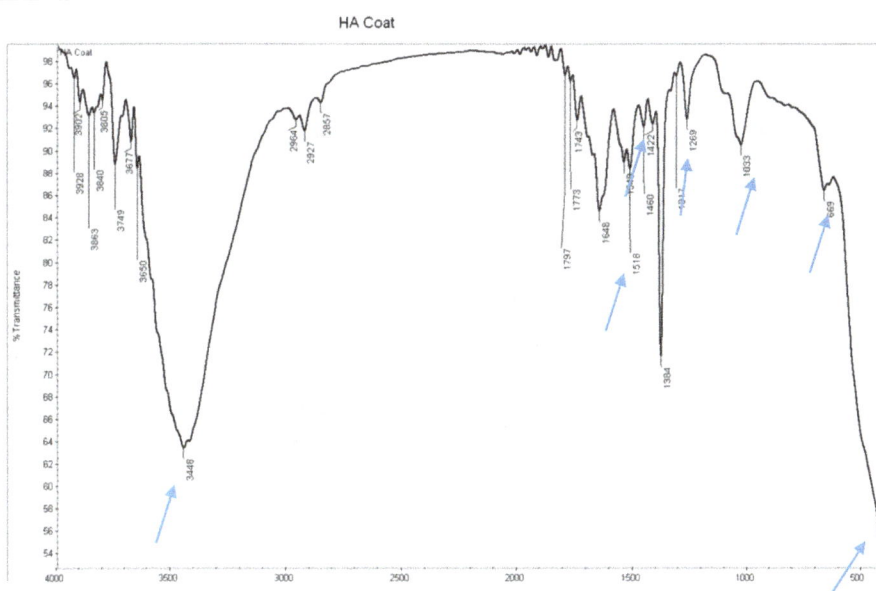

Fig. 3 IR spectra of HA-Zn powder scrapped from coated titanium specimen

pressed against the coating by the use of a pencil eraser for 90 s. The tape is then rapidly removed (without jerk movements) at 180° angle, and the degree of film removal is detected when the tape is pulled off. Because an integral coating with substantial adhesion is often not detached at all, the sternness of the test is typically improved by making a figure X cutting into the coat using a sharp scalpel with enough pressure to reach the metal substrate, then applying the tape and remove it. The denuded area is inspected for removal of coating from the substrate, and then the adhesion is ranked by relating the detached part of the coat versus a recognized rating scale. The test is repeated for three other locations in

the same specimen. Coverage of coated substrate was computed using Matlab (version7.1) [25].

Results
FT-IR results
Figure 2 shows the FT-IR spectra of $Ca(NO_3)_2 \cdot 4H_2O$ with weak sharp absorption peak bands at 742, 821, and 1048 cm^{-1}, a strong broad absorption band at 1354 cm^{-1}, and a strong shoulder absorption band at 1455 cm^{-1}. A wide broad absorption band peak appears at 3442 cm^{-1} due to the presence of water. Figure 3 shows the FT-IR spectra of HA-Zn powder scrapped from CpTi specimens; the band at ~421 cm^{-1} may be

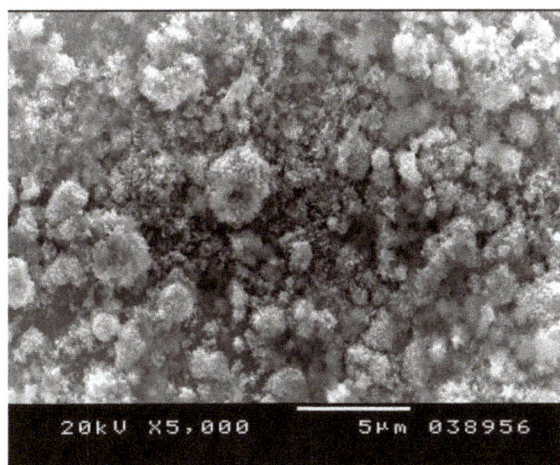

Fig. 4 Scanning electron microphotograph of Cp titanium specimen coated with nano HA- Zn at ×5000

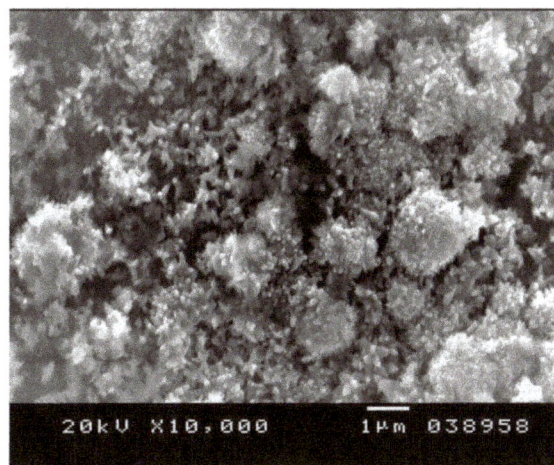

Fig. 5 Scanning electron microphotograph of Cp Titanium specimen coated with HA-Zn at X10,000

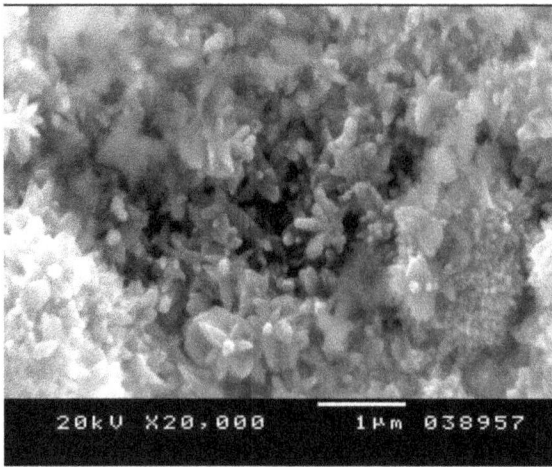

Fig. 6 Scanning electron microphotograph of Cp titanium specimen coated with HA-Zn at ×20,000

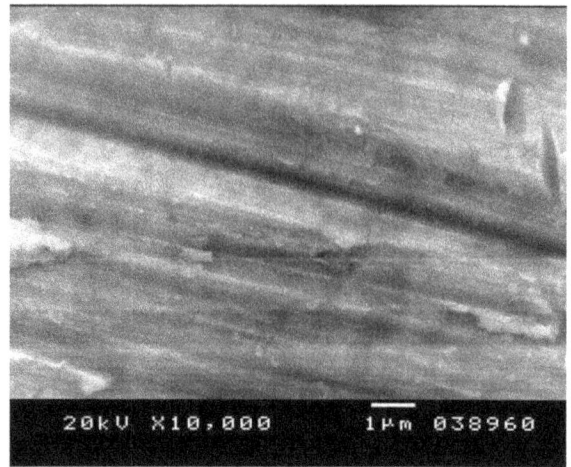

Fig. 8 Scanning electron microphotograph of control Cp titanium specimen at ×10,000

due to the stretching vibrational mode of Zn–O. The absorption bands at 669 cm^{-1} and around 3448 cm^{-1} are due to the stretching vibration and the bending of the O–H bond that contributes in hydrogen bond formation between water molecules adsorbed by hydroxyapatite and potassium bromide used for pellet preparation. The wide broad absorption band in the area of 1033–1269 cm^{-1} wave number is attributed to the stretching vibrations of P–O bonds in the phosphate group (PO$_3$$^{-4}$). The low-intensity band presented in the area of 1422–1518 cm^{-1} wave numbers is attributed to the stretching vibration of the C–O bond of the carbonates (CO$_3$$^{-2}$).

SEM and EDS results

Figures 4, 5, and 6 show the SE microphotographs of CpTi specimens coated with HA-Zn, the specimens'

surface is homogenously covered with evenly distributed globular/rosette-like nano-structures that tend to aggregate in characteristic cluster forms with little intervening porosity. On the other hand, Figs. 7, 8, and 9 show the SE microphotographs of control CpTi specimens with blanc surfaces; only the cutting lines of machining appear. The EDS analysis of HA-Zn shows the presence of zinc, titanium, calcium, and phosphorus; the atomic ratio of Ca/P is 1.67 (Fig. 10). However, the control specimen only contains titanium element (Fig. 11).

Roughness results

Table 1 shows the mean average roughness value of the HA-Zn coated and control specimens; the average roughness is 0.34 μm for the control group and increased significantly to be 1.09 μm for the HA-Zn-

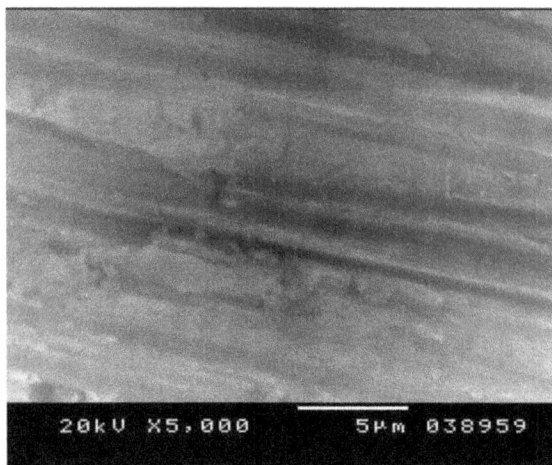

Fig. 7 Scanning electron microphotograph of control Cp Titanium specimen at X 5,000

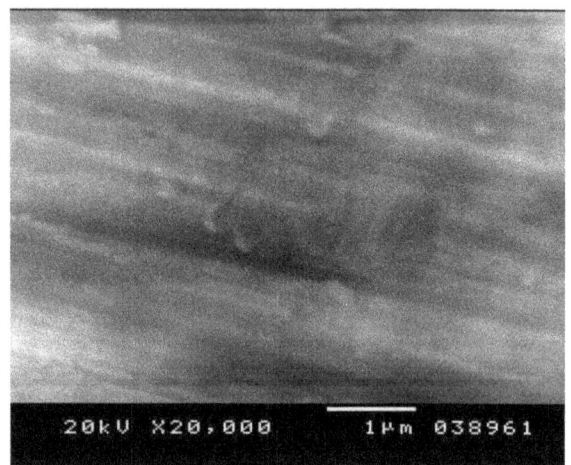

Fig. 9 Scanning electron microphotograph of control Cp titanium specimen at ×20,000

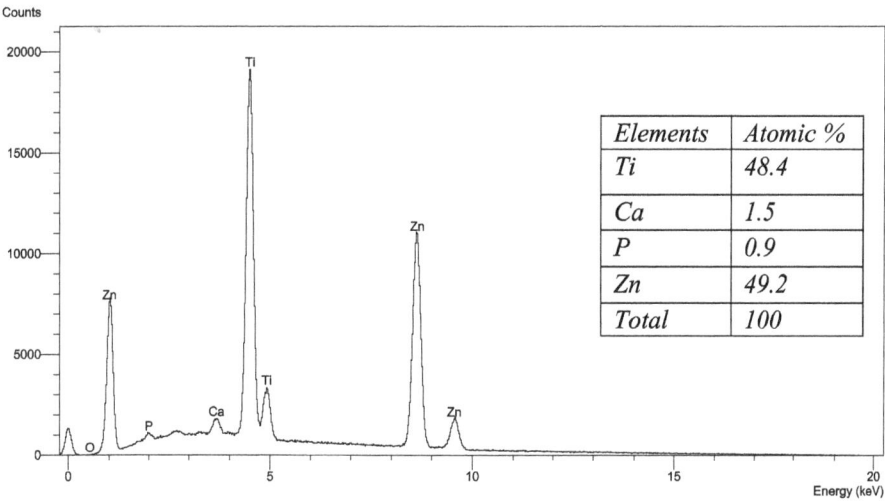

Fig. 10 Energy dispersive spectrum of Cp titanium specimen coated with HA-Zn

coated group ($P = 0.009$) when compared using a pair comparison of the Student t test using SPSS version 20.

Adhesive test results
Following the examination of X cut areas after the adhesive tape removal; the adhesion was rated to be 5A, as no peeling or coat removal occurred along the incisions' length or at their intersection.

Discussion
Metallic orthopedic prosthesis is most commonly used due to its good mechanical properties, but its failure mostly occurs due to the lack of proper bone bonding and/or the occurrence of post-operative infections. Hydroxyapatite is commonly used as a bone filler biomaterial or as a coat for titanium prosthesis due to its decent biocompatibility, osseoconductivity, and bioactivity [26].

However, as a ceramic material, HA still has lower mechanical properties [27]. The biological apatite differs from synthetic apatite because the former contains numerous cationic substitutions, such as Zn^{2+}, Na^+, Mg^{2+}, and has smaller size than synthetic apatite [28, 29]. It was proposed that the addition of zinc to hydroxyapatite had led to a reduction in inflammatory reaction and an improvement of bioactivity [28, 30].

Plasma spraying, sol-gel, and electrophoretic deposition has been all utilized to deposit HA on titanium implants, with some difficulties and worries of suppressing the HA particles' adhesion, anodic polarization of metal substrate, and increasing metals' corrosion risk [19–21]. Electrochemical deposition (ED) is the selected approach in this study due to its simplicity, easiness of parameters control, uniform coating thickness produced, and its applicability for multidimensional implant surfaces [22].

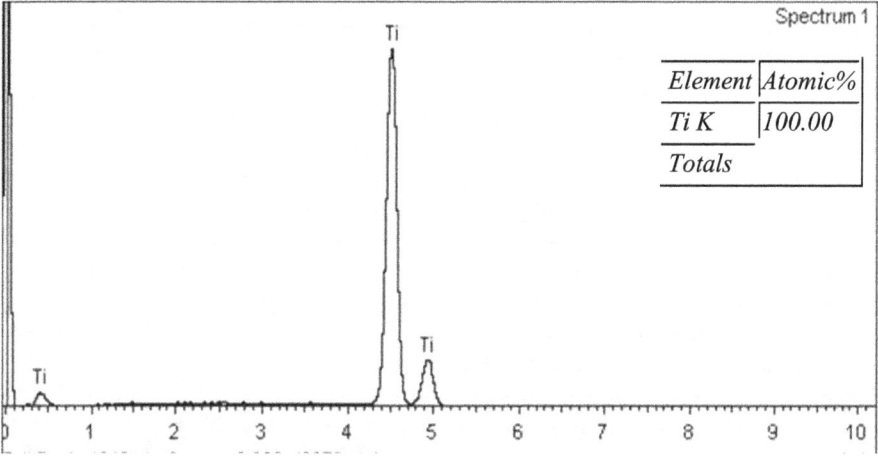

Fig. 11 Energy dispersive spectrum of control Cp titanium specimen

Table 1 The Student t test of the control and coated specimen roughness Ra (μm)

	Number of specimens	Mean ± (SD)	Standard error mean	F value	P value
Control	7	0.34 ± (0.06)	0.02	9.67	0.009*
HA/Zn coated	7	1.09 ± (0.16)	0.60		

In the current study, an electrochemical deposition was applied to prepare nano-HA-Zn coating on titanium metal aiming to improve bioactivity, osseointegration, and preventing peri-implantitis. At this early point of research, the coatings' procedure was accustomed to produce a uniform thickness of HA-Zn coating, characterize its chemical structure, observe its surface morphology, and evaluate the surface roughness and coat adhesive properties.

Recycling of natural-derived resources is a challenging task that may have both environmental and economical profits. Cuttlebone fishery is a naturally derived biomaterial that was used as a source of calcium during the electrochemical deposition process in this study. It was confirmed in the IR spectra (Fig. 2) that $Ca(NO_3)_2·4H_2O$ resulted from the reaction of $CaCO_3$ of cuttlebone and nitric acid [31]. The selected time for electrochemical deposition of HA-Zn coating was 2 h; as by then, the formation of a white detectable coating had occurred and could be scrapped for IR spectral analysis. After preparation of HA-Zn coating, the analyzed powder appeared to still have the HA characterization. Li et al. prepared Zn-HA coatings through a hydrothermal method and found that the FT-IR spectra of Zn-HA has no significant changes than the as-prepared HA [32]; this Zn-HA spectrum paralleled with this study.

Yang et al. prepared a Zn-HA coating on Ti plates by an electrochemical process, and the SEM examination showed irregularly shaped rod-like crystals with hexagonal cross-section; this corresponded well with the current study results. They also concluded that a Zn-HA coating improves proliferation and differentiation of osteoblasts and would enhance implant osseointegration [11].

Ceramic coatings must have good adhesion to the implant to act as a barrier and assure good protection to the substrate. The adhesion test was performed in this study to verify the adequacy of the coating thickness.

An improvement of coating adhesion occurs as their thickness decrease, although very thin coatings may not attain the protection requirements [33]. Contrariwise, it is recognized that thick ceramic coatings may develop cracks after the deposition procedure [34]. The adhesive tape test read the highest score (5A); this might be attributed to the fine homogenous, closely packed, coating particles that appear crack free and highly sintered, as proved by the SEM results in Figs. 4, 5, and 6.

Dental implants do exist with various geometries, different lengths and diameters, and features, such as, pits, pores, vents, and slots. Essentially, a highly rough surface produces better initial stability and anchorage. Moreover, a rough surface with a larger surface area facilitates particles exchange between the implant and surrounding tissues. It could be concluded that such coatings with an increased surface area could have better clinical performance [35]. This developed electro-deposition process, can be applied to deposit a nano-HA-Zr coating to complex implant surfaces and thus increases their surface area, surface roughness, initial stability and clinical performance.

Supplementary, biocompatibility, anti-bacterial activity, and in vivo investigations are required to correlate between the HA-Zn coating properties and their effect on bone formation and osseo-integration.

Conclusions

The electro-chemical method can be employed for HA-Zn coating deposition on titanium metal, where Ca source was a recycled cuttlebone fish to precipitate HA phases. Using a Zn anode on a low-sustained voltage was able to induce an even coat thickness of HA-Zn precipitation and increase the surface roughness significantly.

Acknowledgements
The authors would like to express their gratitude for Dr. Sherif Kishk, Professor of Communication and Electrical Engineering, Faculty of Engineering, Mansoura University, for his help in photographing and analyzing the coating for adhesion test.

Authors' contributions
All authors carried out the experimental study conception and design. FR helped in the experimental part of the study. NA did the data acquisition and interpretation. NE performed the statistical analysis, drafted the manuscript, and revised it critically for important intellectual content. FR had given final approval of the version to be published. All authors read and approved the final manuscript.

Competing interests
El-Wassefy N, Aref N, and Reicha F declare that they have no competing interests.

Author details
[1]Dental Biomaterials Department, Faculty of Dentistry, Mansoura University, 35516 El Gomhoria St., Mansoura, Egypt. [2]Physics Department, Faculty of science, Mansoura University, 35516 El Gomhoria St., Mansoura, Egypt.

References
1. Brunette DM, Tengvall P, Textor M TP, Textor M, Thomsen P. Titanium in medicine: material science, surface science, engineering, biological responses and medical applications. Springer Science & Business Media; 2012. p.13–24.

2. Heydenrijk K, Meijer HJA, van der Reijden WA, Vissink A, Raghoebar GM, Stegenga B. Microbiota around root-formed endosseous implants. A review of the literature. October. 2002;17:829–38.

3. El Hachmi M, Penasse M. Our midterm results of the Birmingham hip resurfacing with and without navigation. J Arthroplasty. 2014;29:808–12.

4. Abu-Amer Y, Darwech I, Clohisy JC. Aseptic loosening of total joint replacements: mechanisms underlying osteolysis and potential therapies. Arthritis Res Ther. 2007;9 Suppl 1:S6.

5. Jasty M. Clinical reviews: particulate debris and failure of total hip replacements. J Appl Biomater. 1993;4:273–6.

6. Schwarz F, Sculean A, Romanos G, Herten M. Influence of different treatment approaches on the removal of early plaque biofilms and the viability of SAOS2 osteoblasts grown on titanium implants. Clin oral. 2005;9:111–7.

7. Tsang CS, Ng HMA. Antifungal susceptibility of Candida albicans biofilms on titanium discs with different surface roughness. Clin Oral Investig. 2007;11:361–8.

8. Phan T, Buckner T, Sheng J, Baldeck JD, Marquis RE. Physiologic actions of zinc related to inhibition of acid and alkali production by oral streptococci in suspensions and biofilms. Oral Microbiol. 2004;19:31–8.

9. Rossi L, Migliaccio S, Corsi A, Marzia M, Bianco P, Teti A, et al. Reduced growth and skeletal changes in zinc-deficient growing rats are due to impaired growth plate activity and inanition. J Nutr. 2001;131:1142–6.

10. Zhao S, Dong W, Jiang Q, He F, Wang X, Yang G. Effects of zinc-substituted nano-hydroxyapatite coatings on bone integration with implant surfaces. J Zhejiang Univ Sci B. 2013;14:518–25.

11. Yang F, Dong W, He F, Wang X, Zhao S, Yang G. Osteoblast response to porous titanium surfaces coated with zinc-substituted hydroxyapatite. Oral Surg Oral Med Oral Pathol Oral Radiol. 2012;113:313–8.

12. Hall SL, Dimai HP, Farley JR. Effects of zinc on human skeletal alkaline phosphatase activity in vitro. Calcif Tissue Int. 1999;64:163–72.

13. Hosea HJ, Taylor CG, Wood T, Mollard R, Weiler HA. Zinc-deficient rats have more limited bone recovery during repletion than diet-restricted rats. Exp Biol Med. 2004;299:303–11.

14. Tsai M-T, Chang Y-Y, Huang H-L, Hsu J-T, Chen Y-C, Wu AY-J. Characterization and antibacterial performance of bioactive Ti–Zn–O coatings deposited on titanium implants. Thin Solid Films. 2013;528:143–50.

15. Hu H, Zhang W, Qiao Y, Jiang X, Liu X, Ding C. Antibacterial activity and increased bone marrow stem cell functions of Zn-incorporated TiO2 coatings on titanium. Acta Biomater. 2012;8:904–15.

16. Burguera-Pascu M, Rodríguez-Archilla A, Baca P. Substantivity of zinc salts used as rinsing solutions and their effect on the inhibition of Streptococcus mutans. J Trace Elem Med Biol. 2007;21:92–101.

17. Holister P, Weener JW, Vas CR, Harper T. Nanoparticles [Internet]. Vol. 3, Technology White Papers. 2003. p. 1–11. Available from: http://www.nanoparticles.org/pdf/Cientifica-WP3.pdf

18. Surmenev RA, Surmeneva MA, Ivanova AA. Significance of calcium phosphate coatings for the enhancement of new bone osteogenesis—a review. Acta Biomater. 2014;10(2):557–79.

19. Kar A, Raja KS, Misra M. Electrodeposition of hydroxyapatite onto nanotubular TiO2 for implant applications. Surf Coatings Technol. 2006;201:3723–31.

20. Manso M, Jiménez C, Morant C, Herrero P, Martínez-Duart J. Electrodeposition of hydroxyapatite coatings in basic conditions. Biomaterials. 2000;21:1755–61.

21. Prasad BE, Kamath PV. Electrodeposition of dicalcium phosphate dihydrate coatings on stainless steel substrates. Bull Mater Sci. 2013;36:475–81.

22. Lu X, Zhao Z, Leng Y. Calcium phosphate crystal growth under controlled atmosphere in electrochemical deposition. J Cryst Growth. 2005;284:506–16.

23. Battistella E, Mele S, Pietronave S, Foltran I, Lesci GI, Foresti E, et al. Transformed cuttlefish bone scaffolds for bone tissue engineering. Adv Mater Res. 2010;89–91:47–52.

24. Specification of ISO E. 4287–Geometrical Product Specifications (GPS)–Surface Texture: Profile Method–Terms, Definitions and Surface Texture Parameters. International Organization for Standardization, Genève. 1997.

25. ASTM Committee D-1 on Paint and Related Coatings, Materials, and Applications. Standard test methods for measuring adhesion by tape test. ASTM International; 2009.

26. Kuo MC, Yen SK. The process of electrochemical deposited hydroxyapatite coatings on biomedical titanium at room temperature. Mater Sci Eng C. 2002;20:153–60.

27. Suchanek W, Yoshimura M. Processing and properties of hydroxyapatite-based biomaterials for use as hard tissue replacement implants. J Mater Res. 1998;13:94–117.

28. Kohli S, Batra U, Kapoor S. Influence of zinc substitution on physicochemical and in vitro behaviour of nanodimensional hydroxyapatite. Asian J Eng Appl Technol. 2014;3:63–7.

29. Ginebra MP, Driessens FCM, Planell JA. Effect of the particle size on the micro and nanostructural features of a calcium phosphate cement: a kinetic analysis. Biomaterials. 2004;25:3453–62.

30. Grandjean-Laquerriere A, Laquerriere P, Jallot E, Nedelec JM, Guenounou M, Laurent-Maquin D, et al. Influence of the zinc concentration of sol-gel derived zinc substituted hydroxyapatite on cytokine production by human monocytes in vitro. Biomaterials. 2006;27:3195–200.

31. Norwitz G, Chasan DE. Application of infrared spectroscopy to the analysis of inorganic nitrates phase I: spectra of inorganic nitrates in acetome and the use of such spectra in analytical chemistry. Philadelphia, Pa; No. FA-T68-7-1 Quality Assurance. 1968. Directorate.

32. Li M, Xiao X, Liu R, Chen C, Huang L. Structural characterization of zinc-substituted hydroxyapatite prepared by hydrothermal method. J Mater Sci Mater Med. 2008;1;19:797–803.

33. Fernandez-Pradas JM, Clèries L, MartmHnez E, Sardin G, Esteve J, Morenza JL. Influence of thickness on the properties of hydroxyapatite coatings deposited by KrF laser ablation. Biomaterials. 2001;22:2171–5.

34. Ribeiro AAA, Balestra RMM, Rocha MNN, Peripolli SBB, Andrade MCC, Pereira LCC, et al. Dense and porous titanium substrates with a biomimetic calcium phosphate coating. Appl Surf Sci. 2013;265:250–6.

35. Lee B-H, Lee C, Kim D-G, Choi K, Lee KH, Do Kim Y. Effect of surface structure on biomechanical properties and osseointegration. Mater Sci Eng C. 2008;28:1448–61.

11

The efficacy of a porcine collagen matrix in keratinized tissue augmentation

C. Maiorana[1], L. Pivetti[2], F. Signorino[2]* (ID), G. B. Grossi[3], A. S. Herford[4] and M. Beretta[2]

Abstract

Background: When keratinized tissue width around dental implants is poorly represented, the clinician could resort to autogenous soft tissue grafting. Autogenous soft tissue grafting procedures are usually associated with a certain degree of morbidity. Collagen matrices could be used as an alternative to reduce morbidity and intra-operatory times. The aim of this study was to assess the efficacy of a xenogeneic collagen matrix as a substitute for soft tissue grafting around dental implants.

Methods: Fifteen consecutive patients underwent a vestibuloplasty and keratinized tissue reconstruction around dental implants, both in the mandible and the maxilla, with a porcine collagen matrix. The so obtained keratinized tissues were measured and evaluated after 6 months and 1, 4, and 5 years.

Results: The average gain of keratinized tissue was 5.7 mm. After 6 months, it was observed a resorption of 37%, after 1 year 48%, and after 5 years 59%. The mean gain of keratinized tissue after 5 years was 2.4 mm. Hemostatic effect and post-operative pain were evaluated too. All subjects referred minimal pain with no bleeding. No adverse reaction nor infection was noted.

Conclusions: The present study showed the efficacy of a porcine collagen matrix in keratinized tissue augmentation. The possibility to use a soft tissue substitute is a great achievement as morbidity decreases and bigger areas can be treated in a single surgery.

Keywords: Collagen matrix, Keratinized tissue, Mucosal grafts, Xenogeneic graft

Background

A variety of factors can lead to teeth loss. From periodontal disease to trauma, the bone remodeling that always follows this event can complicate the subsequent prosthetical rehabilitation [1]. Both removable and implant-fixed restorations require both an adequate quantity of bone and sorrounding soft tissue. Even in severe atrophies of the jaw, nowadays, many bone augmentation techniques are applicable, all with an acceptable long-term stability [2]. Unfortunately, these techniques, especially in major reconstructions, lead to a deficient quantity of soft tissue, above all keratinized mucosa. Whether or not the presence of keratinized tissue around dental implants is necessary, it has been controversial for many years. The lack of evidence in literature regarding implant survival rate in absence of keratinized tissue cannot lead to any conclusion [3]. Nonetheless, the presence of this kind of tissue is desirable for a number of reasons, as shown by many authors. A retrospective study, based on 339 implants, showed that a lack of keratinized tissue around dental implants, especially in the posterior region, led to higher plaque accumulation and mucositis [4]. Thin or narrow (< 1 mm) peri-implant keratinized mucosa was shown to have a higher association with mucosal recessions [5]. At the same time, another retrospective evaluation of 250 implants after 5 to 10 years of functional loading demonstrated a negative correlation between the presence of keratinized tissue and mucosal recessions [6]. Consequently, it is safe to say that sufficient peri-implant keratinized tissue prevents peri-implant plaque accumulation and buccal soft

* Correspondence: fabroski@hotmail.it

[2]Center for Edentulism and Jaw Atrophies, Maxillofacial Surgery and Dentistry Unit, Fondazione IRCCS Cà Granda—Ospedale Maggiore Policlinico, University of Milan, Via della Commenda 10, 20122 Milan, Italy

tissue recessions, accordingly reducing the risk of mucositis and peri-implantitis [7, 8]. A surgical technique based on an apically positioned flap (APF) for vestibuloplasty associated with grafting materials (whether autologous or not) is considered the gold standard for soft tissue augmentation [9]. While a number of autologous grafts have been studied in the past, free gingival grafts from the palatal region are considered the most reliable and effective, in spite of the high morbidity of this type of surgery and extremely poor esthetics [10, 11]. In the past few years, collagen matrices (CM) have been studied as a valid substitute for free gingival grafts, in particular the porcine CM Mucograft (Geistlich Biomaterials GmbH, Baden-Baden, Germany). So far, a number of studies have demonstrated that the Mucograft is reliable and comparable with free gingival graft for what concerns achievements in keratinized tissue augmentation around both teeth or dental implants [12–15]. Additional advantages are a lower patient morbidity due to the absence of a donor site and the high esthetic value, matching texture and color of the adjacent mucosa [11, 15–17]. Concerns about long-term stability of this kind of procedure are more than reasonable, as the majority of papers in literature have short-term follow-ups (< 1 year), while just a few extend over this period. The aim of the present research is to evaluate the efficacy of the Mucograft in a standard APF procedure over 5 years of follow-up.

Methods

The study was designed as a multicentered (Milan University—School of Dentistry/Loma Linda University—School of Dentistry) prospective observational (non-controlled) clinical study according to the STROBE criteria. The participants of the study presented areas of deficient attached and unattached mucosa precluding the construction of effective functioning prosthesis. The study included a total of 15 patients, both female and male, who were candidates for mucosal soft tissue augmentation by means of a xenogeneic CM (Geistlich Mucograft®, Geistlich Pharma AG, Wolhusen, CH). Patients included had to be at least 18 years old, both systemically and periodontally healthy with good oral hygiene; patients who were heavy smokers or bore systemic diseases that could influence bone turnover/wound healing were excluded. The purpose of the surgery was to improve the quantity of attached and unattached mucosa in order to facilitate the final prosthetic rehabilitation. The entire study was reviewed and approved by the Ethics Committee of the IRCCS Ospedale Maggiore Policlinico di Milano, Fondazione Ca' Granda. Written consent was obtained at the recruitment visit from all the participants.

The material

The xenogeneic CM (Mucograft®) is a class III medical device according to the Medical Device Directive 93/42

(EEC definitions: 1.1, long-term implant; 1.2, implantable; 8, resorbable; and 17, porcine origin). Its structure consists of two functional layers: a cell occlusive layer consisting of collagen fibers in a compact arrangement and a thick porous layer. This porous layer provides a space that favors the formation of a blood clot and the ingrowth of tissue from adjacent sites. This xenogenic graft has been cleared by the EU and US Food and Drug Administration for regenerative therapy involving teeth and implants.

The surgical procedure

The surgical procedure, as already described in a previous study, consisted in a standard apically positioned flap with subsequent apposition of the CM, performed under local anesthesia [17]. At first, a midcrestal incision was performed in the residual keratinized band and a split thickness flap was raised. Any muscle fibers and fibrous banding attached in the area were dissected from the periosteum and were reduced toward the depth of the vestibule. In addition, submucosal fatty tissue was also dissected from the periosteum over the bone in the area. The lateral portion of the mucosal flap was sutured to the periosteum in the depth of vestibule. The denuded area of the wound in the vestibule was then covered by the CM. The CM was sutured to the surrounding mucosa anteriorly, posteriorly, and in the vestibular direction. The suturing was by 5–0 nylon. Approximately half of these sutures were allowed to remain in place for a period of 4 to 6 weeks to determine the outline of the original periphery of the incision and "graft" post-operatively. This was important in determining the area of actual re-epithelization of the defect and in determining and quantifying any shrinkage by scarring in the grafted area. Time was taken from the first incision to the last suture to record and compare the surgery length. A previously prepared acrylic splint was placed over the vestibuloplasty site at the time of surgery. This splint remained in place for 10 days at which time it was removed. The patient had to irrigate the area with 0.9% NaCl solution for those 10 days and rinse with 0.2% chlorhexidine.

Specific endpoints and clinical follow-up

The primary endpoints were to evaluate the shrinkage degree of the width of keratinized mucosa and length of the re-epithelization process. The secondary endpoints assessed clinical evaluation of the grafted area, post-operative hemostatic effect, pain level, and length of surgery. Follow-up control visits were scheduled at 3 days after surgery and then 10 days, 2 weeks, 3 weeks, 1 month, 2 months, 6 months, 1 year, and 4 and 5 years as showed by the clinical case reported in Fig. 1. At each examination time point, the width of keratinized tissue (recorded from the crestal to the apical sutures; 3 to 5 measurement from mesial to distal) and vestibular depth

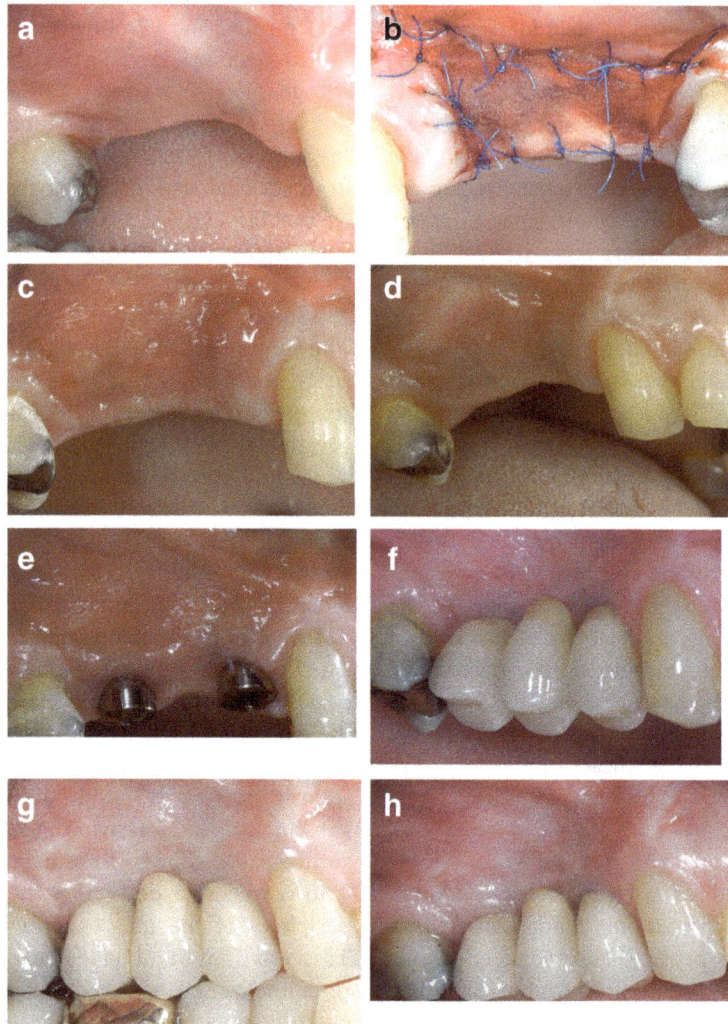

Fig. 1 a Pre-op. **b** Post-op. **c** Two weeks after surgery. **d** Four weeks after surgery. **e** Six months after surgery. **f** One year after surgery. **g** Four years after surgery. **h** Five years after surgery

were recorded by means of a 15-mm North Carolina periodontal probe. Once the implants were placed, measurement was taken from the free gingival margin, at the prosthetical crown's zenith. Re-epithelization was evaluated clinically after 4 weeks on a scale from excellent (100% of the grafted area) to poor (< 40%). The degree of healing and maturation of tissues were observed and compared to the physiological healing time. Digital pictures were taken at each examination for comparison with the adjacent soft tissue. Hemostatic effect and pain level, evaluated using the Mankoski Pain Scale (from 0 to 10 where 0 is "No Pain" and 10 is "Pain makes you pass out"), were recorded until the 10th day (or whenever an increase of discomfort/bleeding was reported by the patient); examination time point in which the protective acrylic splint was removed [18]. Sutures were left in place for 4 weeks in order to facilitate the recording during healing. In all cases, dental implants were placed

2 months after the CM grafting elevating a full-thickness flap accessing the crestal bone. No differences between the original and the newly formed keratinized tissue were clearly appreciable so the flap was designed without any particular modifications. No bone grafting procedures were needed. Healing abutments were placed following a golden standard protocol, consisting in 4 months healing for the maxillary implants and 3 months for the mandibular ones.

Statistical significance

Since a split-mouth design was not feasible and the defects being corrected by the mucosa particularly in the vestibular portion of the study are not usually symmetrical or bilateral, the use of paired subjects was not a reliable format. All the data were analyzed with IBM's SPSS Statistics using ANOVA Repeated Measurements statistical method. Mean values for keratinized mucosal width and probing depth were recorded in millimeters at each examination time point and subsequently expressed in a percentage. First measurement for keratinized tissue, recorded immediately after surgery, was considered as 100%. Less than 20% of contraction was considered as excellent value, while good when less than 50%, fair to poor when higher than 50%, and unsatisfactory when the graft was lost.

Results

A total of 15 patients were enrolled for the study, 12 females and 3 males, aged between 43 and 72 years old. Of these patients, 11 received surgery in the mandible and 4 in the maxilla. No complications were registered during surgeries and the immediate post-operative course was uneventful for all patients. At 1 year, 2 patients dropped out of the study: the first patient experienced a peri-implantitis that was solved with a conventional free gingival graft procedure while the second one developed peri-implant pockets with perimucositis, making the 1-year analysis possible only on 13 patients. No allergic reactions were registered during the clinical trial. The average keratinized tissue width before surgery was 0.4 mm. The initial gain in keratinized tissue (as measured immediately post-op) was 5.7 mm. Constant contraction of the grafted area, and decrease in keratinized tissue width, could be observed throughout 5 years of follow-up (Fig. 2). The initial 6 months were the most critical, with the highest reduction, resulting in a mean of 2.2 mm loss (37%) of value. Another 0.5 mm were lost in the following 6 months (leading to the 1 year examination time point), raising the value of contraction to 48%. After 1 year, the contraction considerably slowed down, with a further 11% width loss over the subsequent 4 years. The total loss after 5 years of follow-up was a mean value of 3.3 mm, corresponding to 59% of the initial measurement (Fig. 3). Clinically, it was assessed that the height of the keratinized tissue was, in any case, lower than the adjacent sites. Re-epithelization was excellent and complete in most patients after 4 weeks

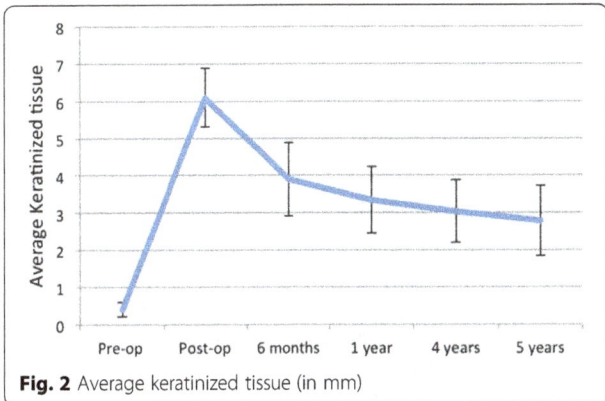

Fig. 3 Shrinkage rate during time

(Fig. 4). The matrix also proved to be a great hemostatic, with no bleeding referred by subjects in the post-op period. The procedure was short, with a mean operative time of 20 min from first incision to last suture, and painless, as referred by patients to the examiners during the first two follow-ups (Mankoski Pain Scale value of 1–2). No visible difference in texture and color could be found, after healing was complete, between the grafted area and surrounding tissue, ensuring a great esthetic outcome over the entire 5 years of follow-up.

Discussion

The study was carried out to evaluate the efficacy of a xenogeneic CM when used as a soft tissue substitute in the reconstruction of an adequate amount (at least 2 mm) of keratinized tissue around dental implants. The xenogeneic CMs have already been investigated in order to check their compatibility and effectiveness as scaffold [19, 20]. One of the first studies was conducted by Schoo and Coppes, who experimented the capacities of a freeze-dried dura mater grafting material in stimulating keratinized mucosa, with very poor results [21]. Two studies by Harris, in 2001, analyzed the usefulness of acellular dermal matrices when positioned upon the

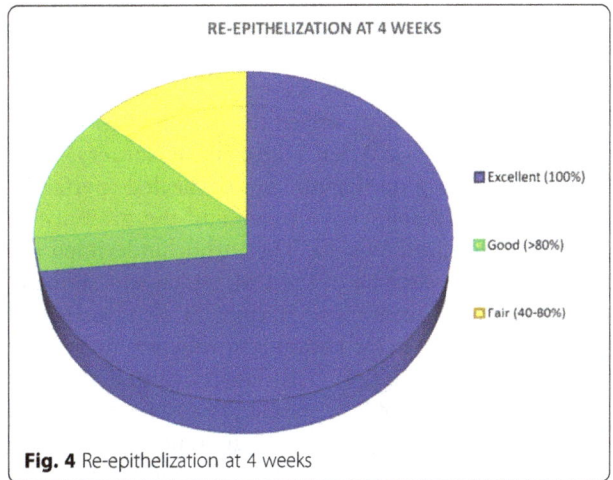

Fig. 2 Average keratinized tissue (in mm)

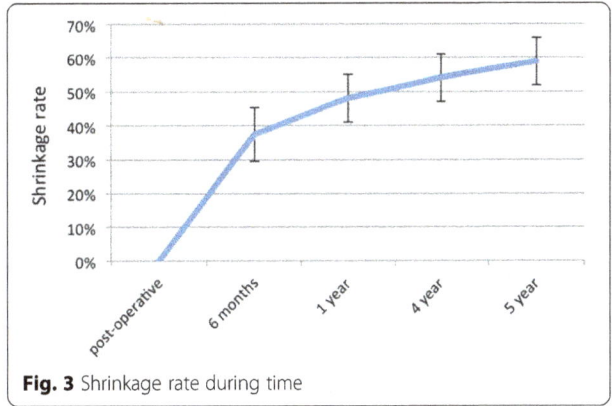

Fig. 4 Re-epithelization at 4 weeks

periosteum and bone [22, 23], without any particular results. Furthermore, in 2001, Wei P. and Laurell L. conducted two studies: one clinical and one histological [24]. Six patients received an autologous graft while the remaining six an allogeneic one. The increment in adherent mucosa was detectable in both groups, but the gain was very little with the allogeneic graft. This was related to an excessive shrinkage of the graft post-operatively. Histologically, it was observed that all grafted sites showed a scar-like tissue, incapable of inducing cellular differentiation. The fast resorption represented a big concern in this technique leading to a disturbed healing and sequentially to a lack of keratinized tissue. Harris et al. underlined the great esthetic outcome in addition to the efficacy of substitutive matrices for soft tissue [25]. Despite the physical and mechanical characteristics of these matrices are still under investigation, it has already been observed how these matrices show statistically significant results confronted with the autologous grafting techniques [26]. Comparable results were observed evaluating not only by keratinized mucosa and thickness and vestibular depth evaluation but also by histological study [27]: during the first week of healing, it has been noticed a tissue remodeling due to phagocytosis of pre-existing collagen fibers by macrophages. After 2 weeks, new collagen fibers were detected as long as neoangiogenesis and re-epithelization on the membrane surface. At 4 weeks, it was difficult to find pre-existing collagen fibers. At 10 weeks, the healing process was complete and the esthetic is already acceptable. Schmitt et al. achieved similar outcomes in their study, which compared free gingival grafts and a porcine CM [16]. At 90 days after surgery, biopsies were harvested for histologic and immunohistologic analyses. It was observed the presence of specific keratinized tissue markers is in the CM grafted areas. CMs were also clinically tested as an alternative option for root coverage. McGuire and Scheyer tested the CM associated to a coronally advanced flap in recession defects [28]. They find out how the porcine CM in combination with a coronal flap represented a satisfactory alternative to autografts for covering dehiscence-type recession defects. They also noticed a reduction of the morbidity due to the absence of soft tissue graft harvesting. Nevins M. et al. tested the porcine CM around a single tooth [11]. After 1 year from surgery, both xenogeneic and autologous grafts healed perfectly, showing mature connective tissue and the presence of enough keratinized mucosa. The author underlined the better esthetic outcome of the CM, which was showing a perfect tissue integration. Herford et al. investigated the efficacy of CMs for keratinized mucosa augmentation in cases of lack [29]. They demonstrated an overall mean shrinkage of 14% (range, 5 to 20%). Sanz et al. confirmed how xenogeneic CMs guarantee predictable and satisfactory results: their primary endpoint was to evaluate the potentiality in gaining keratinized tissue in comparison with an autologous graft [16]. At 6 months, they observed an insignificant statistical variance between the autologous (60% shrinkage) and the xenogeneic (67%). Despite the CM shrinkage range is still very wide (from 14 to 75%), most of the authors observed that the majority of shrinkage occurred in the first month after surgery. In the present study, the highest shrinkage rate was observed in the first 6 months ($P = 0.002$) while the following follow-up at 1, 4, and 5 years. The shrinkage was slower but reached a final value of 59%, which is included in the range observed in the other studies. In the present paper, by analyzing the post-operative course, one factor is particularly highlighted: the great decrease in morbidity. Post-operative pain in autologous grafting is caused by the presence of a second surgical site, the donor site. Most of the patients who underwent this type surgery did not feel any pain at all, except a little nuisance that required a mild analgesic as medication. In the present study, the grafts were additionally covered with a vestibular retention splint. The use of the vestibular retention splint guaranteed a mechanic protection for the grafts. Moreover, it had a preventive effect on re-insertion of vestibular muscle fibers. Despite the influence of the splint on the width of keratinized mucosa has not be taken in consideration in this study, Heberer et al. previously concluded its use after vestibuloplasty reduced the graft shrinkage [30]. Furthermore, they observed a general reduction of time of the surgery and post-op morbidity too. The CM is extremely easy to use, with an average length of surgery of 30 min, excluding anesthesia [16]. Intra-operative and post-operative bleeding was extremely limited. The xenogeneic CM showed an ideal haemostatic effect with no excessive bleeding during surgery and no bleeding at all during post-operative period, similar to other techniques using absorbable collagen sponges in different kinds of treatments [31]. Furthermore, all grafted sites presented, when healing was completed, an optimal integration with the surrounding tissues, as stated by other authors in previous studies [15–17]. Rotundo an Pini-Prato observed the good esthetic of the CM also when used in the coverage of multiple gingival recession [32]. Laino et al. described excellent results of CM in wound repairing when placed after intraoral mucosal biopsy [33]. Recently, Schmitt et al. observed the long-term efficacy of CM when used in vestibuloplasty when compared to free gingival graft [34]. Despite the free gingival group showed lower values of keratinized tissue resorption, the CM showed good stability and better esthetic outcomes. Further studies with a larger sample, investigating the long-term effectiveness of CMs and alternative treatment options, should be performed in the future to better assess a univocal outcome about the topic.

Conclusions

With the limits of this study, it can be assessed that the CM is an effective option for the keratinized tissue augmentation. The percentage of shrinkage of the graft is comparable to data recovered from other studies and does not represent a problem also after 5 years. The CM integration is slow and constant, providing the necessary scaffold to regenerate keratinized mucosa and ensuring a perfect healing. Patients reported no bleeding, and postoperative morbidity was very low. Observing the grafted areas, it is possible to notice the high esthetic result without any dyschromia with the surrounding tissue. This study shows that this type of CM can find major interest in those patients who need a keratinized tissue augmentation around implants with great esthetic outcome or in those who can bear little pain. Further studies will be necessary to assess definitively the efficacy and the applications of this material, eventually gaining statistical value.

Funding
The authors declare no funds for the research.

Authors' contributions
CM and ASH designed the study; MB performed the patient treatment, and LP and FS performed the data collection and edited the manuscript. GBG performed the data analysis. All authors read and approved the final version of the manuscript.

Competing interests
Carlo Maiorana, Luca Pivetti, Fabrizio Signorino, Giovanni Battista Grossi, Alan Scott Herford, and Mario Beretta declare that they have no competing interests.

Author details
[1]Oral Surgery, Center for Edentulism and Jaw Atrophies, Maxillofacial Surgery and Dentistry Unit, Fondazione IRCCS Cà Granda—Ospedale Maggiore Policlinico, University of Milan, Milan, Italy. [2]Center for Edentulism and Jaw Atrophies, Maxillofacial Surgery and Dentistry Unit, Fondazione IRCCS Cà Granda—Ospedale Maggiore Policlinico, University of Milan, Via della Commenda 10, 20122 Milan, Italy. [3]Department of Oral Surgery, School of Dentistry, University of Milan, Milan, Italy. [4]Department of Oral & Maxillofacial Surgery, Loma Linda University, Loma Linda, CA, USA.

References
1. Forman G. Presenile mandibular atrophy: its aetiology, clinical evaluation and treatment by jaw augmentation. Br J Oral Surg. 1976;14(1):47–56.
2. Chiapasco M, Casentini P, Zaniboni M. Bone augmentation procedures in implant dentistry. Int J Oral Maxillofac Implants. 2009;24(Suppl):237–59.
3. Grusovin MG, Coulthard P, Worthington HV, Esposito M. Maintaining and recovering soft tissue health around dental implants: a Cochrane systematic review of randomised controlled clinical trials. Eur J Oral Implantol. 2008;1(1):11–22.
4. Chung DM, Oh TJ, Shotwell JL, Misch CE, Wang HL. Significance of keratinized mucosa in maintenance of dental implants with different surfaces. J Periodontol. 2006;77(8):1410–20.
5. Zigdon H, Machtei EE. The dimensions of keratinized mucosa around implants affect clinical and immunological parameters. Clin Oral Implants Res. 2008;19(4):387–92.
6. Artzi Z, Carmeli G, Kozlovsky A. A distinguishable observation between survival and success rate outcome of hydroxyapatite-coated implants in 5-10 years in function. Clin Oral Implants Res. 2006;17(1):85–93.
7. Brito C, Tenenbaum HC, Wong BK, Schmitt C, Nogueira-Filho G. Is keratinized mucosa indispensable to maintain peri-implant health? A systematic review of the literature. J Biomed Mater Res B Appl Biomater. 2014;102(3):643–50.
8. Lin GH, Chan HL, Wang HL. The significance of keratinized mucosa on implant health: a systematic review. J Periodontol. 2013;84(12):1755–67.
9. Costello BJ, Betts NJ, Barber HD, Fonseca RJ. Preprosthetic surgery for the edentulous patients. Dent Clin N Am. 1996;40(1):19–38.
10. Zucchelli G, Mele M, Stefanini M, Mazzotti C, Marzadori M, Montebugnoli L, et al. Patient morbidity and root coverage outcome after subepithelial connective tissue and de-epithelialized grafts: a comparative randomized-controlled clinical trial. J Clin Periodontol. 2010;37(8):728–38.
11. Nevins M, Nevins ML, Kim SW, Schupbach P, Kim DM. The use of mucograft collagen matrix to augment the zone of keratinized tissue around teeth: a pilot study. Int J Periodontics Restorative Dent. 2011;31(4):367–73.
12. Vignoletti F, Nuñez J, de Sanctis F, Lopez M, Caffesse R, Sanz M. Healing of a xenogeneic collagen matrix for keratinized tissue augmentation. Clin Oral Implants Res. 2015;26(5):545–52.
13. Vignoletti F, Nuñez J, Discepoli N, De Sanctis F, Caffesse R, Muñoz F, et al. Clinical and histological healing of a new collagen matrix in combination with the coronally advanced flap for the treatment of Miller class-I recession defects: an experimental study in the minipig. J Clin Periodontol. 2011;38(9):847–55.
14. Jepsen K, Jepsen S, Zucchelli G, Stefanini M, de Sanctis M, Baldini N, et al. Treatment of gingival recession defects with a coronally advanced flap and a xenogeneic collagen matrix: a multicenter randomized clinical trial. J Clin Periodontol. 2013;40(1):82–9.
15. Schmitt CM, Tudor C, Kiener K, Wehrhan F, Schmitt J, Eitner S, et al. Vestibuloplasty: porcine collagen matrix versus free gingival graft: a clinical and histologic study. J Periodontol. 2013;84(7):914–23.
16. Sanz M, Lorenzo R, Aranda JJ, Martin C, Orsini M. Clinical evaluation of a new collagen matrix (Mucograft prototype) to enhance the width of keratinized tissue in patients with fixed prosthetic restorations: a randomized prospective clinical trial. J Clin Periodontol. 2009;36(10):868–76.
17. Maiorana C, Beretta M, Pivetti L, Stoffella E, Grossi GB, Herford AS. Use of a collagen matrix as a substitute for free mucosal grafts in pre-prosthetic surgery: 1 year results from a clinical prospective study on 15 patients. Open Dent J. 2016;10:395–410.
18. Mankoski A. Mankoski Pain Scale, copyright 1995. 1996.
19. Scarano A, Barros RR, Iezzi G, Piattelli A, Novaes AB. Acellular dermal matrix graft for gingival augmentation: a preliminary clinical, histologic, and ultrastructural evaluation. J Periodontol. 2009;80(2):253–9.
20. Petrauskaite O, PDS G, Fernandes MH, Juodzbaylys G, Stumbras A, Maminskas J, Cicciù M. Biomimetic mineralization on a macroporous cellulose-based matrix for bone regeneration. Biomed Res Int. 2013;2013:452750.
21. Schoo WH, Coppes L. Use of palatal mucosa and lyophilized dura mater to create attached gingiva. J Clin Periodontol. 1976;3(3):166–72.
22. Harris RJ. Gingival augmentation with an acellular dermal matrix: human histologic evaluation of a case—placement of the graft on bone. Int J Periodontics Restorative Dent. 2001;21(1):69–75.
23. Harris RJ. Gingival augmentation with an acellular dermal matrix: human histologic evaluation of a case—placement of the graft on periosteum. Int J Periodontics Restorative Dent. 2004;24(4):378–85.
24. Wei PC, Laurell L, Geivelis M, Lingen MW, Maddalozzo D. Acellular dermal matrix allografts to achieve increased attached gingiva. Part 1. A clinical study. J Periodontol. 2000;71(8):1297–305.
25. Harris RJ. Clinical evaluation of 3 techniques to augment keratinized tissue without root coverage. J Periodontol. 2001;72(7):932–8.
26. Lee KH, Kim BO, Jang HS. Clinical evaluation of a collagen matrix to enhance the width of keratinized gingiva around dental implants. J Periodontal Implant Sci. 2010;40(2):96–101.
27. Lima RS, Peruzzo DC, Napimoga MH, Saba-Chujfi E, Dos Santos-Pereira SA, Martinez EF. Evaluation of the biological behavior of Mucograft® in human gingival fibroblasts: an in vitro study. Braz Dent J. 2015;26(6):602–6.
28. McGuire MK, Scheyer ET. Long-term results comparing xenogeneic collagen matrix and autogenous connective tissue grafts with coronally advanced

flaps for treatment of dehiscence-type recession defects. J Periodontol. 2016;87(3):221–7.

29. Herford AS, Akin L, Cicciu M, Maiorana C, Boyne PJ. Use of a porcine collagen matrix as an alternative to autogenous tissue for grafting oral soft tissue defects. J Oral Maxillofac Surg. 2010;68(7):1463–70.

30. Heberer S, Nelson K. Clinical evaluation of a modified method of vestibuloplasty using an implant-retained splint. J Oral Maxillofac Surg. 2009; 67(3):624–9.

31. Cicciù M, Herford AS, Juodžbalys G, Stoffella E. Recombinant human bone morphogenetic protein type 2 application for a possible treatment of bisphosphonates-related osteonecrosis of the jaw. J Craniofac Surg. 2012; 23(3):784–8.

32. Rotundo R, Pini-Prato G. Use of a new collagen matrix (mucograft) for the treatment of multiple gingival recessions: case reports. Int J Periodontics Restorative Dent. 2012;32(4):413–9.

33. Laino L, Troiano G, Menditti D, Herford AS, Lucchese A, Cervino G, Lauritano F, Serpico R, Cicciù M. Use of collagen matrix to improve wound repair after mucosal biopsy: a multicenter case series. Int J Clin Exp Med. 2017;10(5):8363–8.

34. Schmitt CM, Moest T, Lutz R, Wehrhan F, Neukam FW, Schlegel KA. Long-term outcomes after vestibuloplasty with a porcine collagen matrix (Mucograft®) versus the free gingival graft: a comparative prospective clinical trial. Clin Oral Impl Res. 2016;27:e125–33.

12

Mucositis, peri-implantitis, and survival and success rates of oxide-coated implants in patients treated for periodontitis 3- to 6-year results of a case-series study

Reiner Mengel[1]*[iD], Theresa Heim[2] and Miriam Thöne-Mühling[1]

Abstract

Aim: The aim of this case-series study is to evaluate the prevalence of mucositis, peri-implantitis, and survival and success rates of oxide-coated implants in subjects treated for periodontitis.

Materials and methods: Twenty-four subjects treated for generalized chronic periodontitis (GCP) and five treated for generalized aggressive periodontitis (GAP) were orally rehabilitated with a total of 130 dental implants. Subjects were examined 2 to 4 weeks prior to extraction of non-retainable teeth and at insertion of superstructure. Additional examinations were performed during a 3-month recall schedule over a 3- to 6-year follow-up period. Radiographs were taken after insertion of the superstructure and 1, 3, and 5 years later.

Results: The results showed implant survival rates of 97.1% in GCP subjects versus 96.2% in GAP subjects. The implant success rate was 77.9% in GCP subjects and 38.5% in GAP subjects. In GCP subjects, mucositis was present in 7.7% and peri-implantitis in 12.5% of the implants. In GAP subjects, 28.0% of the implants showed mucositis and 32.0% peri-implantitis. Implant failure, mucositis, and peri-implantitis were more evident in GAP subjects. Peri-implantitis was more prevalent for implants in the maxilla and implants >10 mm. After 5 years, the mean peri-implant bone loss in GAP subjects was 2.89 mm and in GCP subjects 1.38 mm.

Conclusions: Periodontally diseased subjects treated in a supportive periodontal therapy can be successfully rehabilitated with oxide-coated dental implants for a follow-up period of 3- to 6-years. Implants in the maxilla and GAP subjects were more susceptible to mucositis and peri-implantitis, with lower implant survival and success rates.

Keywords: Dental implants, Mucositis, Peri-implantitis, Periodontitis, Survival rate

Background

In recent years, a great number of different implant systems varying in materials, surface structure, and macroscopic design have been introduced to the dental market [1]. In studies using implants with modified surfaces, it was concluded that rough surfaces induce a stronger initial bone response, achieve stability more rapidly, and integrate more fully with extant bone [2–6]. Dental implants with oxide-coated (anodised) surfaces have demonstrated, in histologic and histomorphometric examinations, that the newly formed bone infiltrates the pores of the surface oxide layer and thereby establishes a strong interlock between the bone and oxidized implant [7–9]. The oxide-coated implant surface is categorized as "moderately rough," typically with a thickened titanium oxide layer of high crystallinity and phosphorous content.

A prospective long-term clinical study on implants with oxide-coated surfaces revealed an implant survival rate of 99.2% and mean marginal bone loss of 0.7 ± 1.35 mm after 10 years of function [10]. Only 1.9% of

* Correspondence: mengel@mailer.uni-marburg.de
[1]Department of Prosthetic Dentistry, School of Dental Medicine, Philipps-University, Marburg/Lahn, Germany
Full list of author information is available at the end of the article

the implants showed significant marginal bone loss (> 3 mm) together with bleeding on probing and suppuration. In a retrospective study, no difference could be found when comparing the clinical performance (survival rate, marginal bone loss, presence of bleeding, and probing depth) of turned versus oxide-coated surface implants after 5 years of loading [11]. In a 9-year study with an immediate loading protocol, implants with oxide-coated surfaces achieved a 10% higher survival rate compared to turned surface implants [12].

These results indicate that the survival rate of dental implants in long-term studies seems to be high, irrespective of surface type. However, the influence of the implant surface type on the development and progression of mucositis and peri-implantitis especially in periodontally diseased subjects remains largely unknown. In animal studies, it has been suggested that oxide-coated implants are more susceptible to mucositis and peri-implantitis [13–15]. Whether or to what extent these findings might be translated to humans is yet unknown. A Cochrane review found no evidence of a superior long-term success that could be attributed to any one type of implant surface [1]. Furthermore, the review concluded that there are limited data suggesting that implants with relatively smooth surfaces are less susceptible to peri-implantitis-induced bone loss.

The aim of this long-term clinical study on partially edentulous subjects treated for periodontal disease was to evaluate the prevalence of mucositis and peri-implantitis and to determine the survival and success rates of dental implants with oxide-coated surfaces.

Materials and methods
Study population

A total of 29 partially edentulous subjects were consecutively recruited from the Dental School of Medicine, Philipps-University, Marburg, Germany between April 2010 and April 2013 (Table 1). Subjects were excluded for the following reasons: history of systemic disease (e.g., cardiovascular diseases, diabetes mellitus, osteoporosis), pregnancy, untreated caries, current orthodontic treatment, continuous drug administration, and psychiatric disorders. Systemic diseases were assessed by an internist.

All subjects were treated for periodontitis at the Dental School of Medicine, Philipps-University, Marburg, Germany. Periodontal treatment was followed by a 3-month recall schedule for 3 to 6 years. Each recall session comprised oral hygiene control with motivation and instruction, subgingival scaling, and root planing at tooth surfaces with probing depth (PDs) > 4 mm, and bleeding on probing (BOP). Preceding implant placement, non-retainable teeth were removed and subgingival scaling and root planing were performed for residual

Table 1 Implants in study population

	GCP	GAP
Patient	24	5
Sex		
Female	15	3
Male	9	2
Age		
< 50 years	2	2
> 50 years	22	3
Implant system		
Nobelspeedy Replace RP	49	17
Nobelspeedy Replace NP	16	4
Nobel Replace Straight Groovy	29	5
Nobelspeedy Groovy	10	0
Topography		
Anterior maxilla	26	12
Posterior maxilla	36	10
Anterior mandible	18	0
Posterior mandible	24	4
Superstructure		
Single crowns	52	4
Removable	41	21
Fixed bridges	11	0
Bone quality		
1	3	–
2	97	21
3	4	5
Degree of atrophy		
A	41	12
B	28	14
C	35	–

teeth where necessary. Six months after tooth removal, the residual teeth showed healthy periodontal tissue with PDs ≤ 3 mm and no BOP.

Periodontal disease was diagnosed according to the criteria of the American Academy of Periodontology [16]. The clinical and radiological findings in the recall schedule before insertion of the implants were the basis to distinguish between generalized chronic periodontitis (GCP) and generalized aggressive periodontitis (GAP). Twenty-four subjects (9 males and 15 females; mean age, 63 years) with GCP displaying more than 30% of sites affected, with bone loss < 0.2 mm per year. Five subjects (two males and three females; mean age, 31 years) with GAP displaying more than 30% of sites affected, with bone loss > 0.2 mm per year.

Implant placement and prosthesis

At total, 130 implants with oxide-coated surfaces (Nobel Replace Straight Groovy; Nobel Speedy Groovy; Nobel Speedy Replace, Nobel Biocare, Zürich, Switzerland) were placed with a length of 10 to 15 mm and a diameter of 3.5 or 4 mm. In GCP subjects 104 implants were inserted, and in GAP subjects, 26 implants (Table 1).

In both groups, the bone quality and atrophy of the alveolar bone were classified during implant insertion according to Lekholm and Zarb [17].

Second-stage surgery was performed in the maxilla after 6 months and in the mandible after 3 months. Implant placement and second-stage surgery were performed by a single periodontist (R.M.).

About 4 weeks after the final abutments were placed, GCP subjects were rehabilitated with single crowns, implant-supported bridges, or removable superstructures, according to the Marburg double crown system [18] (Table 1). In GAP subjects, single crowns or removable superstructures (Marburg double crown system) were inserted. All prosthetic appliances were provided at the Dental School of Medicine, Philipps-University, Marburg, Germany. All crowns and bridges were cemented and solely porcelain-fused-to-metal restorations.

Clinical parameters

At each session, the Gingival Index (GI) [19], Plaque Index (PI) [20], PDs, BOP, gingival recession (GR), and clinical attachment level (CAL) were evaluated at four sites (mesial, distal, buccal, and lingual/palatinal) on the teeth and implants. The CAL was measured at the teeth from the cement-enamel junction to the base of the pocket. For implants, the upper edge of the corresponding final abutment served as the top reference point. Trauma to peri-implant tissue was avoided by waiting 1 year after implant placement before measuring probing depths.

The clinical examinations were performed by four examiners (all dentists, formally affiliated with the Dental School of Medicine, Philipps-University, Marburg, Germany) before study initiation, each examiner was calibrated for intra- and interexaminer reproducibility using duplicate measurements of a minimum of 50 sites in at least five subjects. The correlation coefficients were 0.90 to 0.99 for intraexaminer reproducibility and 0.91 to 0.95 for interexaminer reproducibility.

Radiographic examination

Standardized radiographs of the teeth and implants were taken by two persons using the parallel technique [21]. These radiographs were obtained immediately after insertion of the superstructure (baseline for mucositis and peri-implantitis evaluation) and at 1, 3, and 5 years thereafter. The digitized radiographs were evaluated using a computer software (Planmeca Romexis Version 3.0.1, Planmeca, Helsinki, Finland). Bone loss was determined in relative terms at the mesial and distal tooth surfaces by measuring the distance from the CEJ to the apex. The distance from the marginal bone level to the upper edge of the implant was measured (in mm) at the mesial and distal implant surfaces and related to the implant thread. All radiographs were analyzed by an independent masked examiner.

Study follow-up schedule

All patients received a supportive periodontal therapy at the Dental School of Medicine, Philipps-University, Marburg, in the course of the observation period. The first clinical examination was 2 to 4 weeks before the non-retainable teeth were extracted. The periodontally healthy residual dentition and the implants were evaluated immediately after the superstructure was inserted. Subsequently, the subjects were followed up at 3-month intervals for 3 to 6 years. At each follow-up session, the clinical parameters were recorded and subjects were remotivated and reinstructed in effective oral hygiene. In addition, the teeth and implants were cleaned professionally. Supragingival deposits were removed, followed by polishing with rubber cups and polishing paste. Subgingival debridement was performed in the teeth and implants with PDs > 4 mm and BOP positive. In the teeth, conventional stainless-steel curettes and ultrasonic devices were used, whereas in implants, plastic curettes and polyether ether ketone-tips for the ultrasonic device were applied to avoid damage of the implant surface.

A functional analysis and medical history were performed at the beginning of the study and reviewed annually.

Cigarette smoking status was self-reported. Subjects were considered smokers if they had been smoking 10 or more cigarettes a day during the past 5 years [22].

Statistical evaluations

Data analysis was performed with a computerized statistics package (SPSS 12.0.1 for Windows, SPSS). The examined patients were not included in any other publications.

Mean values for clinical and radiologic parameters were determined separately for the implants and the teeth, for both patient groups, and for every visit. Four visits were consolidated for analysis.

The probability of implant loss (implant survival) at a certain time was computed with reference to previously established criteria using a Kaplan-Meier survival curve.

The assessment of implant success, mucositis, and peri-implantitis was performed at the time of radiographic examination 1 year after insertion of the superstructure and 3 and 5 years thereafter.

The implant success rate was defined by the following parameters: no implant movement, no discomfort (pain, foreign body sensation etc.), PDs ≤ 5 mm without BOP, no continuous radiologic translucency surrounding implants, and annual peri-implant bone loss ≤ 0.2 mm 1 year after insertion of the superstructure [23]. Implants that did not meet at least one criterion were considered a failure.

Peri-implant mucositis was defined as PDs ≥ 5 mm with BOP and no bone loss after the first year of loading. Peri-implantitis was defined as PDs > 5 mm with or without BOP and an annual bone loss of > 0.2 mm after the first year of loading.

All technical and surgical complications (e.g., fracture of the abutment screw or superstructure, compromised wound healing) were recorded.

The potential risk factors of gender, implant topography, implant length, type of superstructure, and bone quality and atrophy were analyzed for their correlation with the prevalence of mucositis, peri-implantitis, implant success, and survival. At first, the effect of each risk factor was tested with a univariate regression analysis. A multivariate analysis was performed for risk factors with P values of ≤ 0.05 in the univariate analysis. The extent of the effect of a risk factor was indicated with an odds ratio (OR), with a confidence interval (CI) of 95%.

Results

All 29 subjects were examined over the period of 3 to 6 years (Table 2). For the duration of the observation period, all the remaining teeth were periodontally healthy, with PDs ≤ 3 mm and negative BOP. All subjects were non-smokers, had excellent oral hygiene, attended the follow-up examinations on a regular basis, and had no systemic disease.

Implant survival

In total, four implants (3.1%) were lost during the observation period. In a GAP subject (male), one implant (left upper first bicuspid) was removed during second-stage surgery because of mobility. In two GCP subjects (one male and one female), two implants with single crowns (right upper first bicuspid and left lower first molar) were removed after 53 and 68 months due to peri-

implantitis. One implant with a single crown (right lower first molar) of a GCP subject (female) fractured 27 months after loading. The implant survival rate was 96.2% in GAP subjects and 97.1% in GCP subjects.

Mucositis

Nine subjects (31.0%) showed mucositis in 15 implants (11.6%) (Table 3). Three GAP subjects displayed mucositis in seven implants (28.0%), compared to eight implants (7.7%) in six GCP subjects. In more than 70% of the implants, a mucositis was first diagnosed after 3 years of loading.

In the multivariate implant-related analyses, the risk of mucositis was higher in GAP subjects (OR = 4.672 with $p = 0.012$) and in females (OR = 5.267 with $p = 0.016$).

The uni- and multivariate patient-related analyses did not show significant differences. All other clinical parameters were found to be non-significant in both the implant- and patient-related analyses.

Peri-implantitis

Seven subjects (24.1%) with 21 implants (16.3%) showed peri-implantitis (Table 4). Three GAP subjects displayed peri-implantitis in 8 implants (32.0%) compared to 13 implants (12.5%) in four GCP subjects. In about 60% of the implants, a peri-implantitis was first diagnosed after 3 years of loading.

In the multivariate implant-related analyses, the risk of peri-implantitis was higher in the maxilla (OR = 15.680 with $p = 0.001$) and implants >10 mm (OR = 9.555 with $p = 0.001$). All other clinical parameters were found to be non-significant.

The univariate analyses showed a significantly higher risk for peri-implantitis in GAP subjects (OR = 3.294 with $p = 0.027$) and at implants with bone quality grade 3 (OR = 21.200 with $p = 0.000$). However, these differences were not significant in multivariate analyses.

Both the uni- and multivariate patient-related analyses were non-significant.

Implant success

The implant success rate was 77.9% for GCP implants and 38.5% for GAP implants. Twenty-two implants (21.2%) failed in 10 GCP subjects (41.7%), and 16 implants (61.5%) failed in (all) GAP subjects (100.0%).

Table 2 Observation period (patient and implant related)

Years	Patients (total)	GCP patients	GAP patients	Implants (total)	Implants maxilla			Implants mandible		
					Total	GCP	GAP	Total	GCP	GAP
3	29	24	5	130	84	62	22	46	42	4
4	22	17	5	92	55	34	21	37	33	4
5	20	15	5	84	53	32	21	31	27	4
6	17	12	5	74	50	28	21	24	20	4

Table 3 Risk factors for mucositis

	Mucositis	n	Univariate analyses			Multivariate analyses		
			OR	(95% CI)	P	OR	(95% CI)	P
Subjects								
GAP	3	5	4.500	(0.601; 3.708)	0.138			n.s.
GCP	6	24						
Female	7	18	2.864	(0.473; 17.351)	0.231			n.s.
Male	2	11						
Implants								
GAP	7	25	4.667	(1.504; 4.482)	0.010	4.672	(1.447; 15.080)	0.012
GCP	8	104						
Female	13	76	5.269	(1.135; 4.393)	0.013	5.267	(1.104; 25.122)	0.016
Male	2	53						
Superstructure								
Single crown	6	56	0.897	(0.509; 1.583)	0.708			n.s.
Fixed bridge	1	11						
Removable	8	62						
Bone quality								
1	0	3	2.769	(0.506; 15.168)	0.203			n.s.
2	13	118						
3	2	8						
Degree of atrophy								
A	8	53	1.609	(0.785; 3.298)	0.179			n.s.
B	5	41						
C	2	35						
Topography								
Ant. maxilla	7	38	2.423	(0.647; 9.074)	0.161			n.s.
Post. maxilla	5	45						
Ant. mandible	0	18						
Post. mandible	3	28						
Implant length								
≥ 10 mm	9	81	0.875	(0.291; 2.631)	0.813			n.s.
< 10 mm	6	48						

Logistic regression analyses showed whether differences were significant ($p \leq 0.05$)
CI confidence interval, n.s. non-significant, OR odds ratio, p significance

In the multivariate implant-related analyses, implants placed in the maxilla (OR = 3.241 with $p = 0.022$), and in GAP subjects (OR = 4.218 with $p = 0.006$), had a significantly higher risk of failure.

The multivariate patient-related analyses showed a higher risk of implant failure in GAP subjects (OR = 3.032 with $p = 0.004$) (Table 5).

Radiological evaluation

The mean mesial and distal marginal bone loss after 5 years was 2.19 mm (SD 1.85) in both patient groups. Peri-implant bone loss in GAP subjects was 2.89 mm (SD 1.90) and that in GCP subjects 1.38 mm (SD 1.05).

Complications

Mechanical complications were observed in two implants in two GAP subjects and in six implants in five GCP subjects. One abutment screw fractured, as well as the veneers of four ceramic crowns, and three abutments loosened and unscrewed. Surgical complications were not seen.

Discussion

The present study examines the success rates of oxide-coated implants in subjects with treated periodontal disease. Several long-term clinical studies on periodontally healthy subjects have revealed survival rates of 97.1 to 99.2% for oxide-coated implants [10, 24, 25]. The results of the present study show a comparable implant survival rate (96.2% in GAP and 97.1% in GCP subjects) for subjects with treated periodontal disease.

These findings confirm numerous studies indicating that implants with different surfaces in subjects with generalized chronic periodontitis have a survival rate of over 90% after 5 years [23, 26–31]. In a prospective study with GCP subjects, implants with rough surfaces showed a survival rate of 96.0% after an observation period of 11.6 years [32]. However, the implant survival rate for GAP subjects was 80.0%, after a follow-up period of 8.3 years. The lower survival rate of implants in patients with GAP was also present on implants with turned surfaces. In a prospective 5- to 16-year study, the survival rate was only 83.3% [23].

When reflecting the higher survival rate of implants in GAP subjects in the present study, one has to consider the small number of subjects in this group as well as the short follow up of 6 years. In a systematic review, comparing implant survival rates for GAP subjects in long-term studies, it was shown that survival rates ranged from 97.4 to 100% in studies with a follow-up period of < 5 years, falling to 83.3 to 96.0% for studies with longer observation periods [33].

Although implant survival rates given in different studies are comparable, analyzing mucositis and peri-implantitis prevalence is challenging. In the present study, GCP subjects showed mucositis in 7.7% and peri-implantitis in 12.5% of the implants. The GAP group displayed mucositis in 28.0% and peri-implantitis in 32.0% of the implants. A prospective 10-year study that examined GCP subjects with rough surface implants revealed a slightly higher peri-implantitis rate (28.6%) [31]. In a 3- to 16-year study, GAP subjects with turned surfaces implants displayed a higher mucositis (56.0%) and a comparable peri-implantitis rate (26.0%) [23].

These results from long-term clinical studies indicate that oxide-coated implants achieve equivalent survival rates and prevalence of mucositis and peri-implantitis when compared to implants with other surface characteristics. They support the assumption that the implant surface has little influence on the development of mucositis or peri-implantitis. This was subsequently confirmed in a Cochrane review, where in clinical long-term

Table 4 Risk factors for peri-implantitis

	Peri-implantitis	n	Univariate analyses			Multivariate analyses		
			OR	(95% CI)	P	OR	(95% CI)	P
Subjects								
GAP	3	5	7.500	(0.931; 60.427)	0.054			n.s.
GCP	4	24						
Female	4	18	0.762	(0.135; 4.301)	0.759			n.s.
Male	3	11						
Implants								
GAP	8	25	3.294	(1.186; 9.151)	0.027	2.596	(0.720; 9.352)	0.149
GCP	13	104						
Female	9	76	0.459	(0.178; 1.184)	0.105			n.s.
Male	12	53						
Superstructure								
Single crown	7	56	0.881	(0.538; 1.442)	0.613			n.s.
Fixed bridge	4	11						
Removable	10	62						
Bone quality								
1	0	3	21.200	(3.915; 114.798)	0.000	30.896	(5.178; 0.868)	0.056
2	16	118						
3	6	8						
Degree of atrophy								
A	5	53	0.716	(0.404; 1.269)	0.252			n.s.
B	10	41						
C	6	35						
Topography								
Ant. maxilla	9	38	14.286	(1.849; 110.358)	0.000	15.680	(1.914; 128.455)	0.001
Post. maxilla	11	45						
Ant. mandible	0	18						
Post. mandible	1	28						
Implant length								
≥ 10 mm	9	81	7.048	(1.563; 31.782)	0.002	9.555	(1.900; 48.051)	0.001
< 10 mm	6	48						

Logistic regression analyses showed whether differences were significant ($p \leq 0.05$)
CI confidence interval, n.s. non-significant, OR odds ratio, p significance

studies no evidence could be found that any specific type of implant system or surface modification conferred superior long-term success [1].

The findings of the present clinical study also allow us to put the previous results obtained from animal studies into context [13–15]. These studies analyzed the effects of ligature-induced peri-implantitis in implants with different surface characteristics placed in Labrador dogs. The results revealed increased marginal bone loss and more soft tissue destruction surrounding oxide-coated implants as compared to implants with other surfaces. These animal studies were subject to critical review [34], with the authors identifying shortcomings pertaining to the statistical analyses. Due to the small number of animals examined (six dogs), it is not possible to draw any valid conclusion regarding clinical application in human subjects. It is also apparent that the results of such animal studies are not wholly predictive of the human scenario [35].

Conclusions

The results of the present case series study should be interpreted in a critical light because of the small study population. However, it can be concluded that periodontally diseased subjects treated in a supportive periodontal therapy can be successfully rehabilitated with oxide-coated

Table 5 Implant failure rates

	Failure rate	n	Univariate analyses			Multivariate analyses		
			OR	(95% CI)	P	OR	(95% CI)	P
Subjects								
GAP	5	5	2.400	(1.495; 3.853)	0.006	3.032	(1.131; 8.123)	0.004
GCP	10	24						
Female	11	18	0.364	(0.077; 1.716)	0.194			n.s.
Male	4	11						
Implants								
GAP	16	26	5.964	(2.378; 14.959)	0.000	4.218	(1.515; 1.746)	0.006
GCP	22	104						
Female	23	76	1.128	(0.522; 2.439)	0.758			n.s.
Male	15	54						
Superstructure								
Single crown	15	56	0.952	(0.854; 1.062)	0.368			n.s.
Fixed bridge	5	11						
Removable	18	62						
Bone quality								
1	0	3	4.172	(3.038; 5.731)	0.000			n.s.
2	30	118						
3	9	9						
Degree of atrophy								
A	14	53	0.912	(0.330; 2.496)	0.156			n.s.
B	17	42						
C	8	35						
Topography								
Ant. maxilla	16	38	5.306	(1.901; 14.810)	0.000	3.241	(1.105; 9.512)	0.022
Post. maxilla	17	46						
Ant. mandible	0	18						
Post. mandible	6	28						
Implant length								
≥ 10 mm	9	82	0.485	(0.211; 1.115)	0.080			n.s.
< 10 mm	6	48						

Logistic regression analyses showed whether differences were significant ($p \leq 0.05$)
CI confidence interval, *n.s.* non-significant, *OR* odds ratio, *p* significance

dental implants for a follow-up period of 3 to 6 years. The results suggest that implants in the maxilla and in subjects treated for generalized aggressive periodontitis were more susceptible to developing mucositis and peri-implantitis, with lower implant survival and success rates.

Funding
This study was supported by a research grant from the Philipps-University of Marburg.

Authors' contributions
MTM and RM participated in the design and undertaking of the study as well as the drafting of the manuscript. TH carried out the statistics section and drafting of the manuscript. All authors read and approved the finale manuscript.

Authors' information
RM is a professor at the Department of Prosthetic Dentistry, School of Dental Medicine, Philipps-University, Marburg/Lahn, Germany. TH is a private practicioner in Gruben, Brandenburg, Germany. MT is a researcher at the Department of Prosthetic Dentistry, School of Dental Medicine, Philipps-University, Marburg/Lahn, Germany.

Competing interests
M. Thöne-Mühling, T. Heim, and R. Mengel state that there were no conflicts of interests during the undertaking of the study.

Author details
¹Department of Prosthetic Dentistry, School of Dental Medicine, Philipps-University, Marburg/Lahn, Germany. ²Gruben, Brandenburg, Germany.

References
1. Esposito M, Ardebili Y, Worthington HV. Interventions for replacing missing teeth: different types of dental implants. Cochrane Database Sys Rev. 2014;7: CD003815.
2. Salata LA, Burgos PM, Rasmusson L, Novaes AB, Papalexiou V, Dahlin C, Sennerby L. Osseointegration of oxidized and turned implants in circumferential bone defects with and without adjunctive therapies: an experimental study on BMP-2 and autogenous bone graft in the dog mandible. Int J Oral Maxillofac Surg. 2007;36:62–71.
3. Shibli JA, Feres M, de Figueiredo LC, Iezzi G, Piattelli A. Histological comparison of bone to implant contact in two types of dental implant surfaces: a single case study. J Contemp Dental Pract 2007a;8:29–36.
4. Shibli JA, Grassi S, de Figueiredo, LC, Feres M, Marcantonio EJ, Iezzi G, Piattelli A. Influence of implant surface topography on early osseointegration: a histological study in human jaws. J biomed mat res Applied Biomaterials Part B 2007;80:377–385.
5. Yeo I-S, Han J-S, Yang J-H. Biomechanical and histomorphometric study of dental implants with different surface characteristics, J biomedical materials res. Part B Applied Biomaterials 2008;87:303–311.
6. Xia L, Feng B, Wang P, Ding S, Liu Z, Zhou J, Yu R. In vitro and in vivo studies of surface-structured implants for bone formation. Int J Nanomedicine. 2012;7:4873–81.
7. Schüpbach P, Glauser R, Rocci A, Martignoni M, Sennerby L, Lundgren AK, Gottlow J. The human bone-oxidized titanium implant interface: a light microscopic, scanning electron microscopic, back-scatter scanning electron microscopic, and energy-dispersive x-ray study of clinically retrieved dental implants. Clin Implant Dent Related Res. 2005;7(Suppl 1):36–43.
8. Zechner W, Tangl S, Furst G, Tepper G, Thams U, Mailath G, Watzek G. Osseous healing characteristics of three different implant types. Clin Oral Implants Res. 2003;4:150–7.
9. Huang Y-H, Xiropaidis AV, Sorensen RG, Albandar JM, Hall J, Wikesjo UME. Bone formation at titanium porous oxide (TiUnite®) oral implants in type IV bone. Clin Oral Implants Res. 2005;16:105–11.
10. Östman P-O, Hellman M, Sennerby L. Ten years later. Results from a prospective single-centre clinical study on 121 oxidized (TiUnite®) Brånemark implants in 46 patients. Clin Implant Dent Related Res. 2012;14: 852–60.
11. Jungner M, Lundqvist P, Lundgren S. A retrospective comparison of oxidized and turned implants with respect to implant survival, marginal bone level and peri-implant soft tissue conditions after at least 5 years in function. Clin Implant Dent Relat Res. 2014;16:230–7.
12. Rocci A, Rocci M, Rocci C, Scoccia A, Gargari M, Martignoni M, Gottlow J, Sennerby L. Immediate loading of Brånemark system TiUnite and machined-surface implants in the posterior mandible, part II: a randomized open-ended 9-year follow-up clinical trial. Int J Oral Maxillofac Implants. 2013;28:891–5.
13. Albouy J-P, Abrahamsson I, Berglundh T. Spontaneous progression of experimental peri-implantitis at implants with different surface characteristics: an experimental study in dogs. J Clin Periodontol. 2012;39:182–7.
14. Albouy J-P, Abrahamsson I, Persson LG, Berglundh T. Spontaneous progression of peri-implantitis at different types of implants. An

experimental study in dogs. I: clinical and radiographic observations. Clin Oral Implants Res. 2008;19:997–1002.

15. Albouy J-P, Abrahamsson I, Persson LG, Berglundh T. Spontaneous progression of ligatured induced peri-implantitis at implants with different surface characteristics. An experimental study in dogs II: histological observations. Clin Oral Implants Res. 2009;20:366–71.

16. Armitage GC. Development of a classification system for periodontal diseases and conditions. Ann Periodontol. 1999;4:1–6.

17. Lekholm U, Zarb GA. Patient selection and preparation. In: Brånemark P-I, Zarb GA, Albrektsson T, editors. Tissue integrated prostheses: Osseointegration in clinical dentistry. Chicago: Quintessence Publ. Co; 1985. p. 199–209.

18. Mengel R, Kreuzer G, Lehmann KM, Flores-de-Jacoby L. A telescopic crown concept for the restoration of partially edentulous patients with aggressive generalized periodontitis: a 3-year prospective longitudinal study. Int J Periodontics Restorative Dent. 2007;3:231–9.

19. Loe H, Silness J. Periodontal disease in pregnancy. I. Prevalence and severity. Acta Odontol Scand. 1963;21:533–51.

20. Silness J, Loe H. Periodontal disease in pregnancy II. Correlation between oral hygiene and periodontal condition. Acta Odontol Scand. 1964;22:121–35.

21. Strid KG. Radiographic results. In: Branemark PI, Zarb GA, Albrektsson T (eds). Tissue-Integrated Prostheses. Berlin: Quintessence Books; 1985:187–198.

22. Kinane DF, Radvar M. The effect of smoking on mechanical and antimicrobial periodontal therapy. J Periodontol. 1997;69:467–72.

23. Swierkot K, Lottholz P, Flores-de-Jacoby L, Mengel R. Mucositis, peri-implantitis, implant success, and survival of implants in patients with treated generalized aggressive periodontitis: 3- to 16-year results of a prospective long-term cohort study. J Periodontol. 2012;83:1213–25.

24. Degidi M, Nardi D, Piattelli A. 10-year follow-up of immediately loaded implants with TiUnite® porous anodized surface. Clin Implant Dent Related Res. 2012;14:828–38.

25. Mozzati M, Gallesio G, Del Fabbro M. Long-term (9-12 years) outcomes of titanium implants with an oxidized surface: a retrospective investigation on 209 implants. J Oral Implantol. 2015:437–43.

26. Busenlechner D, Fürhauser R, Haas R, Watzek G, Mailath G, Pommer B. Long-term implant success at the academy for oral implantology: 8-year follow-up and risk factor analysis. J Periodontal Implant Sci. 2014;44:102–8.

27. Mengel R, Behle M, Flores-de-Jacoby L. Osseointegrated implants in subjects treated for generalized aggressive periodontitis: 10-year results of a prospective, long-term cohort study. J Periodontol. 2007;78:2229–37.

28. Mengel R, Flores-de-Jacoby L. Implants in patients treated for generalized aggressive and chronic periodontitis: a 3-year prospective longitudinal study. J Periodontol. 2005;76:534–43.

29. Mengel R, Schroder T, Flores-de-Jacoby L. Osseointegrated implants in patients treated for generalized chronic periodontitis and generalized aggressive periodontitis: 3- and 5-year results of a prospective long-term study. J Periodontol. 2001;72:977–89.

30. Mengel R, Stelzel M, Hasse C, Flores-de-Jacoby L. Osseointegrated implants in patients treated for generalized severe adult periodontitis. An interim report. J Periodontol. 1996;67:782–7.

31. Karoussis IK, Salvi G, Heitz-Mayfield L, Brägger U, Hämmerle C, Lang N. Long-term implant prognosis in patients with and without a history of chronic periodontitis: a 10-year prospective cohort study of the ITI dental implant system. Clin Oral Implants Res. 2003;14:329–39.

32. De Boever AL, Quirynen M, Coucke W, Theuniers G, De Boever JA. Clinical and radiographic study of implant treatment outcome in periodontally susceptible and non-susceptible patients: a prospective long-term study. Clin Oral Implants Res 2009;20:1341–1350.

33. Kim K-K, Sung H-M. Outcomes of dental implant treatment in patients with generalized aggressive periodontitis: a systematic review. J Adv Prosthodont. 2012;4:210–7.

34. Pettersson K, Mengel R. Comments on the statistical analysis of the paper by Albouy et al comparing four different types of implants with respect to 'spontaneous' progression of peri-implantitis. Eur J Oral Implantol. 2011;1:9–10.

35. Esposito M, Nieri M, Lindeboom J. Comments on the letter from Kjell Pettersson and Reiner Mengel by the editorial team of EJOI. Eur J Oral Implantol. 2011;4:11.

13

Sandwich bone graft for vertical augmentation of the posterior maxillary region

Kenko Tanaka[1,2*], Irena Sailer[2], Yoshihiro Kataoka[1], Shinnosuke Nogami[1] and Tetsu Takahashi[1]

Abstract

The loss of teeth followed by bone resorption often lead to defects in the alveolar ridge, making installation of dental implants difficult. Correction of such bone defects, especially lack of height of the ridge, is a difficult problem for all dental surgeons. This report describes the outcome of treatment after alveolar ridge augmentation in the atrophic posterior maxillary region via segmental sandwich osteotomy combined with placement of an interpositional autograft prior to placement of endosseous implants. The technique was successfully used to treat a deficiency in the vertical dimension of the posterior maxillary region. Six months after graft surgery, two implants were successfully placed in accordance with the original treatment protocol, and they survived for 9 years of follow-up.

Keywords: Bone graft, Long-term follow-up, Interpositional bone graft, Sandwich graft

Background

Osseointegrated implants for the replacement of missing teeth have recently become a routine treatment option [1, 2]. However, any tooth loss may be followed by extensive resorption of the alveolar ridge, which usually makes implant placement difficult or impossible because of the lack of bone volume. There are a variety of defect situations with increasing complexity, ranging from fenestrations, to dehiscences, to both horizontal and vertical deficiencies, while combinations of these also occur. Ridge augmentation techniques are available to effectively and predictably increase the width of the alveolar ridge in horizontal deficiencies. If vertical deficiencies are present, including in combination, the predictability of the techniques is usually substantially lower [3]. A significant bone defect is an anatomical limitation that can be overcome using different surgical techniques, including vertically guided bone regeneration. Several techniques are currently employed, using some combination of autologous bone or biomaterials, various vertical guided bone regeneration (GBR) procedures [4, 5], alveolar

distraction osteogenesis [6], titanium mesh [7], and onlay bone graft [8].

While the vertical augmentation of the bone has been demonstrated with different techniques, the number of complications and failures of the augmentation procedure is still too high to recommend a widespread use of such procedures [9–11]. In addition, vertical augmentation procedures on compromised alveolar ridges are technically sensitive and might cause significant postoperative morbidity and complications, such as severe postoperative pain, swelling, or graft resorption. Furthermore, augmentation procedures always increase cost, morbidity, and treatment time [12].

Recently, rough-surface implants made with new technology have demonstrated better mechanical and biologic characteristics than traditional machined-surface implants. Several clinical studies have demonstrated high success rates and predictable clinical outcomes for placement of short implants. Short implants have been proposed as an alternative to avoid the problems associated with vertical augmentation [12–14]. Still, there is a need for more clinical studies to support this recent concept.

In the literature, the technique of segmental osteotomy accompanied by interpositional grafting has been reported as a practical and predictable procedure with a low incidence of complications and a high probability of

---

* Correspondence: k-tanaka@dent.kagoshima-u.ac.jp
[1]Division of Oral and Maxillofacial Surgery, Department of Oral Medicine and Surgery, Tohoku University Graduate School of Dentistry, 4-1 Seiryo-machi, Aoba-ku, Sendai 980-8575, Miyagi, Japan
[2]Division of Fixed Prosthodontics and Biomaterials Clinic of Dental Medicine, University of Geneva, 19 rue Barthélemy-Menn, CH-1205 Geneva, Switzerland

success [15–19]. This approach leaves the soft tissue on the oral side of the midcrestal incision attached to the crestal bone segment. Various studies have shown that alveolar osteotomy associated with interpositional grafting may be an effective alternative to other surgical techniques for increasing vertical bone height in the posterior maxilla and mandible [15–19]. The technique is based on interposing a bone graft between osteotomized bony segments, which act as a "sandwich," offering good vasculature to both the segment and the graft and resulting in less bone resorption compared to the methods described before [15–19].

This case report describes clinical treatment using segmental osteotomy with interpositional bone grafting to rehabilitate the alveolar ridge in the posterior region of the maxilla with 9 years of follow-up.

Case presentation

A 67-year-old male patient sought implant rehabilitation for the purposes of restoration of occlusal support and assistance with chewing difficulties. Clinical and radiological examinations revealed that teeth were absent 26–27. The clearance from the alveolar ridge to the opposing teeth was 20 mm (Fig. 1). A CT scan showed that the distance from the reabsorbed ridge to the floor of the maxillary sinus was approximately 26: 6.1 mm and 27: 7.5 mm, and the width of clearance was approximately 8 mm. The alveolar bone defect in this case was the loss of ridge height with normal ridge width, class II according to the Seibert classification [20]. Additionally, septa and a thickened sinus membrane were evident within the maxillary sinus (Fig. 2).

As a preoperative diagnosis, it was determined that the septa and a thickened sinus membrane meant that sinus lift augmentation was difficult, and bone augmentation to the crown side was required, but the morphology of the alveolar ridge had been well maintained. The treatment options included using short implants, but evidence on their long-term outcome was still limited at that time.

It was determined that the best treatment involved segmental osteotomy and placement of an interpositional graft using the bone removed from the ramus of the mandible to restore the posterior maxillary alveolar ridge, prior to placement of dental implants.

The operative procedure was performed after the induction of general anesthesia using a 1/160,000 xylocaine solution with epinephrine 1:100,000. A linear incision was made 3 mm above the mucogingival junction. The mucoperiosteum was detached, and the vertical and horizontal osteotomies were prepared using micro-saws. Chisels were used to finalize the osteotomies and to mobilize the bony segment. Care was taken not to damage the palatal mucosa. The surgery proceed to the removal of a bone graft

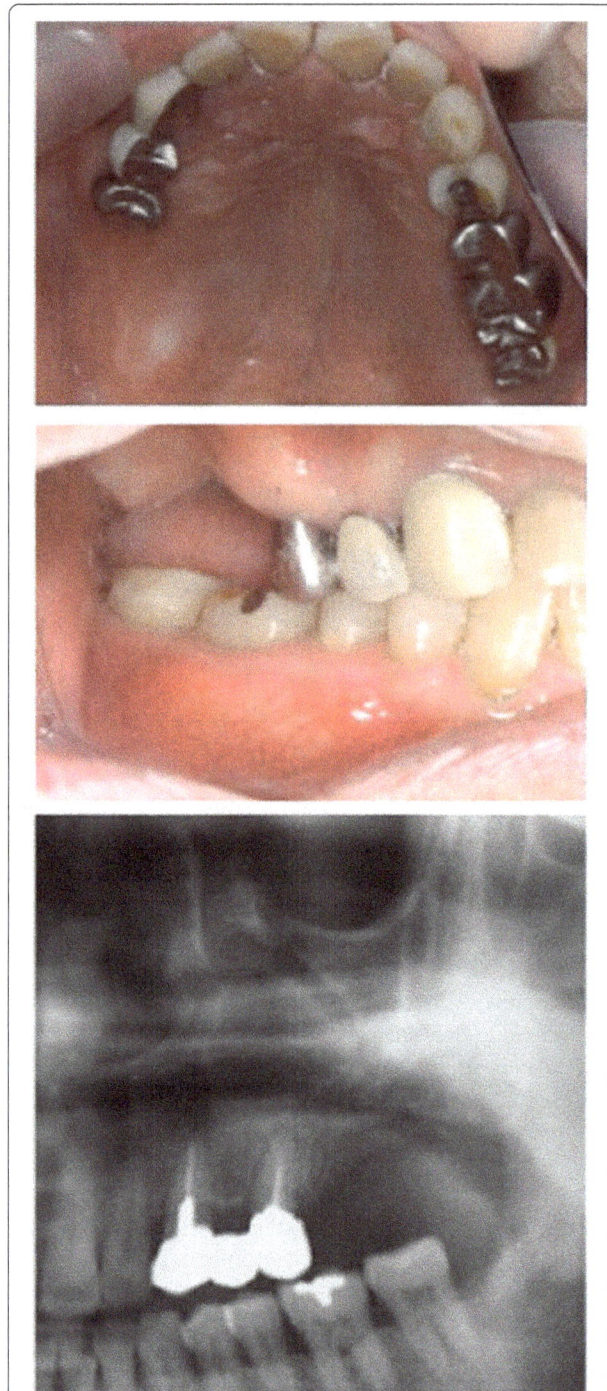

Fig. 1 Preoperative intraoral photograph and radiograph

block (17 × 10 × 4 mm) from the ramus of the left mandible and the adaptation thereof to the recipient site with the cortical portion facing the vestibular side (Fig. 3). The device formed by the mobilized bone segment and the interposed bone graft block was fixed using WY-type microplates and screws (Stryker Japan, Tokyo, Japan). Crushed autologous bone was applied to the region of the graft

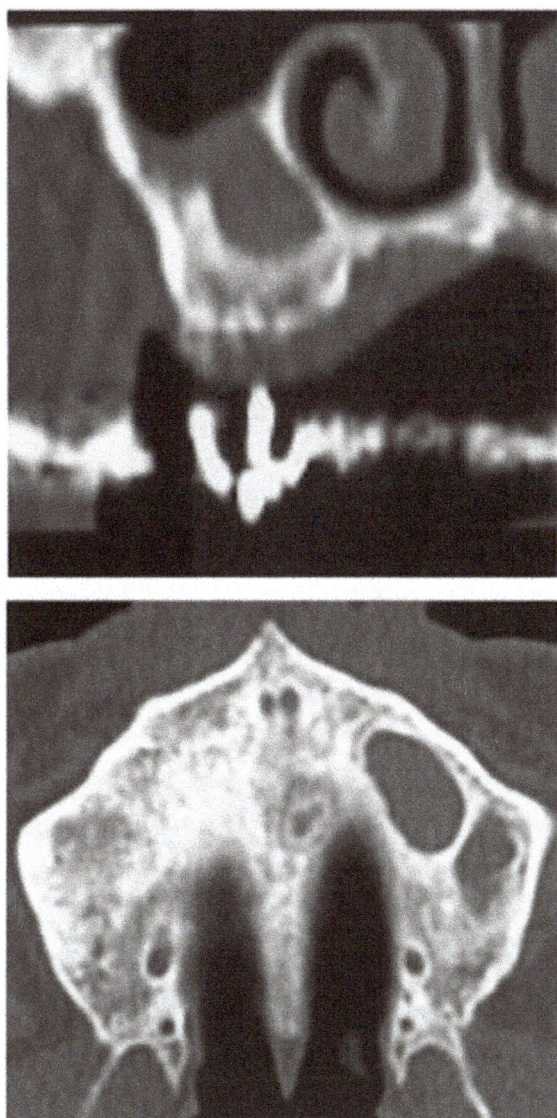

Fig. 2 Septa and thickened sinus membrane within maxillary sinus

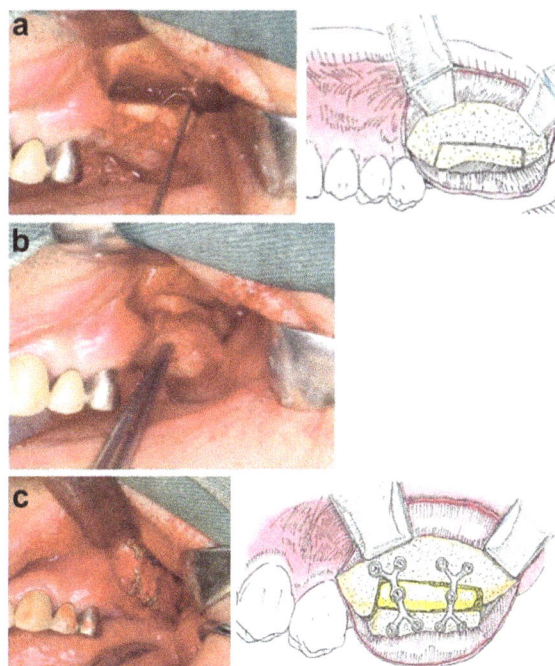

Fig. 3 a A paracrestal incision was made on the buccal side, and horizontal and vertical osteotomies were made with a piezo-electric device. **b** Placement of the ramus bone block as an interpositional graft. **c** Ramus bone graft fixed

(Fig. 3). The procedure was finalized using a running stitch for closure with 5-0 nylon catgut.

Six months after surgery, radiological examinations were carried out and the patient underwent implant placement (Fig. 4). The postoperative bone height had increased to 10.1 mm at position 26 and 12.9 mm at position 27 compared with the preoperative heights of 6.1 and 7.5 mm, respectively. Postoperative clearance was reduced by 11 mm compared with the preoperative clearance. Careful separation of the mucoperiosteum revealed that the fixation device was in the right place, the interpositional bone graft had been incorporated, and gains in the height and thickness of the alveolar ridge had been achieved. The fixation system was removed, and two dental implants (4.5 × 11 mm) (Astra Tech AB, Mölndal, Sweden) were placed in accordance with the

original treatment protocol under the relevant surgical guidance (Fig. 5). Three months after implant surgery, the temporary prosthesis was fixed, and after a further 3 months, the final prosthesis was fixed (Fig. 6). The postoperative course was uneventful for 9 years after surgery (Fig. 7).

Discussion

This paper reports on a segmental osteotomy procedure with an interpositional graft in the posterior maxillary region with 9 years of follow-up.

The techniques used to overcome a lack of alveolar bone height rely on the placement supplemented by various vertical guided bone regeneration (GBR) procedures [4, 5] and the use of alveolar distraction osteogenesis [6], titanium mesh [7], or onlay bone graft [8]. Gains in ridge height of between 3.6 and 9.2 mm depending on the materials used have been reported, and these were associated with 5-year implant survival rates of 97 to 100%, depending on the method employed [3]. On the other hand, it has also been reported the number of complications (e.g., flap dehiscence, barrier exposure) and failures of the augmentation procedure (e.g. infection, graft bone necrosis) [3–8]. Additionally, the biomaterials used as substitutes for the bone require a longer healing time than autologous bone because the substitutes in general are not osteoinductive [3].

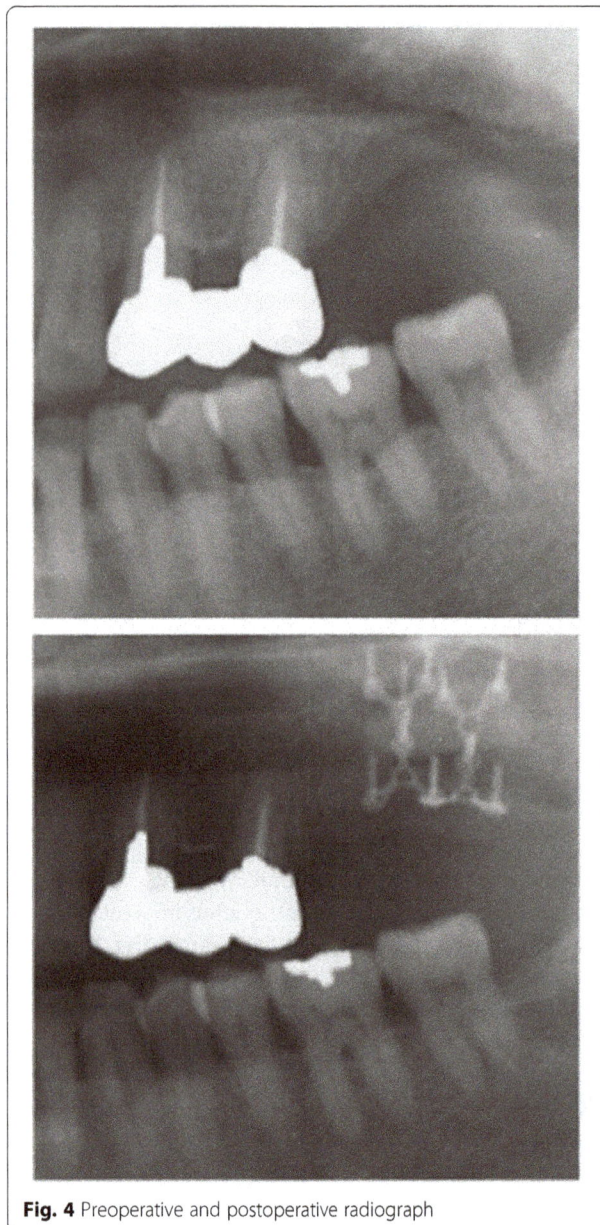

Fig. 4 Preoperative and postoperative radiograph

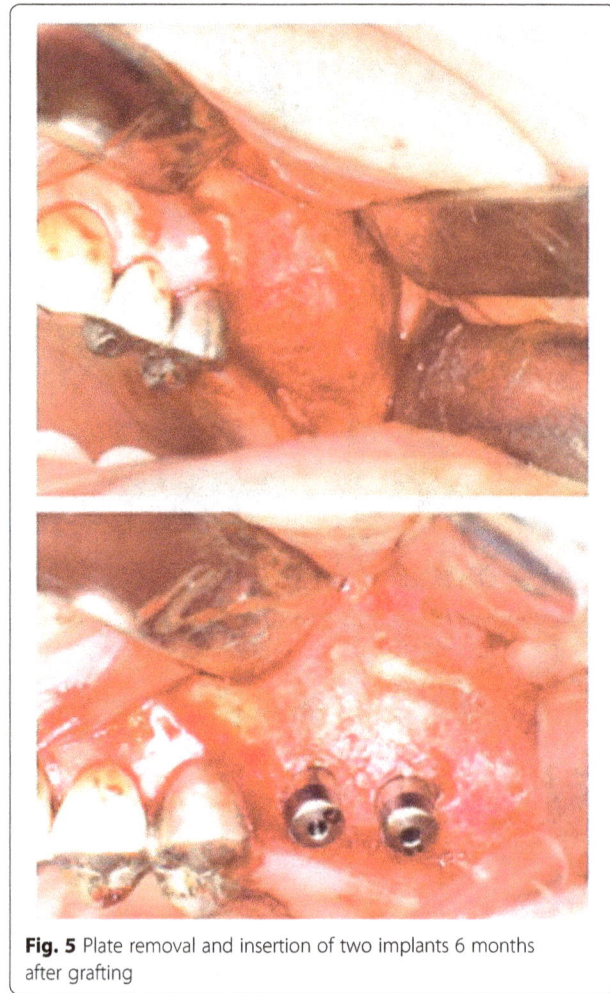

Fig. 5 Plate removal and insertion of two implants 6 months after grafting

Although a certain amount of slow appositional bone growth from the bony walls into the defect is observed, this growth depends on the growth of new blood vessels between each particle. In the alveolar crest, it spontaneously stops at a distance of few millimeters above the defect bone wall. The more distant particles instead heal within fibrous tissue to form a scar. This is expected to have a negative effect on the long-term survival of the restoration [3].

The use of short implants is another possibility when alveolar bone height is inadequate for regular implants. The use of such implants can reduce treatment time, cost, and postoperative morbidity compared to bone augmentation procedures. The first EAO consensus conference (2006) had defined short implants as a device with a design intrabony length of 8 mm or less [21] and had demonstrated high success rates and predictable clinical outcomes for placement of short implants [12–14], but there were still controversies regarding the long-term consequences of peri-implant bone loss around short implants and its impact on the long-term implant success rate at that time.

In this case, the alveolar ridge was Seibert class II, and septa and a thickened sinus membrane were evident within the maxillary sinus. Sinus floor elevation was limited because of the condition of the floor morphology, the presence of septa, and the thickness of sinus floor membrane [22, 23]. Considering these issues, we selected the interpositional bone graft technique using autologous bone in preference to short implants or the use of a biomaterial.

The inlay bone graft technique, first described by Schettler and Holtermann in 1977 [15] which presented the reconstruction of a severely atrophic edentulous mandible, has great potential for bone graft incorporation. The technique is relatively simple and provides satisfactory

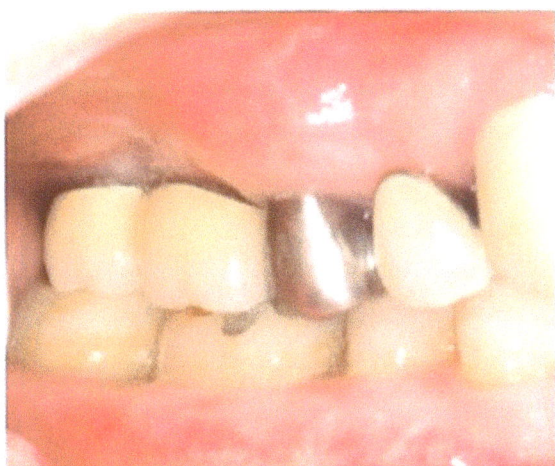

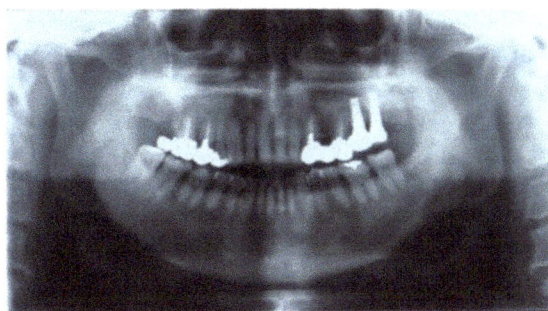

Fig. 7 Nine-year follow-up radiograph of the implants

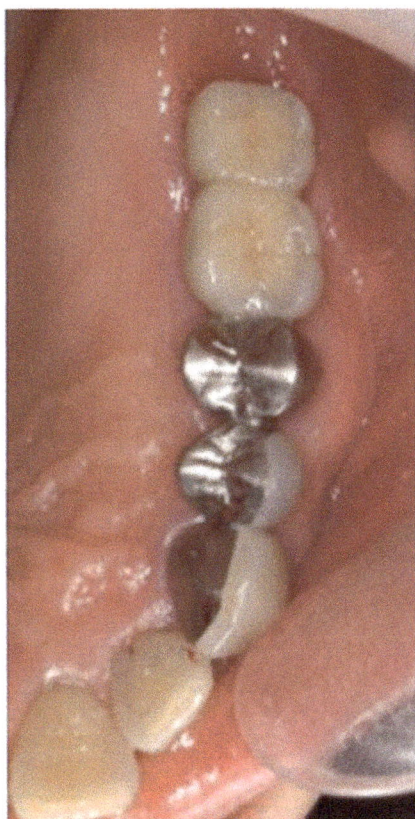

Fig. 6 Application of final fixed prosthesis

results both in terms of surgical success and predictability [15–19]. The technique is predicable because the four walls of the graft are in contact with live tissue, increasing vascularization and reducing resorption [17]. A box-style gap opens between the segments, which borders on an open bone marrow cavity on two sides. This space offers excellent conditions for vascularization of the graft and bone healing. Thus, a temporary prosthesis can be used in the early postoperative period. Since that first report,

several reports on research outcomes, technological progress, and the good results obtained with this technique have been published. This technique is now regarded as a good way to correct vertical deficiencies prior to placement of dental implants [15–19].

On the other hand, alveolar augmentation depends on the operator's experience and is technically sensitive [3]. The most common difficulty is how to manage the soft tissues to preserve the blood supply to the cranial segment; releasing incisions make tension-free closure possible so that the segment does not move palatally.

Nevertheless, in this case, the procedure was carried out successfully, and two regular implants were successfully placed in the alveolar ridge after its enhancement with an autologous bone graft. Those implants survived over 9 years of follow-up.

Conclusions

We described in the present case a vertical lack of the bone from the alveolar ridge to the opposing teeth, the short distance from the reabsorbed ridge to the floor of the maxillary sinus, and the presence of septa and a thickened sinus membrane within the maxillary sinus. A sandwich bone graft was successfully applied and followed up in the long term. The resulting gains in ridge height and increased thickness of the alveolar ridge appear to have been sufficient for effective placement of the implants, given that these implants have been maintained for 9 years since surgery.

Acknowledgements
The authors thank Atumu Kouketu for his figure illustration support and Kouhei Shinmyouzu for the clinical support.

Competing interests
Authors Kenko Tanaka, Irena Sailer, Yoshihiro Kataoka, Shinnosuke Nogami, and Tetsu Takahashi declare that they have no competing interests.

References
1. Adell R, Brånemark PI. A 15-year study of osseointegrated implant in the treatment of the edentulous jaw. Int J Oral Maxillofac Surg. 1981;10:387–416.

2. Albrektsson T, Zarb G, Worthington P, Eriksson AR. The long-term efficacy of currently used dental implants: a review and proposed criteria of success. Int J Oral Maxillofac Implants. 1986;1:11–25.

3. Cordo L, Terheyden H. ITI treatment guide volume 7. Berlin: Quintessence Publishing; 2009. p. 54–55,76.

4. Simion M, Jovanovic SA, Tinti C, Benfenati SP. Long-term evaluation of osseointegrated implants inserted at the time or after vertical ridge augmentation: a retrospective study on 123 implants with 1–5 year follow-up. Clin Oral Implants Res. 2001;12(1):35–45.

5. Chiapasco M, Romeo E, Casentini P, Rimondini L. Alveolar distraction osteogenesis vs. vertical guided bone regeneration for the correction of vertically deficient edentulous ridges: a 1–3-year prospective study on humans. Clin Oral Implants Res. 2004;15:82–95.

6. Chiapasco M, Romeo E, Casentini P, Rimondini L. Alveolar distraction osteogenesis for the correction of vertically deficient edentulous ridges: a multicenter prospective study on humans. Int J Oral Maxillofac Implants. 2004;19:399–407.

7. Roccuzzo M, Ramieri G, Spada MC, Bianchi SD, Berrone S. Vertical alveolar ridge augmentation by means of a titanium mesh and autogenous bone grafts. Clin Oral Implants Res. 2004;15:73–81.

8. Chiapasco M, Zaniboni M, Rimondini L. Autogenous onlay bone grafts vs. alveolar distraction osteogenesis for the correction of vertically deficient edentulous ridges: a 2–4-year prospective study on humans. Clin Oral Implants Res. 2007;18:432–440.

9. Chiapasco M, Casentini P, Zaniboni M. Bone augmentation procedures in implant dentistry. Int J Oral Maxillofac Implants. 2009;24:237–59.

10. Aghaloo TL, Moy PK. Which hard tissue augmentation techniques are the most successful in furnishing bony support for implant placement? Int J Oral Maxillofac Implants. 2007;22:49–70.

11. Milinkovic I, Cordaro L. Are there specific indications for the different alveolar bone augmentation procedures for implant placement? A systematic review. Int J Oral Maxillofac Surg. 2014;43(5):606–625.

12. Thoma DS, Zeltner M, Hüsler J, Hämmerle CH, Jung RE, EAO Supplement Working Group 4 - EAO CC. Short implants versus sinus lifting with longer implants to restore the posterior maxilla: a systematic review. Clin Oral Implants Res. 2015;26:154–169.

13. Lee SA, Lee CT, Fu MM, Elmisalati W, Chuang SK. Systematic review and meta-analysis of randomized controlled trials for the management of limited vertical height in the posterior region: short implants (5 to 8 mm) vs longer implants (>8 mm) in vertically augmented sites. Int J Oral Maxillofac Implants. 2014;29(5);1085–1097.

14. Nisand D, Picard N, Rocchietta I. Short implants compared to implants in vertically augmented bone: a systematic review. Clin Oral Implants Res. 2015;26:170–179.

15. Schettler D, Holtermann W. Clinical and experimental results of a sandwich-technique for mandibular alveolar ridge augmentation. J Maxillofac Surg. 1977;5(3):199–202.

16. Stoelinga PJ, Tideman H, Berger JS, de Koomen HA. Interpositional bone graft augmentation of the atrophic mandible: a preliminary report. J Oral Maxillofac Surg. 1978;36:30–32.

17. Jensen OT, Kuhlke L, Bedard JF, White D. Alveolar segmental sandwich osteotomy for anterior maxillary vertical augmentation prior to implant placement. J Oral Maxillofac Surg. 2006;64:290–296.

18. Jensen OT. Alveolar segmental "sandwich" osteotomies for posterior edentulous mandibular sites for dental implants. J Oral Maxillofac Surg. 2006;64:471–475.

19. Nóia CF, Ortega-Lopes R, Mazzonetto R, Chaves Netto HD. Segmental osteotomy with interpositional bone grafting in the posterior maxillary region. Int J Oral Maxillofac Surg. 2012;41:1563–1565.

20. Seibert JS. Reconstruction of deformed, partially edentulous ridges, using full thickness onlay grafts. Part II. Prosthetic/periodontal interrelationships. Compend Contin Educ Dent. 1983;4(6):549–562.

21. Renouard F, Nisand D. Impact of implant length and diameter on survival rates. Clin Oral Implants Res. 2006;17:35–51.

22. Testori T, Weinstein RL, Taschieri S, Del Fabbro M. Risk factor analysis following maxillary sinus augmentation: a retrospective multicenter study. Int J Oral Maxillofac Implants. 2012;27:1170–1176.

23. Bergh van den JPA, Bruggenkate ten CM, Disch FJM, Tuinzing DB. Anatomical aspects of sinus floor elevations. Clin Oral Implants Res. 2000;11:256–265.

14

Customized SmartPeg for measurement of resonance frequency of mini dental implants

Jagjit Singh Dhaliwal[1,4], Rubens F. Albuquerque Jr[2], Ali Fakhry[1], Sukhbir Kaur[3] and Jocelyne S. Feine[1*]

Abstract

Background: One-piece narrow diameter implants (NDIs) have been recommended as "Single-tooth replacements in the anterior zones, single posterior, multiple-unit fixed dental prosthesis (FDP), edentulous jaws to be rehabilitated with FDP, and edentulous jaws rehabilitation with overdentures in situations with reduced mesiodistal space or reduced ridge width." (ITI consensus 2013). Since NDIs can be immediately loaded, it is important to be able to carry out stability testing. We developed and validated a customized SmartPeg for this type of implant to measure the Implant Stability Quotient (ISQ). The ISQ of mini dental implants (MDIs) was measured and compared with the stability of standard and in a rabbit model.

Objective: The aim of the study is to test the feasibility of a customized SmartPeg for resonance frequency measurement of single-piece mini dental implants and to compare primary stability of a standard and the mini dental implant (3M™ESPE™ MDI) in a rabbit model after 6 weeks of healing.

Methods: Eight New Zealand white rabbits were used for the study. The protocol was approved by the McGill University Animal Ethics Review Board. Sixteen 3M™ESPE™ MDI and equal number of standard implants (Ankylos® Friadent, Dentsply) were inserted into the tibia/femur of the rabbits and compared. Each rabbit randomly received two 3M™ESPE™ MDI and two Ankylos® implants in each leg. ISQ values were measured with the help of an Osstell ISQ device using custom-made SmartPegs for the MDIs and implant-specific SmartPegs™ (Osstell) for the Ankylos®. Measurements were obtained both immediately following implant placement surgery and after a 6-week healing period. Each reading was taken thrice and their average compared using Wilcoxon matched pairs signed-rank tests.

Results: The median ISQ and interquartile range (IQR) values were 53.3 (8.3) at insertion and 60.5 (5.5) at 6 weeks for the 3M™ESPE™MDI and, respectively, 58.5 (4.75) and 65.5 (9.3) for the Ankylos® implant. These values also indicate that both types of implants achieved primary and secondary stability, and this is supported by histological data. ISQ values of both 3M™ESPE™ MDI and Ankylos® increased significantly from the time of insertion to 6 weeks post-insertion ($p < 0.05$).

Conclusions: The new custom-made SmartPeg is suitable for measuring the Implant Stability Quotient of 3M™ESPE™MDIs. The primary stability of 3M™ESPE™MDIs is similar to the primary stability attained by standard implants in the rabbit tibia.

* Correspondence: jocelyne.feine@mcgill.ca
[1]Faculty of Dentistry, McGill University, 2001 McGill College Avenue, Suite 500, Montreal, Quebec H3A 1G1, Canada
Full list of author information is available at the end of the article

Background

Osseointegration refers to the phenomenon for close apposition of the bone to the surface of an implant with no interposing tissue that can be clinically demonstrated by absence of mobility [1, 2]. Obtaining primary stability seems to be a precondition for a successful osseointegration [3]. Dental implants have a success rate of over 90% and are available in various sizes with different surfaces [4, 5]. The diameter of dental implants usually ranges from 3 mm (narrow diameter) to 7 mm (wide diameter), with the majority falling in the "standard diameter" range of 3.7 to 4.0 mm.

Single-piece mini dental implants (MDIs) or narrow diameter implants (NDIs) are being widely used for stabilizing complete dentures [6], orthodontic anchorage [7, 8], single-tooth replacements, and fixing surgical guides for definitive implant placement, and as transitional implants for support of interim removable prosthesis during the healing phase of final fixtures [9–11].

Due to the MDIs' narrower diameter (1.8–2.4 mm) as compared with regular implants, the width of the bone required for their placement is smaller, making the surgery minimally invasive as compared with the surgery for conventional implant insertion [12]. In addition, transmucosal placement is performed using a single pilot drill, reducing the need for sutures and long recovery periods [13]. Mini dental implants can also be immediately loaded and are cost-effective, which makes them an advantageous alternative for mandibular implant overdentures [13, 14]. The success of these implants will depend, however, on their capacity to outstand functional loadings.

Osseointegrated implants are clinically characterized by the absence of mobility, which can be assessed by measuring the primary and secondary implant stability [15, 16]. Some authors have suggested that primary stability is a critical factor in predicting whether an implant will be successful or not, and it is considered of highest importance in the long-term success of dental implants [17, 18]. It has also been reported that micro movements can be detected at an early stage by measuring the primary implant stability and that they are unfavorable to the osseointegration of dental implants [19–21].

Mechanical testing methods like reverse torque, or "pullout test," have been used to study and measure the mechanical interface between implant and bone in various ways [22, 23]. The Branemark group has evaluated the mechanical properties of osseointegrated implants using torsion and pullout tests and lateral loading tests [24, 25]. Presence or absence of mobility and the bone level around the implant can be estimated by non-invasive methods based on resonance frequency analysis (RFA) such as those used by Periotest and Osstell™ devices [26–30].

Resonance frequency analysis has been used to document changes in the bone healing along the implant-bone interface by measuring the stiffness of implant in the bone tissue [31–34]. It has also been used to determine whether implants are ready for the final restoration [35] or ready to be loaded [33] and to identify the implants at "risk" [36]. The first studies using RFA were published in 1996 [37]. In 1997, Meredith et al. suggested a non-invasive method for determining the resonance frequency associated with dental implants by connecting an adapter/transducer onto the abutment in an animal study [38]. The experimented RFA system, base on magnetic pulses, has been commercially produced as Osstell since the year 2000 [19] (Osstell AB, Göteborg, Sweden). Osstell was later followed by Osstell Mentor™ and Osstell ISQ™. It calculates the Implant Stability Quotient (ISQ) converting kilohertz units to ISQ on a scale of 1–100, where 100 signifies the highest implant stability. Increases in ISQ measurements indicate improved bone stiffness and healing around the implant and better implant stability. The Osstell ISQ works by introducing a controlled vibration to the implant by means of a sensor and a rod (SmartPeg) connected to the implant and measuring its frequency. These SmartPegs are usually fabricated for standard diameter implants. The osseointegration potential of single-piece mini dental implants (3M™ESPE™ MDIs) has never been assessed by RFA. The immediate post-surgical ISQ assessment of MDIs is particularly relevant due to their smaller size and surface area in comparison to standard implants.

There are no published studies on the ISQ measurement of mini dental implants, as SmartPegs for these implants are not available till date. Since these are one-piece implants and do not have an internal thread for the SmartPeg's attachment, a custom-made SmartPeg needs to be fabricated for ISQ measurement. Therefore, we developed and tested a customized SmartPeg for 3M™ESPE™ MDIs to measure the ISQ.

Objective

The aim of the study is to test the feasibility of a customized SmartPeg for ISQ measurement of single-piece mini dental implants and to compare the primary stability of a standard and the mini dental implant (3M™ESPE™MDI) in a rabbit model after 6 weeks of healing.

Methods

Development of a customized SmartPeg

Single use Osstell SmartPegs for standard implants are made from a soft metal with a zinc-coated magnet mounted on top of it and attached to the implants or abutments' internal threads. As the company does not provide SmartPegs for one-piece implants, we developed a customized SmartPeg for mini dental implants (3M™ESPE™ MDIs), which do not have internal threads

(Fig. 1). After confirming that the standard SmartPegs™ are fabricated in aluminum, we customized a prototype in the same metal with a square-shaped assembly, which could be tightened with a small screw over the spherical top end of the MDIs. Our SmartPeg prototype was tested for reproducibility verifying the ISQ values on an MDI inserted into a wooden plank made of balsa wood. RFA measurements were taken 50 times, and a standard error of mean of all measurements was calculated.

Animal model and sample size

Eight clinically healthy New Zealand white rabbits weighing >3.5 kg used for the study were housed in the Central Animal House facility. The head of the tibia/femur of the animals were chosen for the implantation of samples because they have been widely used as an animal model, and so, our results could be promptly compared [39–46]. The sample size of this study has been calculated based on the results of a similar study [36]. It was expected that 88% statistical power would be achieved by using sixteen 3M™ESPE™MDIs (experimental) and equal number of regular implants Ankylos®, Dentsply Friadent GmbH (control). Each animal received two implants on each of the hind limbs, i.e., the right and left tibia/femur heads, randomly. Therefore, each animal had a total of four implants, i.e., two experimental and two regular implants, randomly located.

Surgical procedures

The procedures were approved by the institutional animals' ethics review board of McGill University, Montreal, Canada. Adequate measures were taken into consideration

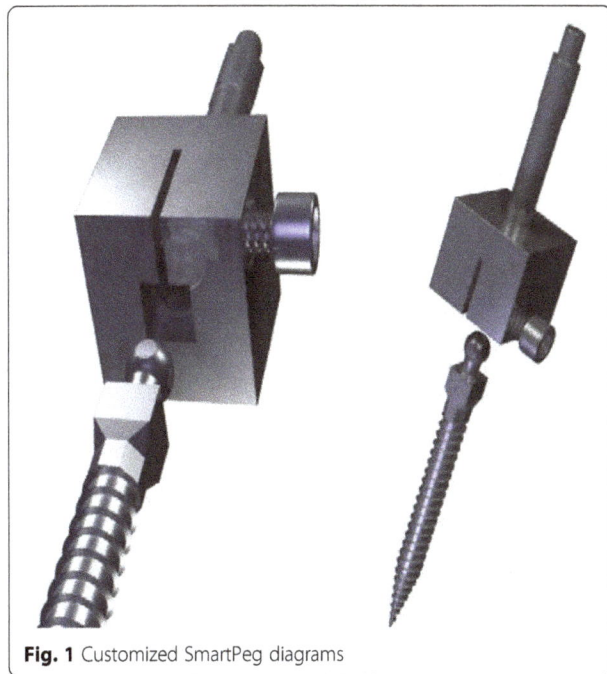

Fig. 1 Customized SmartPeg diagrams

to minimize pain and distress in the animal during the procedure. Animals were anesthetized by intravenous injections of a ketamine hydrochloride-xylazine mixture at 35–50 and 1–3 mg/kg, respectively, according to the method described by Green et al. [47]. Acepromazine was injected subcutaneously at the dosage of 1 mg/kg. Further injections of the mixture were given to maintain anesthesia, if necessary. All surgical procedures were performed in accordance with McGill's standardized operating protocol (SOP).

For the MDIs, a small longitudinal skin incision was made just distal to the tibia/femur joint. The tibia/femur head was exposed subperiosteally, and an osteotomy was performed with the pilot drill under copious irrigation with saline solution, transposing the cortical bone to the depth of 0.5 mm. The implants were aseptically transferred to the bone site and manually rotated clockwise while exerting downwards pressure to start the self-tapping process. When bony resistance was encountered, the winged thumb wrench was used for driving the implant deeper into the bone, if necessary.

Ankylos® implants were inserted in the other tibia/femur head of the animals according to the manufacturer's protocol as follows: After mobilizing the subperiosteal flap and using a 3-mm center punch to register a guiding point for the osteotomy, a twist drill, depth drill series and a conical reamer were used sequentially to complete the osteotomy and to develop a conical shape for accomodation of the implant's body. A counterclockwise rotation was used to compress the bone in case of soft bone. The tap or thread cutter was used to create the threads in dense bones. Following, the implant assembly was aseptically transferred to the osteotomy site, and the implant placement was started manually and finalized using a hand ratchet. If excessive force was experienced, the osteotomy was irrigated, and the depth was checked by retapping.

Resonance frequency assessment

Resonance frequency assessment was performed thrice, just after the insertion of the implants, using the Osstell ISQ™ device. In brief, customized SmartPegs were stabilized onto the head of the 3M™ESPE™ MDIs and Osstell company's specific SmartPeg™ devices were screwed into Ankylos® implants, taking care to ensure that no significant torquing force was applied to the implants, and the RFA was carried out. These procedures were repeated for post-euthanasia RFA.

Post-surgical treatment and euthanasia

The rabbits were given a dose of cephalexin 12 mg/kg 0.5 mL IV once intraoperatively and a postoperative analgesic, i.e., carprofen 2–4 mg/kg SC every 8 h for 3 days, according to McGill's SOP. The animals had a free access to water and food, and routine daily care followed as per McGill's SOP#524.01. The sutures were removed after 7–10 days, and the animals were euthanized at 6 weeks postoperatively. It has been shown by various authors that this period is adequate to develop a "rigid osseous interface" in rabbits [30]. An overdose of pentobarbital sodium 1 mL/kg intravenously was used for this purpose [48].

Statistical analyses

ISQ values were averaged and compared between implant types and times using Wilcoxon's matched pairs signed-rank tests at a significance level of $p < 0.05$. Statistical analysis was performed with the help of SPSS statistical software version 17.

Results

The ISQ values obtained while calibrating the customized SmartPeg were similar to in vivo results. Median ISQ values at insertion and at 6 postoperative weeks were 53.3 (IQR 8.3) and 60.5 (5.5) for the 3M™ESPE™M-DIs, and 58.5 (4.75) and 65.5 (9.3) for the Ankylos® implants, respectively, with no statistical difference (Figs. 2 and 3). The ISQ values of both 3M™ESPE™ MDI and Ankylos® (Figs. 2 and 3) increased significantly from the time of insertion to 6-week post-insertion ($p < 0.05$).

Discussion

It is important to measure the Implant Stability Quotient (ISQ) of single-piece mini dental implants as they are becoming increasingly popular, with the concomitant increase in publications demonstrating their high survival and success rates. Although the clinical use of Osstell devices is also increasing, there is lack of studies on its use with single-piece implants, which do not have internal threads. Implant Stability Quotient (ISQ) is an objective and standardized method for measuring implant stability clinically ranging from 55 to 80, with higher values usually observed in the mandible [49]. The ISQ scale has a non-linear correlation to micro mobility. With more than 700 scientific references, we now know that high stability means >70 ISQ, between 60 and 69 is medium stability, and <60 ISQ is considered as low stability.

The rabbit tibias have been used to determine longitudinal changes in the resonance frequency and measured for over 168 days from the time of implant insertion, and it was observed that resonance frequency values increased over time [38].

However, the relationship between the bone density and ISQ is not significant [50]. Therefore, higher ISQ values are a sign of bone anchorage of implants, but the relationship of resonance frequency analysis with bone structure is unclear [51–53]. ISQ values decline in the first 2 weeks after implant insertion, and these changes may be associated with early bone healing and marginal alveolar bone resorption. Bone remodeling reduces primary bone contact. In the early stage after implant placement, the formation of bony callus and increasing lamellar bone in the cortical bone causes major changes in bone density. Therefore, in the healing process, primary bone contact decreases and secondary bone contact increases [53, 32]. Degidi et al. [54] reported that there may also be a discrepancy as the histological analyses is a two-dimensional picture of the three-dimensional bone-implant contact.

If the initial ISQ value is high, a small drop in stability normally levels out with time. A big drop in stability or decrease should be taken as a warning sign. Lower values are expected to be higher after the healing period.

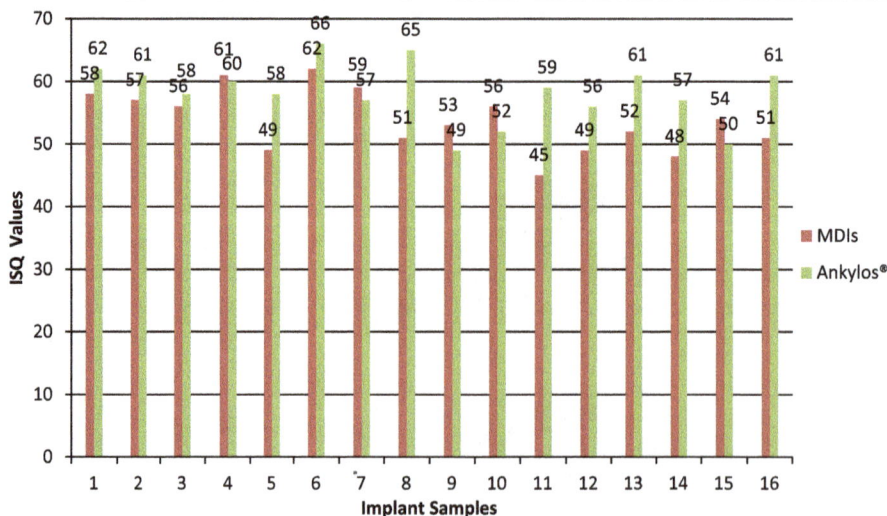

Fig. 2 ISQ values of MDIs and Ankylos® immediately upon insertion

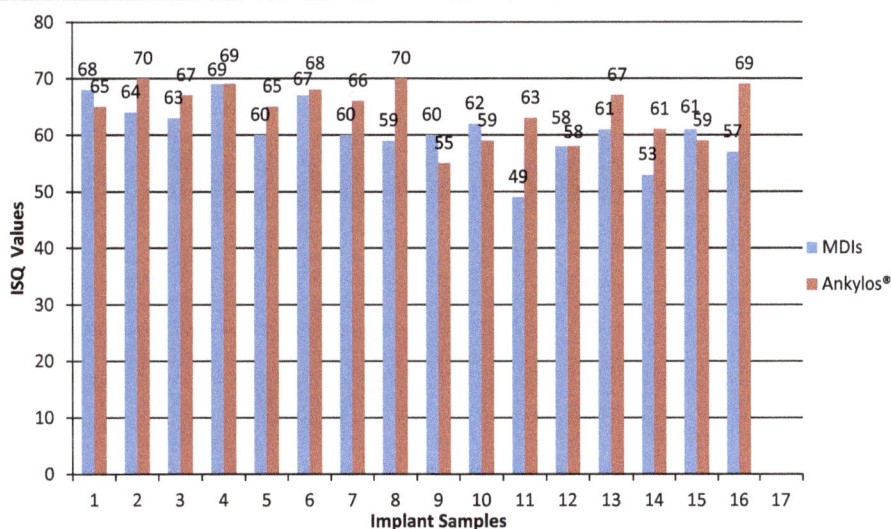

Fig. 3 ISQ values of MDIs and Ankylos® after euthanasia

The opposite could be a sign of an unsuccessful implant, and actions should be taken accordingly.

Studies have shown that the resonance frequency value is greatly associated with the quantity of bone-implant contact [31, 38]. There is a positive correlation between resonance frequency analysis and histomorphometric measurements [37]. In our histological study previously reported, similar findings were demonstrated [55].

Our results indicate that both types of implants achieved primary and secondary stability.

Several measurements may be more dependable than single measures; therefore, it may be important to measure resonance frequency multiple times and average the values in order to obtain the most reliable assessment. While reliability of resonance frequency analysis has not been established in the past for these mini dental implants used for overdentures, studies have shown similar or lower levels of reliability for regular dental implants [56].

In general, there was an increase in the ISQ values in both groups, which may be related to enhancement of rigidity between the implants and neighboring tissues and largely with the changes at the bone-implant interface. It has been demonstrated that there is a development of woven bone surrounding the implants 1 week following placement in the rabbit tibia. This scantily organized bone is resorbed by osteoclasts and slowly remodeled into the lamellar bone and gets more compacted around the implant surface and remodeled to become a mature bone over a period of 42 days [38, 57]. There seems to be minimal changes in the resonance frequency after this period. Our results are in concurrence with the study by Meredith et al. [38].

As there are no studies that provide data based on resonance frequency measurements for single-piece MDIs, the exact RFA threshold values for MDIs may have to be identified with more studies conducted in vivo.

The resonance frequency assessment with a customized SmartPeg would be a useful tool to provide clinically useful information about the condition of the bone-implant interface of 3M™ ESPE™MDIs. Frequently, implant failures are associated with biomechanical reasons; implant stability assessment can reduce this to a great extent. The higher the RFA value, the higher the success in implant treatment and the lower the risk for failure in the future. On the other hand, lower RFA values may indicate greater risk for implant complications. The MDIs are usually immediately loaded. Resonance frequency measurement technique is also of value in evaluating the immediate loading implants [58]. The results of the present study are encouraging and show that it is possible to measure ISQ for these single-piece MDIs. This study is the first of its kind and similar type of studies should be conducted among humans, to make the results more meaningful and generalizable.

Conclusions

The results of this animal study indicate that ISQ measurement of these single-piece MDIs is possible with the help of a custom-made SmartPeg and that 3M™ESPE™MDIs attain primary and secondary stability at the same levels as standard implants in the rabbit tibia.

Authors' contributions
JSD carried out the experiments and drafted the manuscript, RA conceived the study and helped in revising the manuscript, AF contributed to the designing the SmartPeg, SK helped in the data analysis, JSF participated in this study's design and overall coordination. All authors read and approved the final manuscript.

Competing interests

Jagjit Singh Dhaliwal, Rubens F. Albuquerque Jr, Ali Fakhry, Sukhbir Kaur, and Jocelyne S. Feine declare that they have no competing interests.

Author details

[1]Faculty of Dentistry, McGill University, 2001 McGill College Avenue, Suite 500, Montreal, Quebec H3A 1G1, Canada. [2]Faculty of Dentistry of Ribeirão Preto, University of São Paulo, Ribeirão Preto, SP, Brazil. [3]Department of Zoology, Panjab University, Chandigarh, India. [4]PAPRSB Institute of Health Sciences, Universiti Brunei Darussalam, Brunei Darussalam.

References

1. Branemark PI, Adell R, Breine U, Hansson BO, Lindstrom J, Ohlsson A. Intra-osseous anchorage of dental prostheses. I. Experimental studies. Scand J Plast Reconstr Surg. 1969;3(2):81–100. Epub 1969/01/01.
2. Meredith N. Assessment of implant stability as a prognostic determinant. Int J Prosthodont. 1998;11(5):491–501. Epub 1999/01/29.
3. Lioubavina-Hack N, Lang NP, Karring T. Significance of primary stability for osseointegration of dental implants. Clin Oral Implants Res. 2006;17(3):244–50. Epub 2006/05/05.
4. Albrektsson T, Dahl E, Enbom L, Engevall S, Engquist B, Eriksson AR, et al. Osseointegrated oral implants. A Swedish multicenter study of 8139 consecutively inserted nobelpharma implants. J Periodontol. 1988;59(5):287–96. Epub 1988/05/01.
5. Bornstein MM, Valderrama P, Jones AA, Wilson TG, Seibl R, Cochran DL. Bone apposition around two different sandblasted and acid-etched titanium implant surfaces: a histomorphometric study in canine mandibles. Clin Oral Implants Res. 2008;19(3):233–41. Epub 2008/01/08.
6. Bulard RA, Vance JB. Multi-clinic evaluation using mini-dental implants for long-term denture stabilization: a preliminary biometric evaluation. Compend Contin Educ Dent. 2005;26(12):892–7. Epub 2006/01/05.
7. Diedrich P, Fritz U, Kinzinger G, Angelakis J. Movement of periodontally affected teeth after guided tissue regeneration (GTR)—an experimental pilot study in animals. J Orofac Orthop. 2003;64(3):214–27. Epub 2003/07/02.
8. Buchter A, Kleinheinz J, Wiesmann HP, Jayaranan M, Joos U, Meyer U. Interface reaction at dental implants inserted in condensed bone. Clin Oral Implants Res. 2005;16(5):509–17. Epub 2005/09/17.
9. Kwon KR, Sachdeo A, Weber HP. Achieving immediate function with provisional prostheses after implant placement: a clinical report. J Prosthet Dent. 2005;93(6):514–7. Epub 2005/06/09.
10. Kokubo Y, Ohkubo C. Occlusion recording device for dental implant-supported restorations. J Prosthet Dent. 2006;95(3):262–3. Epub 2006/03/18.
11. Ohkubo C, Kobayashi M, Suzuki Y, Sato J, Hosoi T, Kurtz KS. Evaluation of transitional implant stabilized overdentures: a case series report. J Oral Rehabil. 2006;33(6):416–22. Epub 2006/05/05.
12. Campelo LD, Camara JR. Flapless implant surgery: a 10-year clinical retrospective analysis. Int J Oral Maxillofac Implants. 2002;17(2):271–6. Epub 2002/04/18.
13. Shatkin TE, Oppenheimer BD, Oppenheimer AJ. Mini dental implants for long-term fixed and removable prosthetics: a retrospective analysis of 2514 implants placed over a five-year period. Compend Contin Educ Dent. 2007; 28(2):92–9. quiz 100-1. Epub 2007/02/27.
14. Griffitts TM, Collins CP, Collins PC. Mini dental implants: an adjunct for retention, stability, and comfort for the edentulous patient. Oral Surg Oral Med Oral Pathol Oral Radiol Endod. 2005;100(5):e81–4. Epub 2005/10/26.
15. Albrektsson T, Sennerby L. State of the art in oral implants. J Clin Periodontol. 1991;18(6):474–81. Epub 1991/07/01.
16. Atsumi M, Park SH, Wang HL. Methods used to assess implant stability: current status. Int J Oral Maxillofac Implants. 2007;22(5):743–54. Epub 2007/11/03.
17. Davies JE. Mechanisms of endosseous integration. Int J Prosthodont. 1998; 11(5):391–401. Epub 1999/01/29.
18. Romanos GE. Bone quality and the immediate loading of implants-critical aspects based on literature, research, and clinical experience. Implant Dent. 2009;18(3):203–9. Epub 2009/06/11.
19. Cawley P, Pavlakovic B, Alleyne DN, George R, Back T, Meredith N. The design of a vibration transducer to monitor the integrity of dental implants. Proc Inst Mech Eng H J Eng Med. 1998;212(4):265–72. Epub 1998/10/14.
20. Szmukler-Moncler S, Salama H, Reingewirtz Y, Dubruille JH. Timing of loading and effect of micromotion on bone-dental implant interface: review of experimental literature. J Biomed Mater Res. 1998;43(2):192–203. Epub 1998/06/10.
21. Wilmes B, Rademacher C, Olthoff G, Drescher D. Parameters affecting primary stability of orthodontic mini-implants. J Orofac Orthop. 2006;67(3): 162–74. Epub 2006/06/01.
22. Boice GW, Kraut RA. Maxillary denture retention using rare earth magnets and endosteal implants. Int J Oral Implantol. 1991;7(2):23–7. Epub 1991/01/01.
23. Sullivan DY, Sherwood RL, Collins TA, Krogh PH. The reverse-torque test: a clinical report. Int J Oral Maxillofac Implants. 1996;11(2):179–85. Epub 1996/03/01.
24. Branemark R, Ohrnell LO, Nilsson P, Thomsen P. Biomechanical characterization of osseointegration during healing: an experimental in vivo study in the rat. Biomaterials. 1997;18(14):969–78. Epub 1997/07/01.
25. Branemark R, Ohrnell LO, Skalak R, Carlsson L, Branemark PI. Biomechanical characterization of osseointegration: an experimental in vivo investigation in the beagle dog. J Orthop Res. 1998;16(1):61–9. Epub 1998/05/09.
26. Ersanli S, Karabuda C, Beck F, Leblebicioglu B. Resonance frequency analysis of one-stage dental implant stability during the osseointegration period. J Periodontol. 2005;76(7):1066–71. Epub 2005/07/16.
27. Bornstein MM, Chappuis V, von Arx T, Buser D. Performance of dental implants after staged sinus floor elevation procedures: 5-year results of a prospective study in partially edentulous patients. Clin Oral Implants Res. 2008;19(10):1034–43. Epub 2008/10/03.
28. Boronat Lopez A, Balaguer Martinez J, Lamas Pelayo J, Carrillo Garcia C, Penarrocha DM. Resonance frequency analysis of dental implant stability during the healing period. Med Oral Patol Oral Cir Bucal. 2008;13(4):E244–7. Epub 2008/04/02.
29. Quesada-Garcia MP, Prados-Sanchez E, Olmedo-Gaya MV, Munoz-Soto E, Gonzalez-Rodriguez MP, Valllecillo-Capilla M. Measurement of dental implant stability by resonance frequency analysis: a review of the literature. Med Oral Patol Oral Cir Bucal. 2009;14(10):e538–46. Epub 2009/08/15.
30. Guler AU, Duran I, Yucel AC, Ozkan P. Effects of air-polishing powders on color stability of composite resins. J Appl Oral Sci. 2011;19(5):505–10. Epub 2011/09/17.
31. Friberg B, Sennerby L, Meredith N, Lekholm U. A comparison between cutting torque and resonance frequency measurements of maxillary implants. A 20-month clinical study. Int J Oral Maxillofac Surg. 1999;28(4): 297–303. Epub 1999/07/23.
32. Barewal RM, Oates TW, Meredith N, Cochran DL. Resonance frequency measurement of implant stability in vivo on implants with a sandblasted and acid-etched surface. Int J Oral Maxillofac Implants. 2003;18(5):641–51. Epub 2003/10/29.
33. Glauser R, Sennerby L, Meredith N, Ree A, Lundgren A, Gottlow J, et al. Resonance frequency analysis of implants subjected to immediate or early functional occlusal loading. Successful vs. failing implants. Clin Oral Implants Res. 2004;15(4):428–34. Epub 2004/07/14.
34. Sjostrom M, Lundgren S, Nilson H, Sennerby L. Monitoring of implant stability in grafted bone using resonance frequency analysis. A clinical study from implant placement to 6 months of loading. Int J Oral Maxillofac Surg. 2005;34(1):45–51. Epub 2004/12/25.
35. Gallucci GO, Belser UC, Bernard JP, Magne P. Modeling and characterization of the CEJ for optimization of esthetic implant design. Int J Periodontics Restorative Dent. 2004;24(1):19–29. Epub 2004/02/27.
36. Meredith N, Book K, Friberg B, Jemt T, Sennerby L. Resonance frequency measurements of implant stability in vivo. A cross-sectional and longitudinal study of resonance frequency measurements on implants in the edentulous and partially dentate maxilla. Clin Oral Implants Res. 1997;8(3):226–33. Epub 1997/06/01.
37. Meredith N, Alleyne D, Cawley P. Quantitative determination of the stability of the implant-tissue interface using resonance frequency analysis. Clin Oral Implants Res. 1996;7(3):261–7. Epub 1996/09/01.
38. Meredith N, Shagaldi F, Alleyne D, Sennerby L, Cawley P. The application of resonance frequency measurements to study the stability of titanium implants during healing in the rabbit tibia. Clin Oral Implants Res. 1997;8(3): 234–43. Epub 1997/06/01.
39. Steigenga J, Al-Shammari K, Misch C, Nociti Jr FH, Wang HL. Effects of implant thread geometry on percentage of osseointegration and resistance to reverse torque in the tibia of rabbits. J Periodontol. 2004;75(9):1233–41. Epub 2004/11/02.
40. Le Guehennec L, Goyenvalle E, Lopez-Heredia MA, Weiss P, Amouriq Y, Layrolle P. Histomorphometric analysis of the osseointegration of four different implant surfaces in the femoral epiphyses of rabbits. Clin Oral Implants Res. 2008;19(11):1103–10. Epub 2008/11/06.
41. Faeda RS, Tavares HS, Sartori R, Guastaldi AC, Marcantonio Jr E. Evaluation of titanium implants with surface modification by laser beam. Biomechanical study in rabbit tibias. Braz Oral Res. 2009;23(2):137–43. Epub 2009/08/18.
42. Park JW, Kim HK, Kim YJ, An CH, Hanawa T. Enhanced osteoconductivity of micro-structured titanium implants (XiVE S CELLplus) by addition of surface

calcium chemistry: a histomorphometric study in the rabbit femur. Clin Oral Implants Res. 2009;20(7):684–90. Epub 2009/06/06.

43. Yang GL, He FM, Hu JA, Wang XX, Zhao SF. Effects of biomimetically and electrochemically deposited nano-hydroxyapatite coatings on osseointegration of porous titanium implants. Oral Surg Oral Med Oral Pathol Oral Radiol Endod. 2009;107(6):782–9. Epub 2009/02/10.

44. Yildiz A, Esen E, Kurkcu M, Damlar I, Daglioglu K, Akova T. Effect of zoledronic acid on osseointegration of titanium implants: an experimental study in an ovariectomized rabbit model. J Oral Maxillofac Surg. 2010;68(3): 515–23. Epub 2010/02/23.

45. Barros RR, Novaes Jr AB, Muglia VA, Iezzi G, Piattelli A. Influence of interimplant distances and placement depth on peri-implant bone remodeling of adjacent and immediately loaded Morse cone connection implants: a histomorphometric study in dogs. Clin Oral Implants Res. 2010; 21(4):371–8. Epub 2010/02/05.

46. Marin C, Bonfante EA, Granato R, Suzuki M, Granjeiro JM, Coelho PG. The effect of alterations on resorbable blasting media processed implant surfaces on early bone healing: a study in rabbits. Implant Dent. 2011;20(2): 167–77. Epub 2011/03/31.

47. Green CJ, Knight J, Precious S, Simpkin S. Ketamine alone and combined with diazepam or xylazine in laboratory animals: a 10 year experience. Lab Anim. 1981;15(2):163–70. Epub 1981/04/01.

48. Chen J, Zhang Y, Rong M, Zhao L, Jiang L, Zhang D, et al. Expression and characterization of jingzhaotoxin-34, a novel neurotoxin from the venom of the tarantula Chilobrachys jingzhao. Peptides. 2009;30(6):1042–8. Epub 2009/05/26.

49. Morris HF, Ochi S, Orenstein IH, Petrazzuolo V. AICRG, Part V: factors influencing implant stability at placement and their influence on survival of Ankylos implants. J Oral Implantol. 2004;30(3):162–70. Epub 2004/07/17.

50. Manresa C, Bosch M, Echeverria JJ. The comparison between implant stability quotient and bone-implant contact revisited: an experiment in Beagle dog. Clin Oral Implants Res. 2014;25(11):1213–21. Epub 2013/10/10.

51. Alsaadi G, Quirynen M, Michiels K, Jacobs R, van Steenberghe D. A biomechanical assessment of the relation between the oral implant stability at insertion and subjective bone quality assessment. J Clin Periodontol. 2007;34(4):359–66. Epub 2007/03/24.

52. Huwiler MA, Pjetursson BE, Bosshardt DD, Salvi GE, Lang NP. Resonance frequency analysis in relation to jawbone characteristics and during early healing of implant installation. Clin Oral Implants Res. 2007;18(3):275–80. Epub 2007/03/16.

53. Zhou Y, Jiang T, Qian M, Zhang X, Wang J, Shi B, et al. Roles of bone scintigraphy and resonance frequency analysis in evaluating osseointegration of endosseous implant. Biomaterials. 2008;29(4):461–74. Epub 2007/11/07.

54. Degidi M, Perrotti V, Piattelli A, Iezzi G. Mineralized bone-implant contact and implant stability quotient in 16 human implants retrieved after early healing periods: a histologic and histomorphometric evaluation. Int J Oral Maxillofac Implants. 2010;25(1):45–8. Epub 2010/03/09.

55. Dhaliwal J, Albuquerque R, Murshed, M, Tamimi, F, Feine, JS. A histomorphometric comparison of osseointegration with MDIs and standard implants. IADR/AADR/ CADR 91st General Session, Seattle, Washington, USA, March 20–23, 2013

56. Zix J, Hug S, Kessler-Liechti G, Mericske-Stern R. Measurement of dental implant stability by resonance frequency analysis and damping capacity assessment: comparison of both techniques in a clinical trial. Int J Oral Maxillofac Implants. 2008;23(3):525–30. Epub 2008/08/15.

57. Roberts WE, Smith RK, Zilberman Y, Mozsary PG, Smith RS. Osseous adaptation to continuous loading of rigid endosseous implants. Am J Orthod. 1984;86(2):95–111. Epub 1984/08/01.

58. Ostman PO, Hellman M, Albrektsson T, Sennerby L. Direct loading of nobel direct and nobel perfect one-piece implants: a 1-year prospective clinical and radiographic study. Clin Oral Implants Res. 2007;18(4):409–18. Epub 2007/05/16.

15

A novel report on the use of an oncology zygomatic implant-retained maxillary obturator in a paediatric patient

Amit Dattani[1], David Richardson[2] and Chris J. Butterworth[3*]

Abstract

This report details the use of zygomatic oncology osseointegrated implants to support and retain a maxillary obturator in a 13-year-old male patient who underwent a right-sided hemi-maxillectomy (Brown Class 2b) (Brown and Shaw, Lancet Oncol 11:1001–8, 2010) for a myxoid spindle cell carcinoma. At the time of maxillary resection, two zygomatic oncology implants were inserted into the right zygomatic body and subsequently utilised to provide in-defect support and retention for a bar-retained maxillary acrylic obturator prosthesis, which restored the patient's aesthetics and function to a very high level. Close follow-up over 2 years demonstrated ongoing excellent function and disease control with no deleterious effects on facial or dento-alveolar growth clinically. This is the first clinical report of its kind in the published literature detailing the use of a zygomatic implant-retained obturator in a paediatric patient.

Keywords: Zygomatic Implant, Hemi-maxillectomy, Oncology implant, Maxillary obturator, Zygomatic fixtures, Myxoid spindle cell carcinoma

Background

Maxillary defects of acquired [1] or congenital origin produce a communication between the oral and nasal cavities sometimes via an opening into the maxillary antrum and by direct communication into the nose. This in turn can result in masticatory compromise, swallowing and speech impairment, nasal fluid regurgitation and aesthetic concerns. The management of the maxillectomy patient is a complex area where there is still much debate [2], but in the paediatric patient, there is virtually no literature detailing the most appropriate approach. The use of microvascular free-tissue transfer has gained in popularity over time in adults in order to effect a biological closure of the resulting oro-nasal communication, but in the paediatric patient with maxillary malignancy, the use of a prosthetic obturator is more commonly reported [3]. The use of free-tissue transfer in children in the maxillofacial region seems to be mainly restricted to reconstruction of the mandible from the reviewed available literature [4] presumably because prosthetic obturation can offer good results in the maxilla and defer additional complex surgeries to a later date.

An obturator is a custom-made denture prosthesis that is used to close the communication with the antrum/nose in order to allow satisfactory mastication and speech. In the dentate patient, maxillary obturator prostheses may be retained by the natural dentition together with the engagement of undercuts within the maxillary defect itself. The use of osseointegrated implants to assist with the retention of a maxillary obturator has been reported [5]; utilising both dental implants into the residual alveolus and, more recently, the use of zygomatic implants in large maxillectomy defects has also been described [6]. Osseointegrated zygomatic implants provide rigid support and retention for the overlying implant-retained obturator with two, three [7] or four zygomatic implants being used for rehabilitation of a bilateral maxillectomy resection. There is no real information available on the use of zygomatic implants in the support and retention of obturator prostheses for unilateral maxillary defects in the dentate patient, but this situation mandates the use of two implants to allow splinting and

* Correspondence: c.butterworth@liv.ac.uk
[3]Maxillofacial Prosthodontics, Regional Maxillofacial Unit, University Hospital Aintree, Longmoor Lane, Liverpool L9 7AL, UK
Full list of author information is available at the end of the article

bar construction to provide the best available support. Whilst the use of conventional zygomatic implants is possible in this clinical approach, the use of zygomatic implants manufactured specifically for use in maxillectomy situations possess some advantages. The zygomatic oncology implant (Southern Implants Ltd, South Africa) (Fig. 1) has a 20-mm threaded apical portion for engagement in the zygoma bone with the rest of the implant having a polished surface where it extends into the maxillectomy cavity. This improves the patient's ability to clean the implant and the defect and reduces the adherence of nasal secretions and food debris. The 55° angulated implant platform head also facilitates screwdriver access and brings it directly into the line of the prosthodontic arch.

The characteristics of a good obturator will improve swallowing, speech function, minimise nasal fluid leakage from the antrum and nasal spaces, restore facial aesthetics including the teeth and facilitate masticatory function and speech. A surgical obturator can be provided at the time of surgery to facilitate function and haemostasis in the immediate post-operative period, and this can subsequently be replaced with a more definitive prosthesis once the maxillary defect has healed to a more stable condition.

To date, no literature exists on the fabrication of an implant-retained maxillary obturator for a paediatric patient, and this case presentation describes the use of zygomatic oncology implants together with the rationale for their use in a paediatric patient.

Case presentation

A medically fit and well 13-year 11-month-old male was referred to the oral and maxillofacial surgery department at Alder Hey Children's Hospital in Liverpool in regard to an intra-oral swelling of the right palatal region (Fig. 2). An incisional biopsy was initially reported as a pleomorphic adenoma of the premolar region. Subsequently, a CT scan showed no significant bony abnormality, and a wide local excision was carried out with the application of a surgical palatal dressing plate. Histopathology of this resected tissue appeared to show

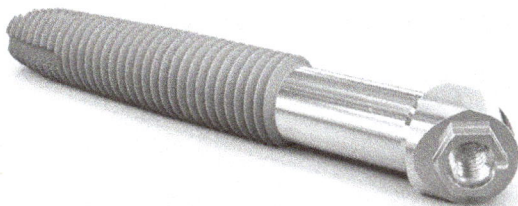

Fig. 1 Zygomatic oncology implant with cleansable polished surface for intra-oral component

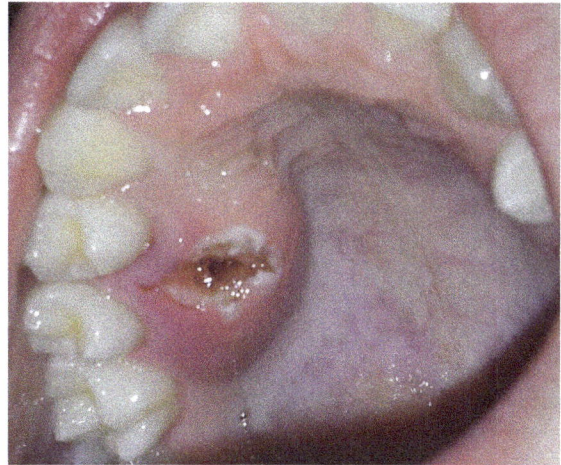

Fig. 2 Palatal swelling (post-biopsy) between upper right first and second premolar teeth

tumour of intermediate malignant grade at the base of the specimen.

Further investigations undertaken to stage the tumour included a repeat CT scan which presented no evidence of significant bony involvement or erosion. An MRI scan showed no significant asymmetry or signal abnormality in the region of the hard palate, and there was no evidence of loco-regional metastasis of this tumour.

Following a discussion of the craniofacial multidisciplinary team and numerous paediatric pathologists, a diagnosis of intermediate-grade sarcoma of the oral mucosa and hard palate was re-affirmed. A partial right-sided maxillectomy was planned to gain adequate tumour clearance, and prior to surgery, the patient attended for dental impressions and counselling regarding the procedures involved, together with instructions regarding the obturator prosthesis.

A low-level right-sided standard hemi-maxillectomy was carried out via an intra-oral approach with preservation of the pterygoid plates (December 2013). The anterior alveolar cut was undertaken through the right lateral incisor socket following the extraction of this tooth in order to maximise the bone support on the maxillary central incisor abutment tooth. The residual zygomatic body on the right side was exposed, and two 37-mm zygomatic oncology implants (Southern Implants Ltd, South Africa) (Fig. 3) were placed with excellent stability, ensuring that the prosthetic heads were positioned beneath the body of the obturator prosthesis and in a useful position for retention of the obturator. The posterior aspect of the cavity was dressed using the buccal pad of fat and the right inferior turbinate removed to facilitate access to the defect for the obturator. An interim prosthetic obturator was fitted and relined with silicone putty material and retained by dental clasps and a single

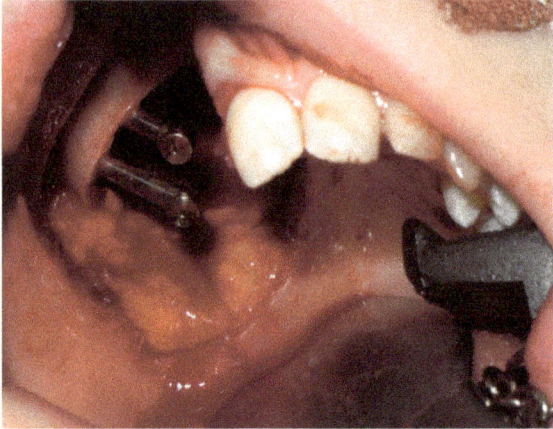

Fig. 3 Low-level right-sided maxillectomy with the insertion of two zygomatic oncology implants at time of surgery

bone screw into the midline of the remaining palatal bone. Recovery from the procedure was uneventful, and the patient was discharged home the following day. Histopathology confirmed the diagnosis of myxoid spindle cell carcinoma of the right maxilla excised with good margins with no need for adjuvant treatment.

Four weeks later, the patient was returned to the operating room for removal and modification of the obturator. The cavity was healing well, and both implants were firm with no evidence of infection. The initial obturator was modified with the application of a soft lining material and the patient subsequently discharged with instructions on the insertion and removal of the obturator.

At the 12-week review (Fig. 4), it was noted the patient had a degree of mucosal polypoidosis in the antral cavity, most probably plaque induced, where the

patient found it difficult to clean around the implants. Oral hygiene instruction was reiterated, and construction of the definitive implant bar-retained obturator was commenced.

Four months following surgery (April 2014), a definitive implant bar-retained maxillary obturator was fitted utilising precision attachments (Rhein attachments, Rhein83, NY, USA.) (Figs. 5 and 6). The retention and support given by the obturator was excellent, and the patient and parents were very pleased with the aesthetic and functional outcome (Figs. 7, 8, 9 and 10) provided by this prosthetic rehabilitation. The patient was put on a regular maintenance programme of review at 6-month intervals and continued to display an excellent standard of oral hygiene around the implants and to report a high degree of oral functioning using it. All mucosal polyposis resolved very quickly following the patient's improved hygiene measures. He continued under review with no evidence of recurrence or problems with the implants or prosthesis in the 22 months since the surgery. The plastic Rhein female attachments were replaced at 18 months, but no other modifications have been required to this obturator since it was fitted. A recent radiographic review (Fig. 11) demonstrated no significant peri-implant bone resorption, and clinically, there had been no alteration in facial growth or appearance (Fig. 12) of this young patient who was 16 years of age at the time of his final review (February 2017). He continues under regular review.

Discussion

The paediatric population rarely suffer malignant disease of the oral cavity requiring any form of maxillectomy, and there is little published evidence around the rehabilitation and restorative management of children undergoing such procedures. The seemingly most common approach for a limited low-level maxillary resection in a child would be to consider resection and simple prosthetic obturation as this allows relatively simple

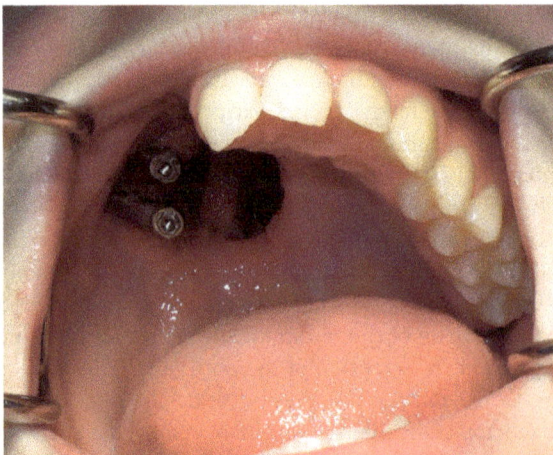

Fig. 4 Twelve-week review post-surgery prior to definitive impressions for the implant-supported prosthesis

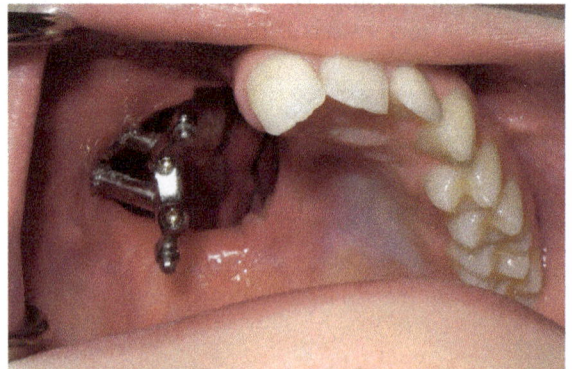

Fig. 5 Zygomatic implant bar utilising Rhein attachments for retention

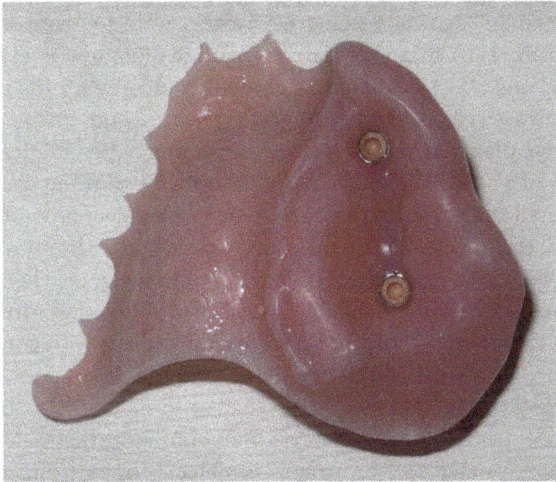

Fig. 6 Intaglio surface of definitive acrylic obturator with bar attachments in place. Note the absence of any other retaining clasps and the simple nature of this prosthesis

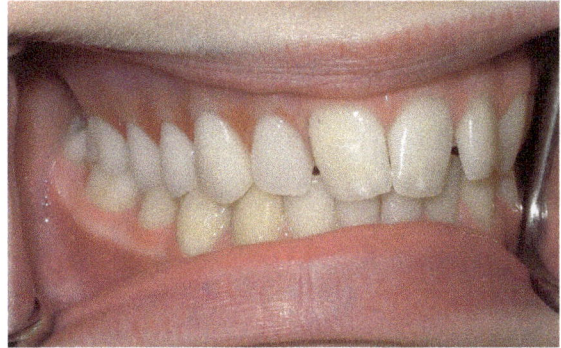

Fig. 8 Anterior view of definitive obturator prosthesis in occlusion

management of the tumour from a surgical point of view as well as immediate functional and aesthetic rehabilitation with a prosthesis. It also allows for full histopathological examination of the resected specimen to ensure complete resection of the tumour before committing the patient to any form of complex surgical reconstruction which could be planned at a later date should the patient wish. The delivery of a maxillary obturator improves quality of life significantly by primarily restoring aesthetic and functional modalities. It also serves as a purpose to allow correct phonation of speech, prevent nasal discharge of masticatory contents and facilitate swallowing. The aesthetic and psychological benefits of facial restoration are paramount in a child undergoing such a procedure. The use of microvascular reconstruction techniques have allowed for autogenous tissue reconstruction

of maxillary defects with either soft or hard tissue. The use of a soft-tissue-only reconstruction such as a radial forearm flap in this clinical situation would prevent successful dental rehabilitation as the soft tissue flap provides no support for the dental prosthesis and, apart from the separation of the oral and nasal cavities, provides no advantage for the patient. The use of a composite-bone-containing flap such as the fibula flap has the potential to provide oro-nasal separation as well as bone to support an implant-retained prosthesis, and with the latest digital technologies, this can be provided rapidly in carefully selected cases [8], although this mode of rapid rehabilitation is not available in many centres. However, there is no published data on this mode of dental rehabilitation in a growing child currently, and this approach should probably be deferred until all mandibular growth has been completed. The use of microvascular reconstruction, in addition, carries with it significant clinical risks as well as potential donor site morbidity and flap failure as well as the potential for fibrous union and loss of individual bony segments where multiple osteotomies are required.

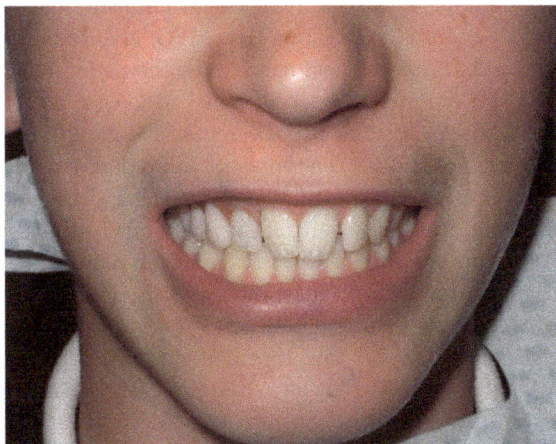

Fig. 7 Smile view of definitive implant-retained obturator at initial fitting (April 2014)

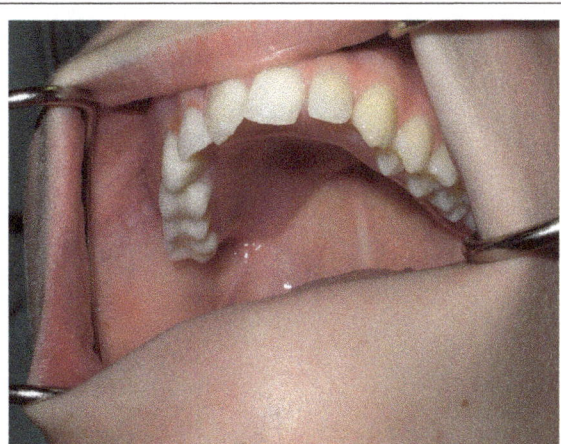

Fig. 9 Palatal view of definitive implant-retained obturator at initial fitting (April 2014)

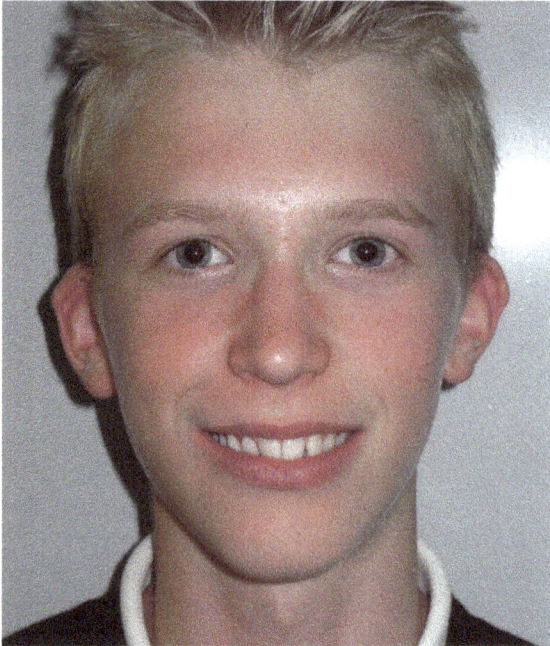

Fig. 10 Full facial view of definitive implant-retained obturator at initial fitting (April 2014)

The difficulty of restoration with a maxillary obturator prosthesis depends on the extent of the surgical resection, with the acceptance that resections with an increasing horizontal component provide a much greater prosthodontic challenge. The number of remaining teeth is a key

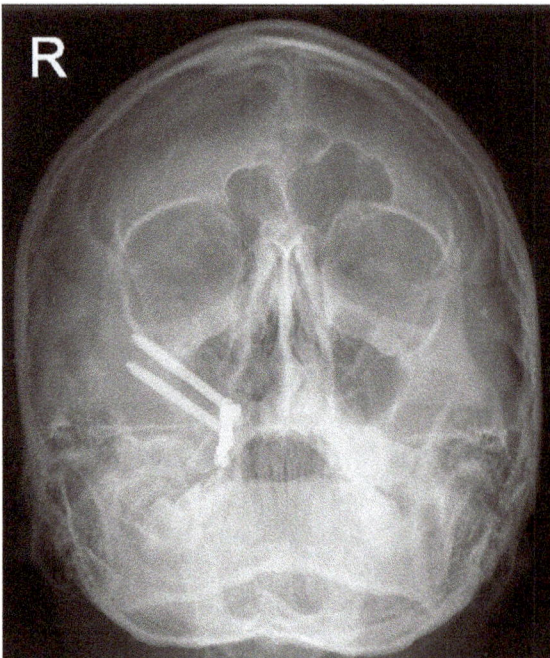

Fig. 11 Facial radiograph at 22-month follow-up

component in conventional obturator design [9] with the remaining dentition being used exclusively to retain the prosthesis by means of clasps which are often in the visual field and affect the resulting aesthetic outcome for the patient as well as placing significant forces onto them. In conventional maxillary defect preparation, the additional use of a split skin graft into the lateral aspect of the cheek is used to provide a scar band to aid with defect retention, and this brings added morbidity to the procedure especially for a paediatric patient. In conventional hemi-maxillectomy cases, gaining some form of retention from the defect is essential in providing the patient with confidence in the use of the prosthesis, and the discomfort associated with this can make paediatric patients anxious about placing and removing the obturator themselves. The advantages of providing "in-defect" support and retention by means of zygomatic implant placement addresses all of these potential difficulties and allows the construction of a simple highly polished acrylic prosthesis that does not require clasping of the teeth in the aesthetic zone, requires very little extension into the defect to affect a peripheral seal and most of all provides good support when the patient masticates on the defect side. No additional skin grafting is required, and the placement and retrieval of the prosthesis is comfortable and atraumatic. Maintenance of the prosthesis is simple with modifications to the peripheral seal as required at the chair side and replacement of the bar attachments from time to time.

In a paediatric patient, the development and subsequent growth of facial skeleton is an added concern, although by age 13/14, the major mid-face growth will be largely completed [10]. Certainly in this case, the bone volume of the zygomatic body was more than adequate for the placement of the implants. In terms of ongoing facial growth, Min Kim et al. report a case where an 11-year-old male underwent a hemi-maxillectomy and a modified functional obturator (MFO) prosthesis was successfully used to obturate the defect and restore aesthetics and function. After 18 months of wearing the MFO, the result was stable, and at 3 years post-operatively, the patient's facial profile was reported as near normal. In the case reported here, it was felt that due to the removable nature of the obturator prosthesis, the implant technique employed would allow for the construction of a new maxillary obturator in the event of any significant continued mid-facial/maxillary growth, which so far has not been required.

The use of modified zygomatic implants (Fig. 1) allows improved hygiene by the patient of the implants within the maxillary defect. The threaded portion of the implants is fully engaged into the bone with only the smooth portion protruding into the defect. Clearly this ongoing hygiene by the patient is of utmost importance in preventing peri-implant soft and hard tissue changes, but the implant design here has facilitated that

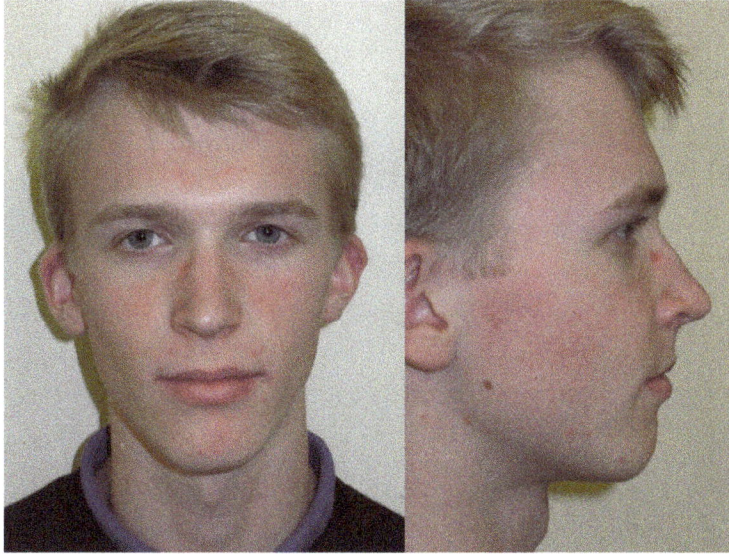

Fig. 12 Facial photograph views at 22-month follow-up

extremely well in this young patient, and no additional professionally directed hygiene measures to maintain excellent peri-implant health have been required to date.

The evidence for loading zygomatic implants immediately is very clear in the literature [11] in a cross-arch manner but not in a unilateral situation as has been utilised in this case. Whilst the stability of the implants achieved at surgery was excellent, it was decided to adopt a delayed loading approach which also gave time for the maxillectomy defect to stabilise prior to the construction of the definitive prosthesis.

Conclusions

The use of zygomatic implants to supplement the stability and retention of the maxillary obturator in this case has improved the function of the prosthesis and provided for a very high-quality rehabilitation for the patient reported with no evidence of disruption to facial growth in the 22 months following surgery.

Authors' contributions
DR and CB carried out the treatment of the patient referred to in this case report. AD carried out the literature review and initial draft of the manuscript. DR helped to draft the manuscript, and CB coordinated the case report, revised and edited the manuscript. All authors read and approved the final manuscript.

Competing interests
Amit Dattani (AD), David Richardson (DR) and Chris Butterworth (CB) declare that they have no competing interests.

Author details
[1]Oral and Maxillofacial Surgery, Regional Maxillofacial Unit, University Hospital Aintree, Liverpool, UK. [2]Maxillofacial Surgery, Regional Craniofacial Unit, Alder Hey Children's Hospital, Liverpool, UK. [3]Maxillofacial Prosthodontics, Regional Maxillofacial Unit, University Hospital Aintree, Longmoor Lane, Liverpool L9 7AL, UK.

References
1. Brown JS, Shaw RJ. Reconstruction of the maxilla and midface: introducing a new classification. Lancet Oncol. 2010;11(10):1001–8.
2. Breeze J, Rennie A, Morrison A, Dawson D, Tipper J, Rehman K, et al. Health-related quality of life after maxillectomy: obturator rehabilitation compared with flap reconstruction. Br J Oral Maxillofac Surg. 2016;54(8):857–62.
3. Kim SM, Park MW, Cho YA, Myoung H, Lee JH, Lee SK. Modified functional obturator for the consideration of facial growth in the mucoepidermoid carcinoma pediatric patient. Int J Pediatr Otorhinolaryngol. 2015;79(10): 1761–4.
4. Ducic Y, Young L. Improving aesthetic outcomes in pediatric free tissue oromandibular reconstruction. Arch Facial Plast Surg. 2011;13(3):180–4.
5. Leles CR, Leles JL, de Paula SC, Martins RR, Mendonca EF. Implant-supported obturator overdenture for extensive maxillary resection patient: a clinical report. J Prosthodont. 2010;19(3):240–4.
6. Celakil T, Ayvalioglu DC, Sancakli E, Atalay B, Doganay O, Kayhan KB. Zygoma implant-supported prosthetic rehabilitation of a patient after bilateral maxillectomy. J Craniofac Surg. 2015;26(7):e620–2.
7. D'Agostino A, Antonio D, Procacci P, Pasquale P, Ferrari F, Trevisiol L, et al. Zygoma implant-supported prosthetic rehabilitation of a patient after subtotal bilateral maxillectomy. J Craniofac Surg. 2013;24(2):e159–62.
8. Runyan CM, Sharma V, Staffenberg DA, Levine JP, Brecht LE, Wexler LH, et al. Jaw in a day: state of the art in maxillary reconstruction. J Craniofac Surg. 2016;27(8):2101–4.
9. Okay DJ, Genden E, Buchbinder D, Urken M. Prosthodontic guidelines for surgical reconstruction of the maxilla: a classification system of defects. J Prosthet Dent. 2001;86(4):352–63.
10. Lux CJ, Conradt C, Burden D, Komposch G. Three-dimensional analysis of maxillary and mandibular growth increments. Cleft Palate Craniofac J. 2004; 41(3):304–14.
11. Chrcanovic BR, Albrektsson T, Wennerberg A. Survival and complications of zygomatic implants: an updated systematic review. J Oral Maxillofac Surg. 2016;74(10):1949–64.

16

Comparison of three different methods of internal sinus lifting for elevation heights of 7 mm: an ex vivo study

Aghiad Yassin Alsabbagh[1]* , Mohammed Monzer Alsabbagh[1], Batol Darjazini Nahas[2] and Salam Rajih[3]

Abstract

Background: Various techniques are available for elevating the sinus membrane. The aim of this study is to evaluate three methods of indirect sinus floor elevation regarding elevation heights of 7 mm on the outcomes of membrane perforation, length of perforation, and time required to perform the procedure.

Methods: Three different methods for indirect sinus lifting, bone added osteotome sinus floor elevation (BAOSFE), sinus floor elevation with an inflatable balloon, and crestal approach system (CAS kit) from OSSTEM, were assessed for their ability to lift the sinus without causing laceration of the Schneiderian membrane. The study was performed on 18 freshly slaughtered sheep heads (36 sinus lifts were done, 12 for each method). CBCT images of the heads were taken to assess the best location for the sinus lift. Then, the heads were bisected and the membrane was exposed from the medial aspect. After that, each method was performed. The intended elevation height was 7 mm. If the 7 mm were not reached, the maximum height of elevation was measured.

Results: The method used was significantly associated with the occurrence of perforation (p value = 0.014) where BAOSFE was associated with the largest number of perforations (58.4%, n = 7) compared to 8.3% and 8.3% for the balloon and CAS kit methods, respectively. The odds ratio for perforation occurrence from BAOSFE compared to the CAS kit was significant (OR = 0.091, p = .022). No significant odds ratio was found for the balloon method compared to CAS kit. Additionally, the method used was significantly associated with time of operation and with the length of perforation (p value < 0.001) where CAS kit required the longest time and BAOSFE caused the biggest perforations.

Conclusions: The study shows that both the balloon and the CAS kit were superior to the BAOSFE in terms of safety in elevating the sinus membrane. Further, in vivo studies have to prove these findings.

Keywords: Maxillary sinus, Schneiderian membrane, Sinus floor elevation, Balloon elevation, Elevation height, CAS kit

Background

More than half of the implants placed in the posterior maxilla require sinus floor elevation (SFE) [1]. The need for this procedure is explained by continuous ridge resorption in an apical direction after tooth extraction combined with progressive sinus pneumatization in addition to poor bone quality that is frequently seen in the maxilla [2].

Sinus membrane perforation is considered the most common complication during sinus floor elevation procedures, and its percentage varies according to the method used. Perforations happen either while fracturing the floor of the sinus or during the elevation of the mucosa [3, 4].

Crestal approach to the sinus kit (CAS kit) was introduced by OSSTEM implants (Osstem Implant Co., Busan, Korea) as a safe and effective method for sinus elevation with the advantage of using a reamer (the CAS drill) to perform the osteotomy in a conical shape and break the bony floor; however, only one questionnaire

* Correspondence: aghiad88@gmail.com
[1]Department of Periodontology, Damascus University Dental School, Damascus, Syrian Arab Republic
Full list of author information is available at the end of the article

that assessed the satisfaction of dentists using the CAS KIT is available in the literature on this method [5]. Using an inflatable balloon for indirect sinus floor elevation has been shown to be successful in elevating the mucosa for elevation heights of up to 10 mm [6, 7]. However, few studies in the literature compared this technique to others.

Lopez-Nino et al. studied the lamb as an ex vivo model for training in sinus floor elevation and concluded that the model is useful because of the similarities in the thickness of the lateral wall of the maxillary sinus and the thickness of the Schneiderian membrane between the models and the human standards [8].

Cone beam computed tomography (CBCT) can precisely visualize the sinus complexity in 3D, with low irradiation to the patient. In implant dentistry, recent guidelines recommend the use of CBCT for three-dimensional treatment planning, especially prior to SFE for evaluating both residual alveolar and sinus conditions [9, 10].

Therefore, the two working hypotheses of our study were "the CAS-Kit is safer than BAOSFE in breaking the sinus floor and the balloon is safer than BAOSFE in elevating the Schneiderian membrane" for elevation heights of 7 mm.

Methods
The sample
To achieve our purposes, an experimental ex vivo study was carried. This research project was approved by the University of Damascus Local Research Ethics Committee (UDDS-3045PG.) and was funded by the Damascus University Postgraduate Research Budget (97687027834DEN). The sinus floor elevations were done on 18 bisected heads of lambs aged between 6 and 12 months that were slaughtered in a maximum of 4 h before the procedures began. CBCT images of the heads were taken using the Picasso® Pro CBCT system (Vatech™, Seoul, South Korea) set at a voxel size of 0.2 mm, tube current of 5 mA, tube voltage of 83 KV with gray scale of 16 bit per pixel. A standardized position of the lamb's heads was maintained by the correct head orientation in accordance with the 3D intersecting planes of the red beam. Then, the images were analyzed for the best location to perform the sinus elevation where remaining bone height (RBH) is less than 5 mm on 3DOnDemand® programme (CyberMed, Finland) (Fig. 1). The RBH was measured from the apical tip of the buccal root on the third premolar which will be extracted to the floor of the sinus. The sample was randomized by generating random numbers using Research Randomizer software (http://www.randomizer.org/) [11] making sure that the same method was not done on the same lamb twice.

Visual assessment
After the extraction of the third premolar, the mesial side of the sinus was exposed (Fig. 2) in order to check the sinus for any perforations. The elevation height was measured using a depth gauge, and the intended

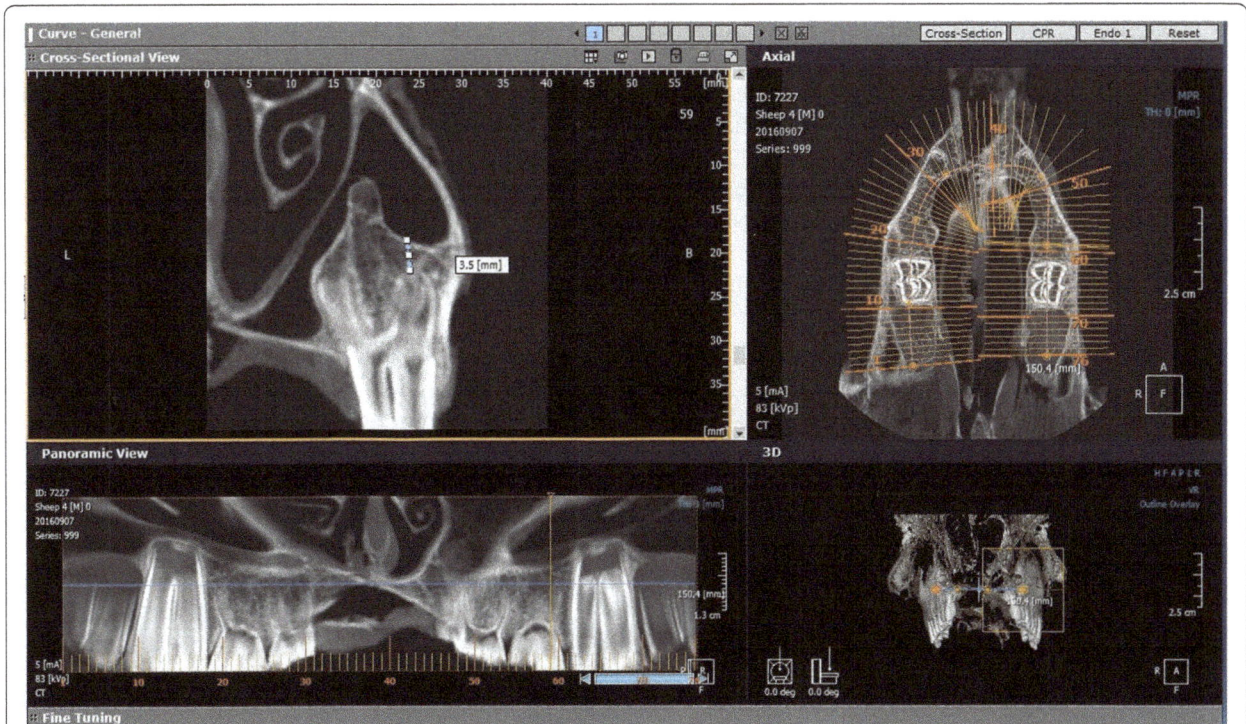

Fig. 1 Determination of the remaining bone height (RBH) on the CBCT image

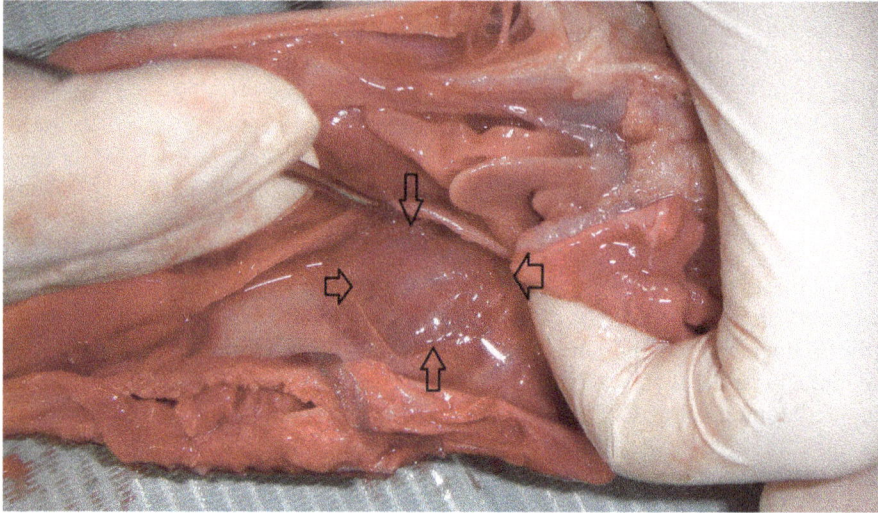

Fig. 2 The exposed mesial aspect of the sinus

elevation height was 7 mm. If this height was not achieved, the maximum elevation was recorded. When a perforation of the membrane was present, its length was measured using a periodontal probe.

Sinus floor elevation methods
BAOSFE

Bone blocks were harvested from the lamb's head and made into soft bone particles using ACE bone mill®(ACE surgical Supply Co., Inc., Brockton, Ma, USA). For this technique, the osteotomy started with a pilot drill for 2 mm followed by burs with increasing diameter up to 3.2 mm. Then, osteotomes (FRIALIT-2 bone expander, Friadent, DENTSPLY Implants) were used to expand the osteotomy and to break the sinus floor after the addition of bone. The 4.5 mm osteotome was used to break the sinus floor and push continuous insertions of bone particles. Every use of the osteotome to pack the bone is expected to lift the sinus membrane for 1 mm [12].

Balloon sinus lift

This approach starts like BAOSFE. The osteotomy is enlarged to 5.0 mm before the balloon (Zimmer Sinus Lift Balloon, Zimmer Dental Inc., California, USA) is inserted (Fig. 3). The sinus floor was broken with the 5 mm osteotome after the addition of bone. The sleeve of the balloon was inserted 1 mm beyond the sinus floor. The saline was injected slowly from the syringe into the balloon, so the balloon would inflate progressively (Fig. 4). The balloon was deflated, and the desired elevation was checked if the elevation was not reached. The balloon was inserted again, and the process is repeated until the desired 7 mm are reached. One cubic centimeter of saline is expected to lift the membrane for 6 mm [13].

CAS kit

The CAS kit consists of a set of safe end drills, metal stoppers, a depth gauge, a hydraulic lifter, bone graft

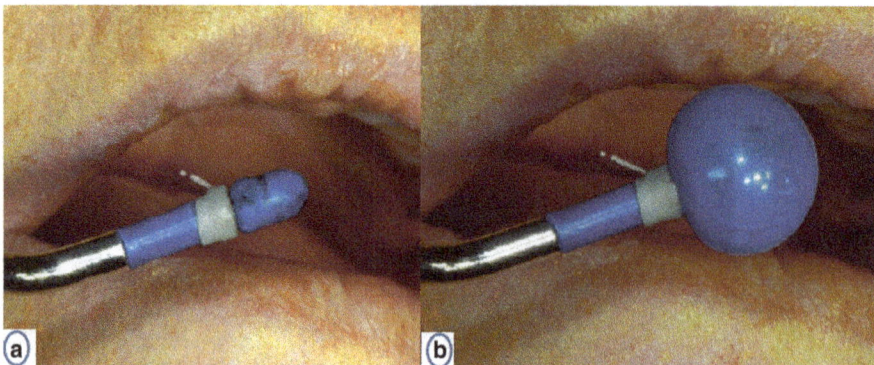

Fig. 3 a The balloon in a resting position. **b** The inflated balloon [12]

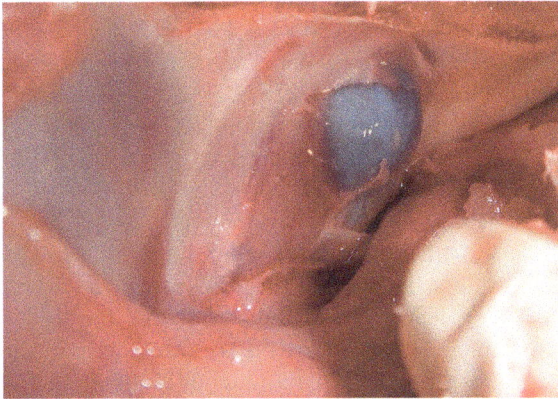

Fig. 4 The inflated balloon while elevating the sinus membrane (The balloon is seen from the medial.)

carrier, condenser, and a bone spreader (Fig. 5). The procedure started with a 2-mm twist drill. The drills were used to enlarge the osteotomy and are stopped 1 mm short of the sinus floor. The sinus floor was broken with the 3.6 mm bur without going through the floor; a depth gauge was used to check the membrane integrity and to slightly lift the membrane. Then, the hydraulic lifter was inserted and stabilized (Fig. 6) and the saline solution is injected. 0.30 mL can elevate the membrane up to 3 mm [5]. The saline is drown out then injected again until the desired elevation is reached.

Statistics

Chi-square test was used to test the association between the three techniques and the occurrence of perforation whereas ANOVA (analysis of variance) was used to assess the association between method used and the two outcomes of the length of the perforation and the time of operation. Logistic regression of method used on the occurrence of perforation was employed to evaluate the odds of perforation for each method. P values equal to or smaller than .05 were considered to be significant. All calculations were made using SPSS version 16 for Windows (SPSS®, Chicago, IL, USA).

Results

For the entire sample, the mean perforation length was (0.711 mm, SD = 1.4) and the mean time required to perform the procedure was (5.65 min, SD = 2.26), and out of the entire sample (N = 36), perforations happened in nine cases for a percentage of 25%.

Chi-square test showed a significant association between method used and the occurrence of perforation (chi-square statistic = 8.585, df = 2, p value = 0.014), as shown in Table 1. Also, ANOVA test showed a significant association between method used and the length of perforation (F = 11.031, df = 2, 33, p value < 0.001) where the BAOSFE caused the largest mean length of perforations (3.42 mm) followed by the CAS kit and the balloon (0.5, 0.5 mm). As for the time required to perform the procedures ANOVA test showed a significant association between method used and the time required to perform it (F = 1221.2, df = 2,33, p value < 0.001); CAS kit required the longest time (8.486 min) followed by the balloon then BAOSFE (5.393, 3.073 min) (Table 1).

Table 2 shows the results of logistic regression of method used on the occurrence of perforation, the odds ratio showed significant differences between the balloon technique and the BAOSFE (OR = 0.091, p value = 0.022), and between the CAS kit and the BAOSFE (OR = 0.091, p value = 0.022); however, no significant differences were found between the balloon and the CAS kit (OR = 1,0, p value = 1). It should be noted that the CAS kit was only able to lift the membrane for a maximum of 5 mm.

Discussion

Although the lateral sinus floor elevation is a proven clinically successful technique [14], the indirect SFE approach is favorable among clinicians because it does not require a second surgery site and hence cause less trauma and discomfort for the patient [14–16]. However,

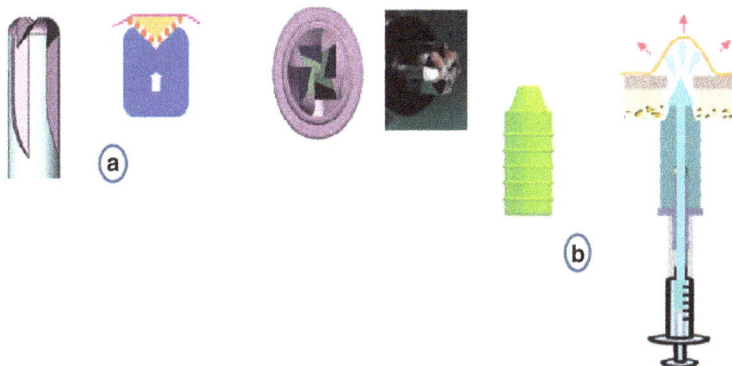

Fig. 5 a The CAS drill has four blades and an inverse conical shape. **b** The hydraulic lifter

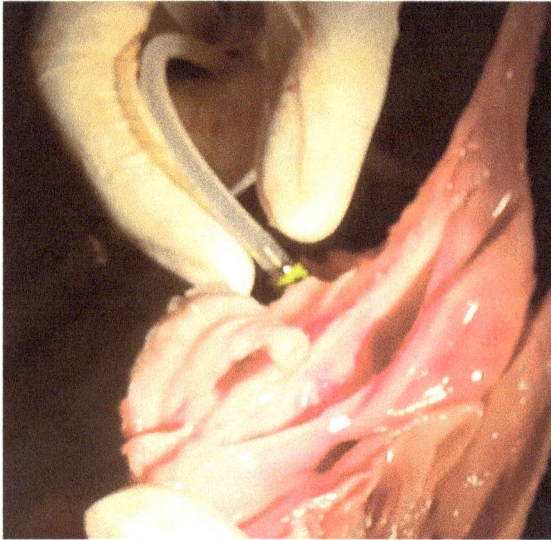

Fig. 6 The hydraulic lifter stabilized in the osteotomy before injecting the saline

this method has its drawbacks, such as a higher risk of membrane perforation, a decreased space for using surgical instruments, and limitation in elevation heights when using the conventional techniques [3, 16, 17].

The osteotome technique originally described by Tatum 1994 has been shown microscopically to elevate the sinus floor for 5 mm without causing perforations [18]. Thus, this technique should not be used when the intended elevation height is more than 5 mm [19]. Therefore, a need for transalveolar approach that can elevate the membrane safely and for elevation heights greater than 5 mm has risen, Tatum described a modified approach to his osteotome technique in which bone particles are pushed in the sinus. The addition of bone will prevent direct contact between the instruments and the membrane [20]. Recently, many methods for SFE have been described as an alternative for the osteotome technique. Most of this techniques fall under two categories: using an inflatable device such as a balloon or using hydraulic pressure, both of which have been shown to reduce the rate of membrane perforation [6, 7, 13, 21, 22]. Soltan and Smiler described the use of the balloon and concluded that it is a highly successful and easy to perform procedure [6]. Recently, many systems have been developed which rely on hydraulic pressure to lift the sinus mucosa including the

Jeder-System (Jeder GmbH, Vienna, Austria) which consists of a drill with a chamber which is filled with saline solution. After the initial drilling is done, the drill is connected to a pump that produces high hydraulic pressure; the pressure is used to break the sinus floor and to lift the membrane [23]. Also, OSSTEM implants introduced the CAS kit as a method for preparing the osteotomy and elevating the membrane through hydraulic pressure.

Using a reamer instead of the osteotomes for breaking the sinus floor has the advantage of creating a thin bone shell that prevents direct contact between the drill and the Schneiderian membrane [24]. Moreover, using a reamer has been shown to cause less discomfort and nausea when compared to the osteotome technique as a result of the constant tapping of the osteotomes [25]. As a result, the CAS kit has the advantage over the BAOSFE and the balloon in preparing the osteotomy and breaking the sinus floor safely and with less complications. Moreover, it was noted during our study that using a drill gives better feedback to the surgeon when breaking the sinus floor compared to the osteotome.

However, in our study, the CAS-kit was able to lift the membrane for a maximum of 5 mm. We believe that the saline pressure injected through the hydraulic lifter from a syringe is small and decreases gradually after leaving the lifter, whereas a study on the Jeder system showed a height gain of (9.2 ± 1.7 mm). This could be attributed to the high hydraulic pressure from the Jeder pump which is a machine that control the hydraulic pressure [23]. On the other hand, in our study, the balloon was able to lift the membrane for 7 mm in all cases; therefore, the balloon was better in elevating the mucosa.

Our study compared between three techniques for SFE for elevation heights of 7 mm. The 7 mm elevation height was chosen as a previous study by Stelzle et al. 2011 showed that BAOSFE caused perforations in the mucosa in all samples for perforation heights of 10 mm [7]. Therefore, we tried to set a threshold that might be achieved with internal sinus lifting techniques and be feasible in clinical practice. Perforations were checked using the three different methods: the mesial window, using a depth gauge, and the injection of saline solution through the osteotomy, which allowed for accurate recording of perforations.

Table 1 The association between the methods used the following variables: occurrence of perforation, length of perforation, and the time of operation

	BAOSFE	BALLOON	CAS kit	Total	Stats	p value
Occurrence of perforation	7 (58.4%) $N = 12$	1 (8.3%) $N = 12$	1 (8.3%) $N = 12$	9 (25%) $N = 36$	$\times 2 = 8.585^a$	0.014
Length of perforation (mean)	3.42 mm	0.5 mm	0.5 mm	0.711 mm	$F = 11.031$	0.0001
Time of operation (mean)	3.073 min	5.393 min	8.486 min	5.651 min	$F = 1221$	0.0001

F ANOVA test
[a]Chi-square test

Table 2 The results of logistic regression of method used on the occurrence of perforation

Methods	BAOFSE		BALLOON		CAS kit	
Number of cases	12		12		12	
Number of perforations	7		1		1	
Percentage	58.4%		8.3%		8.3%	
Comparison of methods regarding perforations (odds ratio)						
	Balloon\BOAFSE		Balloon\CAS kit		CAS kit\BAOFSE	
Odds ratio	0.091		1		0.091	
p value	0.022		1		0.022	
Confidence interval	Lower	Upper	Lower	Upper	Lower	Upper
	1.437	160.972	0.55	18.085	1.437	160.972
Reference group	BAOSFE		BAOSFE		CAS kit	

The BAOSFE technique caused perforations in the membrane in 7 out of 12 cases with a percentage of 58.4. This result is consistent with many previous studies which state that this technique has a high rate of perforations when the RBH is less than 5 mm [2, 7, 26]. Also, all the perforations happened during the elevation process; however, this percentage is different than that reported by Steltzle (100%) in a similar study as the intended elevation height was less by 3 mm in our study [7].

For the balloon technique, only one perforation happened during the elevation process and the balloon was able to lift the membrane for 7 mm in all successful cases. This result supports various studies that showed a high success rate for this technique [6, 7, 13]; however, the osteotomy should be enlarged to 5 mm before inserting the balloon and this might limit the indications for this technique in thin ridges.

The CAS kit caused perforation of the Schneiderian membrane in one of the 12 cases (8.3%) which happened during the osteotomy. This is the first study to our knowledge to assess the CAS kit form OSSTEM implants since we found one published article that was a questionnaire sent to dentists who used the system to assess their satisfaction with the CAS kit, The study reported a membrane perforation rate of 4.1%. This percentage is smaller than that reported in our study (8.3%); however, we believe that our method of checking perforations is more accurate. Also, the difference in sample size may have contributed to the outcome [5].

Conclusions

Within the limitation of this study and that of an ex vivo study, we can accept our hypotheses that the balloon is better than the BAOSFE in elevating the membrane mucosa and the CAS kit is better than the BAOSFE in preparing the osteotomy and breaking the sinus floor for elevation heights of 7 mm. Further, in vivo studies need to be taken to prove these findings.

Authors' contributions
YSA conceived the study, held surgical procedures, and drafted the manuscript. AMM supervised the surgical procedures, reviewed, and approved the manuscript. DNB was responsible for the interpretation of the CBCT images and reviewed the manuscript. RS did the statistical analysis and reviewed the manuscript.

Competing interests
Aghiad Yassin Alsabbagh, Mohammed Monzer Alsabbagh, Batol Darjazini Nahas, and Salam Rajih declare that they have no competing interests.

Author details
[1]Department of Periodontology, Damascus University Dental School, Damascus, Syrian Arab Republic. [2]Department of Orthodontics, Damascus University Dental School, Damascus, Syrian Arab Republic. [3]Temple university, Philadelphia, USA.

References
1. Seong WJ, Barczak M, Jung J, Basu S, Olin PS, Conrad HJ. Prevalence of sinus augmentation associated with maxillary posterior implants. The Journal of oral implantology. 2013;39(6):680–8.
2. Cawood JI, Howell RA. A classification of the edentulous jaws. Int J Oral Maxillofac Surg. 1988;17(4):232–6.
3. Tan WC, Lang NP, Zwahlen M, Pjetursson BE. A systematic review of the success of sinus floor elevation and survival of implants inserted in combination with sinus floor elevation. Part II: transalveolar technique. J Clin Periodontol. 2008;35(8 Suppl):241–54.
4. Cho SC, Wallace SS, Froum SJ, Tarnow DP. Influence of anatomy on Schneiderian membrane perforations during sinus elevation surgery: three-dimensional analysis. Pract Proced Aesthet Dent. 2001;13(2):160–3.
5. Kim YK, Cho YS, Yun PY. Assessment of dentists' subjective satisfaction with a newly developed device for maxillary sinus membrane elevation by the crestal approach. Journal of periodontal & implant science. 2013;43(6):308–14.
6. Soltan M, Smiler DG. Antral membrane balloon elevation. The Journal of oral implantology. 2005;31(2):85–90.
7. Stelzle F, Benner KU. Evaluation of different methods of indirect sinus floor elevation for elevation heights of 10 mm: an experimental ex vivo study. Clin Implant Dent Relat Res. 2011;13(2):124–33.
8. Lopez-Nino J, Garcia-Caballero L, Gonzalez-Mosquera A, Seoane-Romero J, Varela-Centelles P, Seoane J. Lamb ex vivo model for training in maxillary sinus floor elevation surgery: a comparative study with human standards. J Periodontol. 2012;83(3):354–61.
9. Benavides E, Rios HF, Ganz SD, An C-H, Resnik R, Reardon GT, et al. Use of cone beam computed tomography in implant dentistry: the International Congress of Oral Implantologists consensus report. Implant Dent. 2012;21(2):78–86.
10. Harris D, Quirynene M. Guidelines for the use of diagnostic imaging in implant dentistry: update of the EAO clinical oral implants research. 2012.

11. Urbaniak GC, Plous S. Research randomizer (Version 4.0) [Computer software], http://www.randomizer.org/2015. Available from: http://www.randomizer.org/. 2013.

12. Younes R, Nader N, Khoury G. Sinus grafting techniques: a step-by-step guide 2015.

13. Hu X, Lin Y, Metzmacher AR, Zhang Y. Sinus membrane lift using a water balloon followed by bone grafting and implant placement: a 28-case report. Int J Prosthodont. 2009;22(3):243–7.

14. Zitzmann NU, Scharer P. Sinus elevation procedures in the resorbed posterior maxilla. Comparison of the crestal and lateral approaches. Oral Surg Oral Med Oral Pathol Oral Radiol Endod. 1998;85(1):8–17.

15. Esposito M, Felice P, Worthington HV. Interventions for replacing missing teeth: augmentation procedures of the maxillary sinus. The Cochrane database of systematic reviews 2014(5):CD008397.

16. Schwartz-Arad D, Herzberg R, Dolev E. The prevalence of surgical complications of the sinus graft procedure and their impact on implant survival. J Periodontol. 2004;75(4):511–6.

17. Emmerich D, Att W, Stappert C. Sinus floor elevation using osteotomes: a systematic review and meta-analysis. J Periodontol. 2005;76(8):1237–51.

18. Engelke W, Deckwer I. Endoscopically controlled sinus floor augmentation. A preliminary report. Clin Oral Implants Res. 1997;8(6):527–31.

19. Sendyk W, Sendyk C. Reconstrução óssea por meio do levantamento do assoalho do seio maxilar. São Paulo: Santos. 2002:109–22.

20. Summers RB. The osteotome technique: part 3—less invasive methods of elevating the sinus floor. Compendium. 1994;15(6):698, 700, 2–4 passim; quiz 10.

21. Pommer B, Watzek G. Gel-pressure technique for flapless transcrestal maxillary sinus floor elevation: a preliminary cadaveric study of a new surgical technique. Int J Oral Maxillofac Implants. 2009;24(5):817–22.

22. Sotirakis EG, Gonshor A. Elevation of the maxillary sinus floor with hydraulic pressure. The Journal of oral implantology. 2005;31(4):197–204.

23. Jesch P, Bruckmoser E, Bayerle A, Eder K, Bayerle-Eder M, Watzinger F. A pilot-study of a minimally invasive technique to elevate the sinus floor membrane and place graft for augmentation using high hydraulic pressure: 18-month follow-up of 20 cases. Oral surgery, oral medicine, oral pathology and oral radiology. 2013;116(3):293–300.

24. Bae OY, Kim YS, Shin SY, Kim WK, Lee YK, Kim SH. Clinical outcomes of reamer- vs osteotome-mediated sinus floor elevation with simultaneous implant placement: a 2-year retrospective study. Int J Oral Maxillofac Implants. 2015;30(4):925–30.

25. Ahn SH, Park EJ, Kim ES. Reamer-mediated transalveolar sinus floor elevation without osteotome and simultaneous implant placement in the maxillary molar area: clinical outcomes of 391 implants in 380 patients. Clin Oral Implants Res. 2012;23(7):866–72.

26. Toffler M, Toscano N, Holtzclaw D. Osteotome-mediated sinus floor elevation using only platelet-rich fibrin: an early report on 110 patients. Implant Dent. 2010;19(5):447–56.

17

Primary peri-implant oral intra-epithelial neoplasia/carcinoma in situ: a case report considering risk factors for carcinogenesis

Makoto Noguchi[1*], Hiroaki Tsuno[1], Risa Ishizaka[1], Kumiko Fujiwara[1], Shuichi Imaue[1], Kei Tomihara[1] and Takashi Minamisaka[2]

Abstract

Background: Major risk factors for oral squamous cell carcinoma (SCC) are tobacco smoking, a betel quid chewing habit, and heavy alcohol consumption. However, around 15% of oral SCCs cannot be explained by these risk factors. Although oral SCC associated with dental implants is quite rare, there has been a recent gradual accumulation of reports about it. Here, we report a case of primary peri-implant oral intra-epithelial neoplasia/carcinoma in situ (OIN/CIS) in a woman without the major risk factors for oral SCC.

Case presentation: A 65-year-old woman was referred to our clinic with a tumor in the right lower gingiva. She had no history of tobacco smoking and only drank socially. Ten years previously, mandibular right posterior teeth had been replaced with an implant-supported porcelain-fused-to-metal restoration in a dental clinic. About 7 years later, she noticed swelling on the lingual side of the gingiva around the implant-supported restoration, and was eventually referred to our clinic with the suspicion of a neoplasia around the dental implant. The upper part of the implant body was exposed on the implant corresponding to the first molar of the right side of the mandible; this was associated with painless, elastic soft, and relatively well circumscribed gingival swelling on the lingual site. A panoramic radiograph showed slight vertical bone resorption around the implants. An incisional biopsy was conducted under the suspicion of neoplasia. Pathological microscopic examination of the biopsy specimen revealed thickened squamous epithelia with slight nuclear atypism and disorders of the epithelial rete pegs. Immunohistochemical findings showed positive staining for keratin 17 and a negative staining mosaic pattern for keratin 13. High p53, p63, and Ki-67 reactivity was also observed. From these findings, OIN/CIS of the gingiva was pathologically diagnosed, and a wide local excision with rim resection of the mandible, including the implants, was performed. The pathological findings for the resected specimen were same as those for the biopsy specimen. After 1 year of follow-up, there was no evidence of recurrence.

Conclusion: In this case, prolonged peri-implant mucositis or peri-implantitis may have been a plausible risk factor for carcinogenesis.

Keywords: Dental implant, Oral intra-epithelial neoplasia/carcinoma in situ, Peri-implantitis, Risk factor for oral carcinogenesis

* Correspondence: mnoguchi@med.u-toyama.ac.jp
[1]Department of Oral and Maxillofacial Surgery, Graduate School of Medicine and Pharmaceutical Sciences for Research, University of Toyama, 2630 Sugitani Toyama city, Toyama 9300194, Japan
Full list of author information is available at the end of the article

Background

Oral cancer ranks sixth among the malignancies in terms of worldwide prevalence, with more than 90% being pathologically squamous cell carcinoma (SCC) [1]. Oral SCC generally develops via multistep carcinogenesis. The squamous epithelium goes into irreversible change, including epithelial dysplasia and oral intra-epithelial neoplasia/carcinoma in-situ (OIN/CIS) [2], finally resulting in the development of invasive carcinoma through the accumulation of genetic abnormalities caused by persistent exposure to a carcinogen. Risk factors for oral SCCs are smoking, tobacco and betel quid chewing habits, and heavy alcohol consumption. In addition, chronic inflammation, including periodontitis, has been regarded as a possible risk factor for oral SCCs. Laprise et al. [3] conducted a case control study to estimate the extent to which high levels of periodontal disease were associated with oral cancer risk, using a comprehensive adjustment approach for confounding that involved a large set of life course variables. The authors concluded that their findings supported the hypothesis that high levels of periodontal disease increase the risk of oral cancer.

A recent report made a bold statement that dental implants also can be a cause of cancer by providing a "route of entry for squamous cell carcinoma" [4], and another report stated that dental implants can lead to SCC in at-risk patients [5]. The incidence of malignances associated with dental implants seems to be extremely low. Bhatavadekar [6] calculated the theoretical standardized incidence ratio (SIR) to be 0.0017 per million per year. However, recently, case reports of oral malignancies associated with dental implants have gradually been accumulating [7]. Raise et al. [8] pointed out that the number of such cases in the literature has increased sharply in the last decade.

In this study, we report a case of intra-epithelial neoplasia arising from peri-implant mucosa in a woman without a history of tobacco smoking or excessive alcohol consumption, and without predisposing factors for oral SCC, including leukoplakia, erythroplakia, or previous oral cancer.

Case presentation

A 65-year-old woman was referred to our clinic with a tumor in the right lower gingiva. Her medical history included breast cancer without metastatic lesion, diabetes mellitus, hyperlipidemia, and hypertension. She had taken orally aspirin, amlodipine, pravastatin, and bepotastine for 2 years. She drank alcohol socially, but she had no history of tobacco smoking habit.

About 10 years prior to her attendance at our clinic, her mandibular right posterior teeth had been replaced with an implant-supported porcelain-fused-to-metal restoration (three endosseous hydroxyapatite-coated titanium implants) in a dental clinic. The postoperative clinical course was uneventful, and the implant-supported restoration had functioned well. The patient had discontinued her regular follow-up for the maintenance of oral hygiene several months after the completion of the restoration. After about 7 years, she noticed a swelling on the lingual side of the gingiva around the three implants, and she visited a dental clinic. Following conservative treatment with nonsurgical measures for around 2 years, under a diagnosis of peri-implantitis, flap surgery to her lesion was performed in the dental clinic. However, the lesion around the central of the three implants did not improve, and changes to its surface properties were observed, leading to the suspicion of transformation to neoplasia. She was then referred to our clinic 3 months after the flap surgery.

The upper part of the implant body was exposed on the implant corresponding to the first molar of the right side of the mandible; this was associated with painless, elastic soft, and relatively well circumscribed gingival swelling on the lingual site. No pus drainage from the gingival sulcus was observed (Fig. 1). Periodontal disease or peri-implant disease, including peri-implantitis and peri-implant mucositis, were not observed in other regions, including the contiguous implants to the relevant middle implant. Lymphadenopathy in the neck was not detected. A panoramic radiograph showed slight vertical bone resorption around the three implants in the right side of the mandible (Fig. 2). An incisional biopsy was conducted under the suspicion of neoplasia after considering not only the clinical findings, but also the clinical course. Pathological microscopic examination of the biopsy specimen revealed thickened squamous epithelia with slight nuclear atypism and disorders of the epithelial rete pegs accompanied by moderate grade inflammatory cell infiltration. Immunohistochemical findings

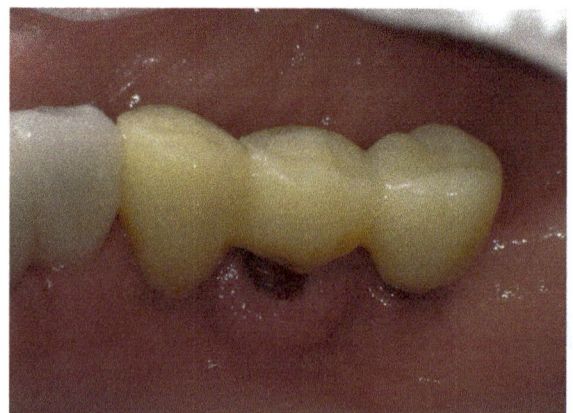

Fig. 1 Well-circumscribed gingival swelling on the lingual side of the right side of the mandible

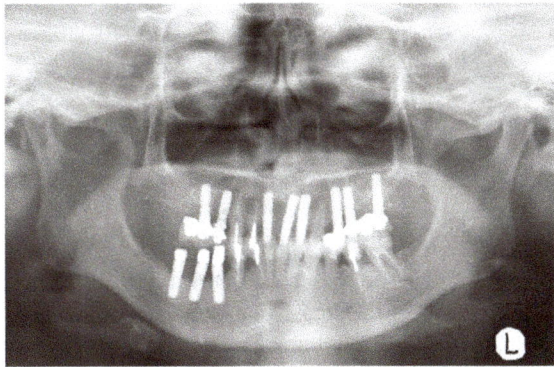

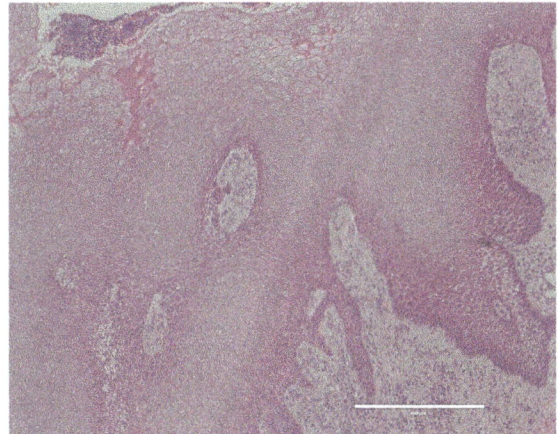

Fig. 3 Pathological microscopic examination reveals thickened squamous epithelia with slight nuclear atypism and disorders of the epithelial rete pegs accompanied by moderate grade inflammatory cell infiltration (HE staining, bar: 400 μm)

showed positive staining for keratin 17 (k17) and a negative staining mosaic pattern for keratin 13 (k13). High p53, p63, and Ki-67 reactivity was also observed in the basal cell layer, but negative staining for p16 (Table 1). These findings indicated to OIN/CIS. Thus, a wide local excision with rim resection of the mandible, including the three implants, was performed under general anesthesia. The postoperative clinical course was uneventful but the patient experienced paresthesia of the lower lip and mental region of the affected side. The pathological diagnosis of the resected specimen confirmed the OIN/CIS found in the biopsy specimen (Figs. 3, 4 and 5). The surgical margin was involved with epithelial dysplasia but free of OIN/CIS. After 1 year of follow-up, there was no evidence of recurrence (Fig. 6).

Discussion

OIN/CIS can sometimes be difficult to distinguish pathologically from epithelial dysplasia on hematoxylin-and eosin-staining sections; this has proved challenging for oral pathologists [9]. Recently, it has been reported that combined immunohistochemistry for k13 and k17 was useful for the differential diagnosis [9, 10]. K13 is a marker for cellular differentiation toward prickle cells in normal stratified squamous epithelia, and its loss or attenuation is observed in oral SCC. Conversely, k17 is not expressed in normal stratified squamous epithelia or

specifically localized in SCCs. Our case showed a partial reduction in k13 expression and a mosaic-like pattern as well as being positive for k17 expression, leading to a diagnosis of OIN /CIS.

In the irreversible multistep carcinogenesis, most cases of invasive oral SCC that break through the basement membrane develop as the next pathological stage into OIN/CIS following severe epithelial dysplasia. Such precancerous lesions are clinically observed to be leukoplakic, erythroplakic, or a combination of these. Oral SCCs are frequently accompanied by such precancerous lesions which spread out around them.

Raiser et al. [8] reviewed 42 cases of oral malignancy in which dental implants were implicated, retrieved from a literature search of PubMed and Google Scholar. From the analysis, the affected individuals tend to be elderly adults (mean age, 68 years). The gender distribution shows a clear 1:1.5 female predominance opposed to the characteristic male predominance of oral cancer in general. They also found that 45.3% of cases occurred in a population with recognized risk factors for oral cancer;

Table 1 Summary of immunohistochemical findings of the present case

Antibody	Sorce	Clone	Staining
Keratin 13	DAKO	DE-K13	Positive
Keratin 17	DAKO	E3	Negative mosaic pattern
p16	Roche	E6H4	Negative
p53	DAKO	DO-7	Positive in the basal cell layer
p63	Nichirei	4A4	Positive in the basal cell layer
Ki-67	Nichirei	SP6	Positive in the basal cell layer

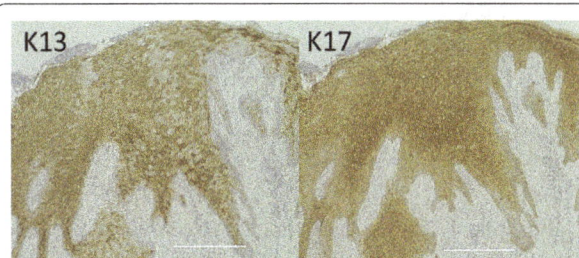

Fig. 4 Immunohistological findings show a negative staining mosaic pattern for keratin 13 (k13) and positive staining for keratin 17 (k17) (immunohistological staining, bar 400 μm)

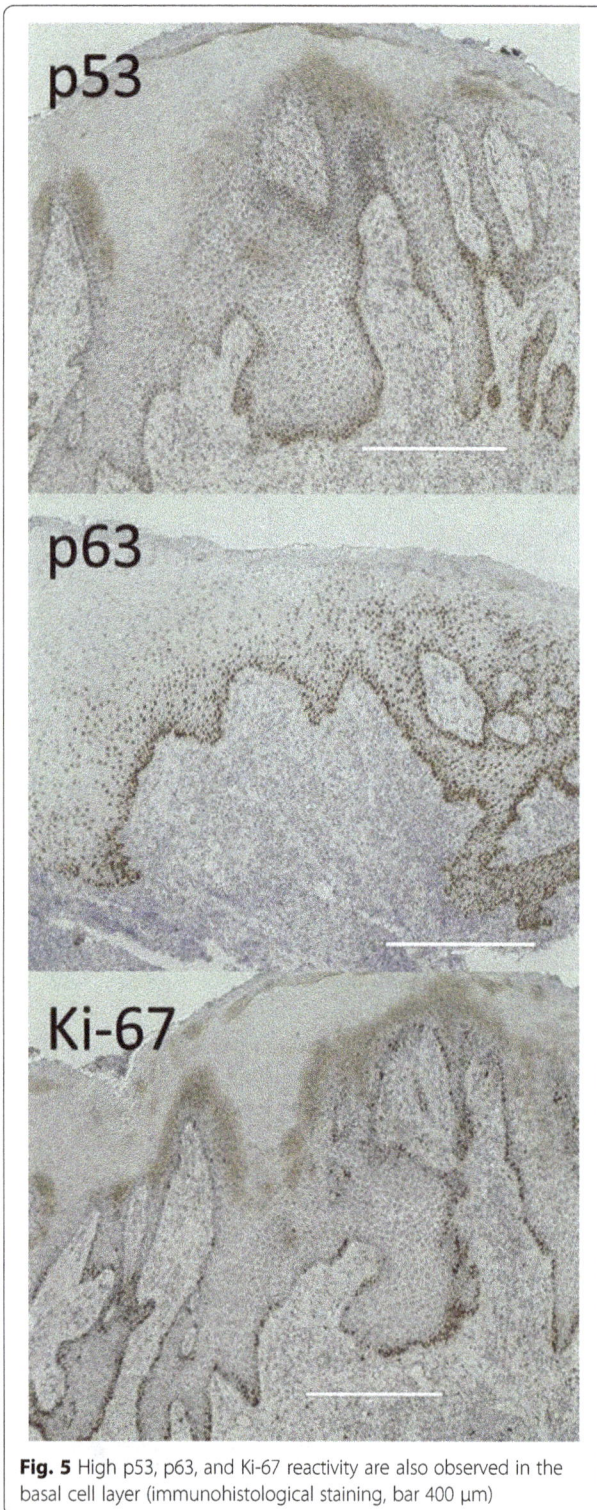

Fig. 5 High p53, p63, and Ki-67 reactivity are also observed in the basal cell layer (immunohistological staining, bar 400 μm)

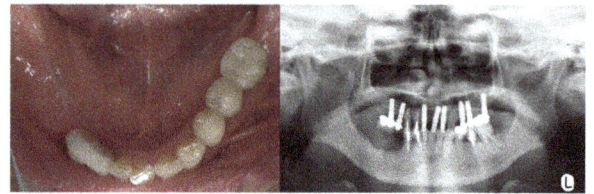

Fig. 6 Postoperative intraoral finding and radiograph

smoking habit or heavy alcohol consumption, nor were further predisposing factors for oral cancer, such as a precancerous lesion or previous oral cancer observed in her oral cavity, including around the OIN/CIS lesion. Thus, she did not fit with the concept of "field cancerization" in the development of oral cancer, which has been accepted by most oral pathologists since being proposed in 1953 by Slaughter et al. [11].

The latest evidence implies that the human papilloma virus (HPV) may be responsible for carcinogenesis in the oral cavity [12, 13]; however, its role is debatable. The interaction of the HPV's E6 and E7 oncoproteins with cell cycle proteins disturbs the cell cycle mechanism and subsequent alteration in the expression of proteins such as p53, p63, and Ki-67 [14]. In our case, the immunohistochemical examination of these cell cycle-related proteins demonstrated overexpression in the basal cell layer, which might be implicated in HPV infection and carcinogenesis. p16 has been regarded as one of the useful markers for HPV-associated carcinogenesis as well as other cell cycle proteins. Particularly in oropharyngeal SCCs, overexpression of p16 notably demonstrates a strong correlation with HPV infection, although it has failed to reveal such strong correlation with oral SCCs [15]. In our case, negative expression of p16 was observed, suggesting negative for HPV infection.

The relationship between the oral microbiome and oral SCC has increasingly been reported since the 1998 study by Nagy et al. [16], which found significantly higher levels of Porphyromonas species and Fusobacterium species on oral SCC, compared with the adjacent healthy mucosa. Recently, Gallimidi et al. [17] indicated that the periodontal pathogens *Porphyromonas gingivalis* and *Fusobacterium nucleatum* stimulated tumorigenesis via direct interaction with oral epithelial cells through toll-like receptors.

Evidence that persistent chronic inflammation may be a causative factor for carcinogenesis has accumulated from preclinical and clinical studies since Virchow proposed a close relationship between chronic inflammation and tumorigenesis [18]. It has been shown that chronic infection and related inflammation contributed to almost 20% of all malignancies worldwide. Various mechanisms for carcinogenesis related to chronic inflammation have been suggested. Inflammatory cells excrete a number of

in addition, 47.5% of cases had experienced a previous oral malignancy, and 19% exhibited the histology of a non-oral malignancy that could metastasize to the jaws or gingiva. Our patient did not have any of the recognized risk factors for oral cancer, including a tobacco-

cytokines and growth factors that promote the survival of neoplastic cells and prevent their apoptosis [19]. Reactive oxygen and nitrogen species induced by chronic inflammation could cause damage to cellular deoxyribonucleic acid (DNA), contributing to malignant cell transformation [20]. Furthermore, a recent study suggested that inflammation could initiate cancer-specific epigenetic changes, including DNA methylation alterations in epithelial cells [21].

Conclusions

In our case, the persistence of peri-implant mucositis or peri-implantitis around the dental implant was implicated as being a plausible risk factor for carcinogenesis. Regular follow-up to ensure the maintenance of oral hygiene after dental implant therapy has again been shown to be important for preventing peri-implantitis, a plausible risk factor for carcinogenesis.

Abbreviations
DNA: Deoxyribonucleic acid; HPV: Human papilloma virus; OIN/CIS: Oral intra-epithelial neoplasia/carcinoma in situ; SCC: Squamous cell carcinoma

Funding
None.

Authors' contributions
MN participated in the design and coordination of the study, drafted the manuscript, and is the corresponding author. HT participated in the design and coordination of the study and helped draft the manuscript. RI, KF, and Si performed the surgery and patient's treatment. KT analyzed the histological data and helped draft the manuscript. All authors read and approved the final manuscript.

Competing interests
Makoto Nogchi, Hiroaki Tsuno, Risa Ishizaka, Kumiko Fujiwara, Shuichi Imaue, and Kei Tomihara declare that they have no competing interests.

Author details
[1]Department of Oral and Maxillofacial Surgery, Graduate School of Medicine and Pharmaceutical Sciences for Research, University of Toyama, 2630 Sugitani Toyama city, Toyama 9300194, Japan. [2]Department of Diagnosis Pathology, Graduate School of Medicine and Pharmaceutical Sciences for Research, University of Toyama, Toyama, Japan.

References
1. Sah JP, Johnson NW, Batsakis JG. Oral cancer. London: Informa Healthcare; 2011. p. 3–32.
2. Japan Society for Oral Tumors. General rules for clinical and pathological studies on oral cancer. 1st ed. Tokyo: Kanehara-shuppan Co; 2010. p. 44–7.
3. Laprise C, Shahl HP, Madathil SA, et al. Periodontal diseases and risk of oral cancer in Southern India: results from the HeNCe Life Study. Int J Cancer. 2016;139:1512–9.
4. Schache A, Thavaraj S, Kalavrezos N. Osseointegrated implants: a potential route for squamous cell carcinoma of the mandible. Br J Oral Maxillofac Surg. 2008;46:397–9.
5. Kwok J, Eyeson J, Thompson I, et al. Dental implants and squamous cell carcinoma in the at risk patient—report of 3 cases. Br Dent J. 2008;205:543–5.
6. Bhatavadekar NB. Squamous cell carcinoma in association with dental implants: an assessment of previously hypothesized carcinogenic mechanisms and a case reports. J Oral Implantol. 2012;38:792–8.
7. Jeelani S, Rajkumar E, Mary GG, et al. Squamous cell carcinoma and dental implants: a systemic review of case reports. J Pharm Bioallied Sci. 2015;7:378–80.
8. Raiser V, Naaj IAE, Shlimi B, et al. Primary oral malignancy imitating peri-implantitis. J Oral Maxillofac Surg. 2016;74:1383–90.
9. Mikami T, Cheng J, Maruyama S, et al. Emergence of keratin 17 vs. loss of keratin 13: Their reciprocal immunohistochemical profiles in oral carcinoma in situ. Oral Oncol. 2011;47:497–503.
10. Nobusawa A, Sano T, Negishi A, et al. Immunohistochemical staining patterns of cytokeratins 13, 14, and 17 in oral epithelial dysplasia including orthokeratotic dysplasia. Pathology International. 2014;64:20–7.
11. Saughter DP, Southwick HW, Smejkal W. Field cancerization in oral stratified squamous epithelium: clinical implications of multicentric origin. Cancer. 1953;6:963–8.
12. Bouda M, Gorgoulis VG, Kastrinakis NG, et al. "High risk" HPV types are frequently detected in potentially malignant and malignant oral lesions, but not in normal mucosa. Mod Pathol. 2000;13:644–53.
13. Jayaprakash V, Reid M, Hatton E, et al. Human papillomavirus types 16 and 18 in epithelial dysplasia of oral cavity and oropharynx: a meta-analysis. Oral Oncol. 2011;47:1048–54.
14. Vasilescu F, Ceauşu M, Tänsen C, et al. P53, p63 and ki-67 assessment in HPV-induced cervical neoplasia. RJME. 2009;50:357–61.
15. Ndiaye C, Mena M, Alemany L, et al. HPV DNA, E6/E7 mRNA, and p16INK4a detection in head and neck cancers: a systematic review and meta-analysis. Lancet Oncol. 2014;15:1319–31.
16. Nagy K, Sonkodi I, Szöke I, et al. The microflora associated with human oral carcinoma. Oral Oncol. 1998;34:304–8.
17. Gallimidi AB, Fischman S, Revach B, et al. Periodontal pathogens Porphyromonas gingivalis and Fusobacterium nucleatum promote tumor progression in an oral-specific chemical carcinogenesis model. Oncotarget. 2015;6:22613–23.
18. Balkwill F, Mantovani A. Inflammation and cancer: back to Virchow? Lancet. 2001;357:539–45.
19. Francuz T, Czajka-Francuz P, Cisoń-Jurek S, et al. The role of inflammation in colon cancer pathogenesis. Postepy Hig Med Dosw. 2016;27:360–6.
20. Kundu JK, Surth YJ. Inflammation: gearing the journey to cancer. Mutat Res. 2008;659:15–30.
21. Maiuri AR, O'Hagan HM. Interplay between inflammation and epigenetic changes in cancer. Prog Mol Biol Trabsl Sci. 2016;144:69–117.

18

Comparison of access-hole filling materials for screw retained implant prostheses: 12-month in vivo study

Rémy Tanimura[1]*🆔 and Shiro Suzuki[2]

Abstract

Background: Screw retained implant prostheses seem to be an efficient restorative method to prevent peri-implantitis caused by cement excess around the abutment. The drawback of the screw-retained prostheses is the difficulty to realize an efficient access-hole filling functionally and aesthetically. Up to now, few in vitro and in vivo studies were reported in the literature. The aim of this study was to evaluate clinical performances of two direct filling materials through a period of 12 months.

Methods: To pursue a previous in vitro evaluation, this in vivo 12 months prospective study followed up and compared the access-hole filling integrity of a modified 4-META (4-methacryloxyethyl trimellitate anhydride)/MMA-TBB (methyl methacrylate-tri-*n*-butyl borane) – based resin (M4M) and a photo-polymerizing nano-hybrid composite resin (CR).

Twenty-eight access-holes were filled with both materials respectively, then impressions and intra-oral photographs were taken at $T = 0$, $T = 1$ M (month), 3, 6, and 12 M. The access-hole surface measurement and the margin analysis (depth and angle) were carried out. The VAS (visual analogue scale) value on marginal discoloration and integrity at the baseline $T = 0$ and $T = 12$ M was recorded.

Results: The mean values of the surface areas changes from $T = 1$ to $T = 12$ M were $83.3 \pm 11.5\%$ for group CR and $77.1 \pm 13.1\%$ for group M4M, respectively. (Mann-Whitney test $p < 0.05$, $p = 0.046$). The mean marginal depth at $T = 12$ M for group CR were 141.2 ± 125.5 μm and 132.1 ± 107.8 μm for the group M4M, respectively. (Mann-Whitney test $p > 0.05$, $p = 0.58$). The mean values of the angle formed at the margin ($T = 12$ M) were for group CR $39.5 \pm 19.4°$ and $28.2 \pm 17.2°$ for group M4M, respectively (Mann-Whitney test $p < 0.0001$). The photographical analysis by VAS values showed no significant difference between CR and M4M groups (Mann-Whitney test $p > 0.05$, $p = 0.848$).

Conclusions: Based on intra- and extra-oral evaluations with the limitation, both CR and M4M combined with a ceramic primer are indicated as promising materials to fill the access-hole. Further long-term investigation is necessary to confirm this finding.

Keywords: Dental implant, Screw-retained, Access-hole, Wear, 4-META

Background

The retention of implant-supported prostheses is provided by the use of a screw or cement. Recently, it was demonstrated that cement-retained prostheses had a higher rate of technical and biological complications [1], despite a better passive fit than the screw-retained restorations [2]. The CAD/CAM development of the implant-supported prostheses allows a better passively fit with screw-retained prostheses [3], and the development of the mechanics of screws reduced screw-loosening complications [4]. Screw retained prostheses can be retrievable and seem to be an efficient restorative method to prevent peri-implantitis caused by cement excess around the abutment [5, 6]. Nevertheless, these restorations have some disadvantages due to the presence

* Correspondence: implant75@gmail.com
[1]8, place du Général Catroux, 75017 Paris, France

of an access-hole opening that can alter the occlusal morphology and reduce the fracture resistance of the ceramic [7, 8]. It is reported that the integrity of the access-hole filling is in relation with the ceramic fracture resistance [9]. The esthetic outcome of the access hole filling is also influenced by the marginal integrity and the long-term stability of the filling material [10, 11].

An in vitro evaluation of a modified 4-META (4-methacryloxyethyl trimellitate anhydride)/MMA-TBB (methyl methacrylate-tri-n-butyl borane) – based resin (M4M) was conducted to compare the wear behavior to a photo-polymerizing nano-hybrid composite resin (CR), and the results were quite promising [12].

The aim of this in vivo study was to compare the access-hole filling integrity of two different filling materials, M4M and CR, during 12 months. The null hypothesis was that superficial and marginal deterioration of M4M and CR would not be significantly different.

Methods

A total of 60 access-holes in 14 patients (5 male and 9 female) aging from 34 to 69 were restored and observed during 12 months. All subjects were informed about the study, and their written consent to participate in the study was taken.

The materials used in this study are presented in Table 1. They include a phosphoric acid monomer ceramic primer (CP): UCP (Super-Bond Universal Ceramic Primer, Sun Medical, Moriyama, Japan), a photo-polymerizing nanohybrid composite (FS): (Fantasista, shade A2, Sun Medical) and its accompanying photo-polymerizing bonding agent (BA):(Hybrid Bond, Sun Medical) and a modified 4-META/TBB-MMA resin (M4M) :(Bondfill SB, Sun Medical).

Access-hole fillings were divided into CR and M4M groups.

Prior to the filling, the bottom of the access holes was filled with a PTFE (polytetrafluoroethylene) film (GEB SAS, Roissy CDG, France) to protect the screw. The thickness of this protective layer was approximately 2 mm.

CR group

CP was applied and immediately air blown. BA was applied for 20 s, air blown for 5 s and then photo-polymerized using a polymerizing unit (Kerr Demi™plus, KavoKerr Group, Washington DC, USA) for 3–5 s. FS was placed by an incremental technique with less than 1 mm thickness for each layer until covering the top of the access hole. Each layer was photo-polymerized for 20 s. The occlusal adjustment was carried out with a diamond bur (Komet 368EF.204.023, Gebr. Brasseler GmbH & Co. KG, Lemgo, Germany), and the polishing was performed using a series of silicone polishers (Komet 9400, 9401, and 9402) with a 5000-rpm speed under water irrigation.

M4M group

CP was applied and air blown. Then, the base liquid of M4M was activated by adding the TBB initiator (3:1 ratio), and a powder/liquid mixture was applied, using a brush-dip technique until the filling of the access hole was completed (Fig. 1). The resin was left for 10 min to complete auto-polymerization. The occlusal adjustment was carried out with the same manner, and the polishing was performed using silicone polishers (Komet 9557, 9553) under the same condition.

Patients who received a metal framed ceramic screw retained implant crown or bridge were included in this study. These access holes were delimited only by ceramic. Those with metal surface exposure were excluded from this study. Patients with edentulous arch or section, full or partial denture as antagonists were excluded from the study. During the evaluation period, 2 patients (male) dropped out from this study. One access-hole (AMB/22) with an atypical shape (non-circular) causing a noticeable overfilling of the M4M was excluded from this study. Finally, 12 patients with a total of 56 access-holes were examined (28 access holes for both groups, CR and M4M). For each patient, access-holes were randomly divided in right and left sides to get equivalent numbers for both materials. All the fillings (CR and M4M groups) were performed by a single operator.

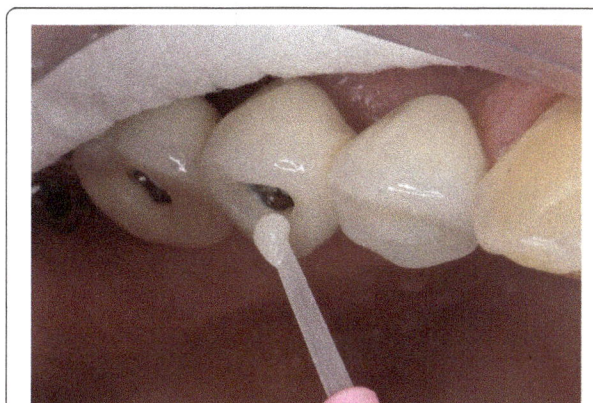

Fig. 1 Brush-dip technique

Table 1

Materials	Product names	Batch numbers	Manufacturer
Ceramic primer	Super-bond UCP	FX1	Sun Medical
Composite	Fantasista	GF11	Sun Medical
Bonding agent	Hybrid bond	FS1/GL1	Sun Medical
Adhesive composite	Bondfill SB	FT2/FS2/FS12	Sun Medical

For each access-hole, the contact patterns of antagonistic cusp in the centric occlusion were recorded intra-orally. They included; A: contact in the center, B: contact on the border of the access-hole and C: no contact close to the border (Fig. 2). At the time of the restoration ($T = 0$), followed by 1, 3, 6, and 12 months ($T = 1$, 3, 6, and 12 M), impressions were taken with polysiloxane impression materials (President, Light Body, (lot: G01914), Soft Putty (lot: G08568), Coltène/Whaledent AG, Switzerland) in a double mixed method. Epoxy casts (Devcon ET, Lot: 350402, ITW PP&F, Japan) were made from these impressions, and the fillings were examined using a motorized digital microscope (DSX510, Olympus KeyMed Ltd, USA) with a 1 µm accuracy under ×30 digital magnification.

For each clinical recall ($T = 0$ to $T = 12$ M), intra-oral photographs of the access hole fillings were taken.

Surface areas changes of access-hole filling

The surface areas of access holes could not be compared as the configuration of access-holes varied in each case. It was therefore necessary to compare longitudinal changes of the surface areas. At the time of $T = 0$, margin of the filling could not be clearly identified, thus, the measurement was fixed to begin at $T = 1$ M. For each

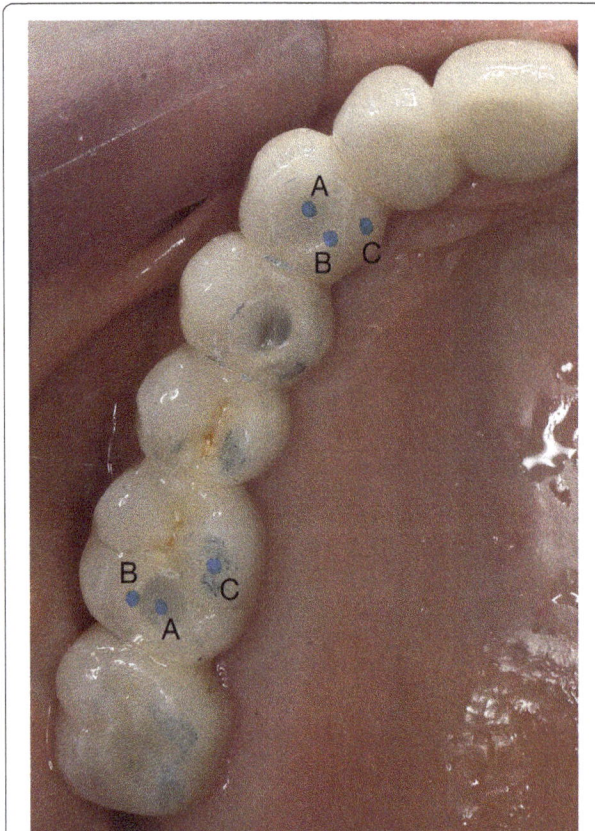

Fig. 2 Occlusal contact point

sample, from $T = 1$ M to $T = 12$ M, the surface areas of access-hole filling were measured perpendicular to the vertical surface of the hole using the same digital microscope. The surface at $T = 1$ M was considered as 100%, and compared with the $T = 3$, 6, and 12 M of identical filling (Fig. 3a–e).

Marginal analysis (depth and angle)

The marginal depth of the access-hole filling at $T = 0$, $T = 1$ M, $T = 3$ M, and $T = 6$ M could not be defined successfully because of the overfilling phenomenon which disrupted the measurement of marginal gap depth and angle (Fig. 3a–e). Only the marginal depth and angle at $T = 12$ M could be measured with the same digital microscope, and the mean value for each group was calculated. Each access-hole was divided into four areas including mesio-buccal, disto-buccal, mesio-palatal and disto-palatal surfaces (Fig. 4) to measure the distance of marginal discrepancy at resin/ceramic interface with a 1 µm accuracy (Fig. 5). With this value, a "marginal discrepancy pattern" could be extrapolated for each group (Fig. 7a, b).

Photographical analysis

For each access hole, an occlusal photograph was taken at the time of $T = 0$, $T = 1$ M, $T = 3$ M, $T = 6$ M, and $T = 12$ M, respectively. The marginal integrity was evaluated and recorded at the baseline and 12 months, according to an esthetical scale VAS (visual analogue scale) described by Weininger et al. [11]. Results were recorded by the authors and summarized in Table 2.

Results

Among the 56 access holes, no filling was dislodged during 12 months, and no complaint was registered from the patients regarding functional and aesthetical aspects.

Surface areas changes

The results for surface areas changes of access-hole fillings at respective intervals were summarized in Table 3 and Fig. 6. The mean values of the change from $T = 1$ M to $T = 12$ M were $77.1 \pm 13.1\%$ for group M4M and $83.3 \pm 11.5\%$ for group CR, respectively. They were not statistically different (Mann-Whitney test $p < 0.05$, $p = 0.046$).

Contact mode and the surface areas changes

The contact distribution was as follows; $A = 2$, $B = 14$, and $C = 40$. The access-hole distributions were 24(CR) and 24(M4M) for the premolar/molar region, 4(CR) and 4(M4M) for the incisor/canine region, respectively. Among 16 access-holes, 11 of M4M and 5 of CR presented "B" (14) or "A" (2) occlusal contact mode. The

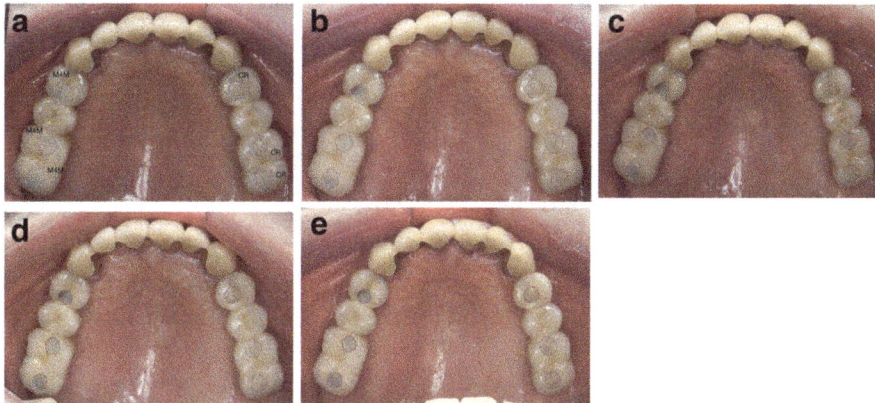

Fig. 3 a–e (Filling surface changes): **a** (ROG, $T = 0$). **b** (ROG, $T = 1$ M). **c** (ROG, $T = 3$ M). **d** (ROG, $T = 6$ M). **e** (ROG, $T = 12$ M)

average of the 11 (M4M) changes of the filling surface area at the time of $T = 12$ M was 77.1%. By pure coincidence, this mean value was identical to that of the 28 (M4M). For the 5 CR, the filling surface at $T = 12$ M was 85.3%. The average of the 28 CR was 83.3%.

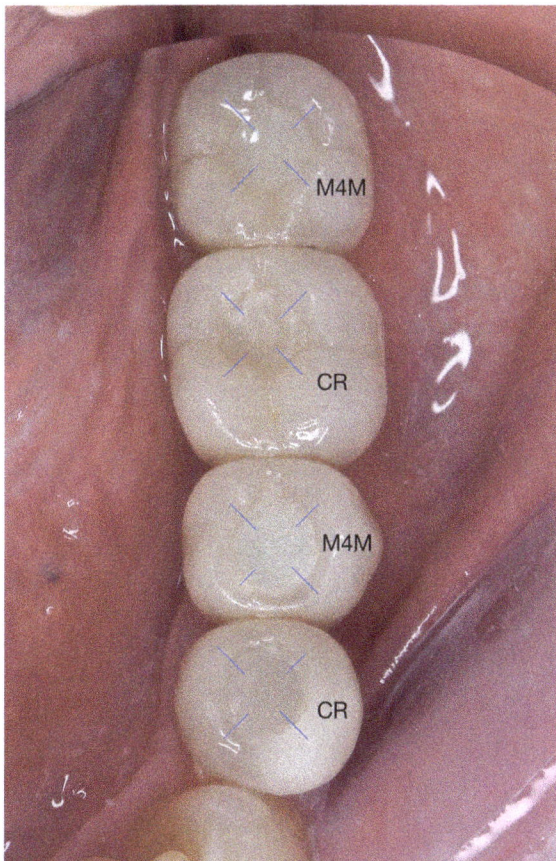

Fig. 4 Margin depth measurement localization (example: TRA, $T = 12$ M)

Marginal discrepancy: depth and angle analysis

The marginal depths of each access-hole (4 points) at $T = 12$ M were measured. The mean values for group CR were 141.2 ± 125.5 μm and 132.1 ± 107.8 μm for the group M4M, respectively. There was no significant difference between groups CR and M4M (Mann-Whitney test $p > 0.05$, $p = 0.58$).

The mean values of the angle at $T = 12$ M for group CR were $39.5 \pm 19.4°$ and $28.2 \pm 17.2°$ for group M4M, respectively. There was a significant difference (Mann-Whitney test $p < 0.0001$) between the groups CR and

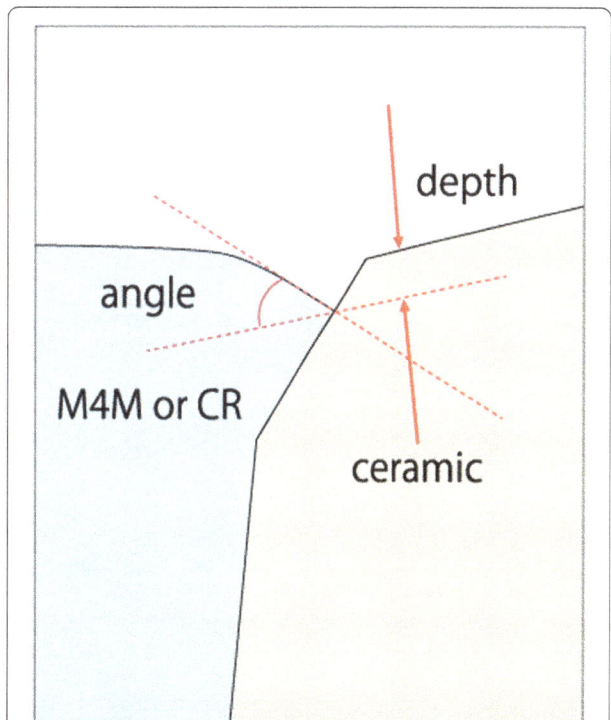

Fig. 5 Depth and angle at the margin

Table 2 Aesthetical Outcomes at T = 12 M (VAS Score)

Patients	Position CR	T = 0	T = 12	Patients	Position M4M	T = 0	T = 12
AMB	13	10	7	AMB	23	10	7
	14	6	5		24	8	3
	16	8	8		26	8	5
	17	10	10		27	8	5
ROG	24	10	7	ROG	14	10	6
	26	10	10		16	10	7
	27	10	10		17	10	7
NEU	11	4	3	NEU	21	6	5
	13	8	7		23	6	5
	16	8	7		25	10	10
POU	36	10	9	POU	27	10	10
TRA	34	10	8	TRA	35	10	10
	36	10	10		37	10	10
PHU	21	4	3	PHU	11	6	5
	25	10	5		14	8	8
	26	8	5		16	10	9
	27	8	5		17	10	9
ORT	15	10	7	ORT	14	10	10
					16	10	7
SUG	45	10	8	SUG	35	8	8
	47	10	10		37	8	8
KAI	46	8	6				
FRA	45	8	8	FRA	25	10	10
	46	10	10		26	8	8
	47	10	10		27	6	6
SHI	37	6	4	SHI	16	8	6
HAS	35	10	10	HAS	45	10	10
	36	8	8		46	8	8
	37	8	8		47	8	8
Average		8.64	7.43	Average		8.71	7.50
SD		1.81	2.23	SD		1.46	2.00

(T = 0)–(T = 12 M): CR 1.21 (SD = 1.37), M4M 1.21 (SD = 1.52) Mann-Whitney p > 0.05 (p = 0.848)
0: Filling completely dislodged
1: Filling partially dislodged
2: Access hole appearance and poor masking
3: 40% masking, with a marginal staining
4: 40% masking, no marginal staining
5: 60% masking, with a marginal staining
6: 60% masking, no marginal staining
7: 80% masking, with a marginal staining
8: 80% masking, no marginal staining
9: Total masking, with a marginal staining
10: Total masking, no marginal staining

Table 3 Surface areas changes of access-hole filling. Unit: %

	T = 1 M	T = 3 M	T = 6 M	T = 12 M
CR	100	93.2	87.6	83.3
M4M	100	91.1	83.2	77.1

Photographical analysis

Discoloration of the filling material as well as the marginal integrity was recorded at $T = 0$ and $T = 12$ M (Table 2). For the CR group, the mean VAS values were 8.64 at $T = 0$ and 7.43 at $T = 12$ M. The difference was 1.21 ± 1.37. For the M4M group, the mean VAS values were 8.71 at $T = 0$ and 7.50 at $T = 12$ M. The difference was 1.21 ± 1.52. No significant difference was found in CR and M4M groups (Mann-Whitney test $p > 0.05$, $p = 0.848$).

Discussion

Nowadays, implant screw-retained prosthesis becomes a popular mode of implant supra-structure restoration. Cement retained implant restoration has issues including irretrievability and difficulty of controlling the cement excess beyond the abutment joint. The cement excess can be a major cause of peri-implantitis [13–15]. Screw-retained implant restoration has also some disadvantages including the difficulty to get a right positioning of the access-hole compatible with a suitable aesthetic appearance and the aesthetic result of the access-hole restoration [16]. Inclined abutment or angling the screw channel can be an option to ameliorate the aesthetical outcomes [17, 18]. Moving the access hole to an occlusal or palatal/lingual zone would increase the indication of screw retained implant restoration. The development of the computer-assisted implant surgery increases the use of the screw-retained prosthesis compared to the cement retained method [19, 20]. Nevertheless, the integrity of the filling of the access hole is necessary to preserve to

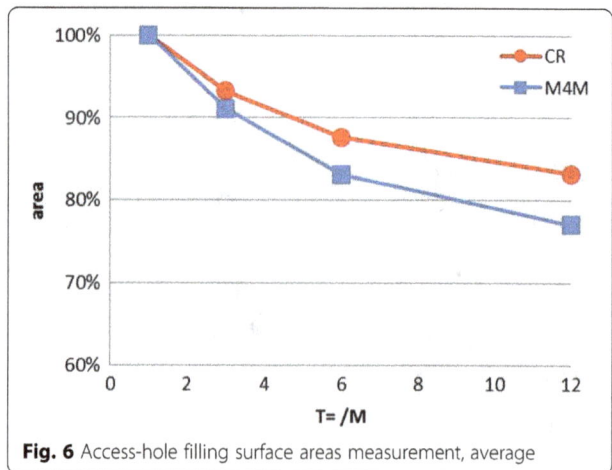

Fig. 6 Access-hole filling surface areas measurement, average

M4M. The marginal discrepancy patterns for both groups CR and M4M were different and shown in Fig. 7a, b.

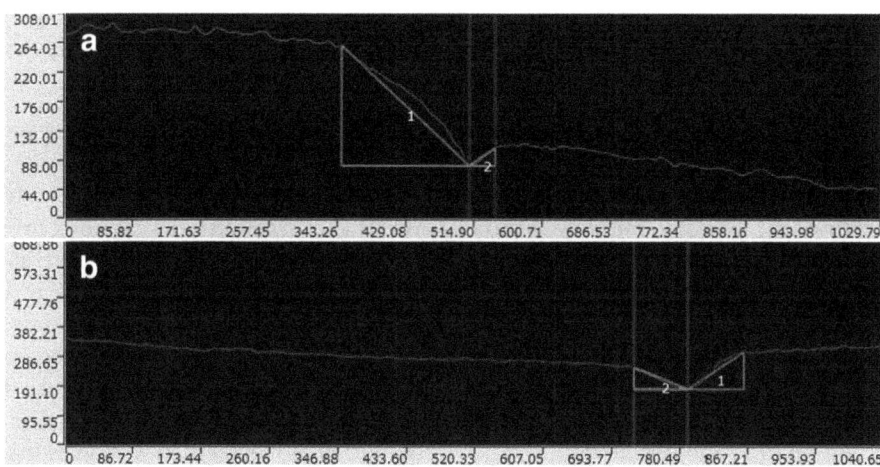

Fig. 7 a, **b** (The marginal discrepancy pattern for group CR and M4M). **a** Group CR (1: Ceramic surface, 2: CR surface) Units of the axis are in μm. **b** Group M4M (1: Ceramic surface, 2: M4M surface) Units of the axis are in μm

occlusal function and the aesthetic outcomes. Moreover, the access hole filling contributes to reinforce the surrounding ceramic [9].

In this context, access-hole filling is a common clinical procedure, but studies are quite limited in the literature. Photo-polymerizing resin composites have been widely used to fill the ceramic access holes, but unfortunately, the prognoses were less favorable [21–23]. The use of an efficient ceramic primer (CP) containing phosphoric acid monomer is mandatory to ensure durable adhesion to the feldspathic ceramic surface [24, 25]. In the previous in vitro study [12], ceramic access-hole specimens filled without ceramic pre-treatment showed no bond strength regardless of the use of the bonding agent. For this reason, in this in vivo study, the CP was used for groups CR and M4M.

Ceramic surfaces can be modified by silicate blasting or acid etching procedures to achieve a reliable adhesion [26, 27]. Hydrofluoric acid treatment has also been recommended but demands considerable precautions [28]. Clinically, decontamination by ultrasonic device during these procedures cannot be done easily [29]. It is also important to reduce clinical steps for access-hole filling.

The in vivo evaluation is quite different from that of the in vitro analysis. In the previous study, all the specimens were calibrated to a flat surface with 2.5 mm diameter. In present study, each access hole had a different dimension and configuration. The filling surfaces were often ø3 to 4 mm in diameter. Access-holes located in the occlusal groove area or in the inclined cusp surface induced an overfilling (Fig. 3a–e).

In clinical situations, masticatory stresses are quite different from the standard three-body generalized wear test [30]. Factors associating with wear processes

including occlusal force, direction and speed of food excursion are individually different according to the location of the access-hole. Therefore, in this study, both filling groups were arranged in a symmetrical random way. For these reasons, the evaluation of changes in surface areas, marginal wear pattern, and marginal depth of fillings were selected.

Surface areas changes

The surface areas of filling were reduced with time due to the wear of overflowed material that occurs systematically in a clinical situation. At the baseline ($T = 0$), M4M group presented the overfilling more frequently compared to the CR group possibly due to the low viscosity of the material during the setting time. M4M is much more fluid than CR, and the setting time duration is longer. The surface reduction by the occlusal wear seems to be smaller when the filling surface comes closer to the vertical inner wall of the access hole (Figs. 3a–e and 6). This particularity is the main difference with the previous in vitro study [12].

This surface reduction due to the wear might have a threshold value in relation with the material thickness at the margin and the toughness of the material regarding the compressive strength against the occlusal loading. A long-term analysis should be conducted to determine if this surface reduction will decrease with time.

Focusing on numbers of access-hole showing a disappearance of the overfilling in an early period (up to T = 3 M), groups CR and M4M exhibited 82% (23/28) and 39.3% (11/28), respectively (Table 4). This can be explained by the differences of mechanical properties of both materials. The elastic moduli of M4M and CR are 1.9 and 7.9 MPa, respectively. Flexural strength of M4M is 66 MPa which is comparable to

Table 4 Disappearance of the overfilling. Unit: %

	$T = 1$ M	$T = 3$ M	$T = 6$ M	$T = 12$ M	No disappearance
CR	53.5% (15/28)	28.5% (8/28)	7.1% (2/28)	3.6% (1/28)	7.1% (2/28)
M4M	28.6% (8/28)	10.7% (3/28)	28.5% (8/28)	28.5% (8/28)	3.6% (1/28)

that of an acrylic resin (60 MPa) and almost half compared to CR (115 MPa) [31, 32]. The low flexural strength of M4M possibly absorbed the occlusal stresses, and the overfilling stayed longer compared to CR.

According to the results of contact mode and the surface areas changes, it was suggested that there were no correlations among the occlusal contact modes and the surface areas reduction up to 12 months in vivo.

Marginal depth analysis

As mentioned in the previous study [12], the margin of M4M group had a better adhesion to the surrounding access hole ceramic and no gap formation was observed between the cavity and the filling material, due to the specific polymerization mode (TBB initiator). The bond strengths on the glazed feldspathic ceramic were 7.6 ± 2.2 MPa for group CR, and 8.6 ± 1.0 MPa for group M4M. In some cases, adhesive failure mode was detected at the margin with group CR. The polymerization shrinkage of the CR might have deteriorated the adhesion quality at the margin [33].

The elastic modulus of a filling material and its flexural strength influence the wear resistance at the marginal zone [31]. The difference of the polymerization mode modifies the stress distribution at the marginal areas. M4M is polymerized with the TBB auto-polymerizing catalyst; therefore it shows low shrinkage at the marginal surface and possesses an advantage of minimizing gap formation [34]. The marginal areas of CR might receive stress concentration, and subsequent micro-gap formation possibly occurred due to polymerization shrinkage during the photo-polymerization. The wear values of filling material itself influence the wear pattern. The 3-body wear values are 1.5 mm [3] for the acrylic resin, 0.9 mm [3] for the M4M and 0.3 mm [3] for the CR. The toothbrush wear test shows the same tendency [34]. Although, CR contains greater amounts of filler (TMPT fillers) compared to M4M (CR:71.5 wt%, M4M:<10 wt%), M4M has an aptitude for lower brittleness compared to CR as its matrix consists of acrylic resin which possesses flexibility [35].

Photographical analysis

The analysis for the ratio of access-hole with or without marginal staining at the time of $T = 12$ M showed that the results in group CR (12/16) and in group M4M (12/16) were the same. For this reason, the marginal discrepancy pattern, different in both groups did not influence the aesthetical result. The occlusal contact point (A, B, or C) was compared to the marginal staining rate. Among the access-holes with A or B contact point, 6 out of 16 presented the marginal staining at the time of $T = 12$ M. For C contact point, 18 out of 40 presented the marginal staining at the time of $T = 12$ M. No correlation was admitted between the occlusal contact mode and the marginal staining.

An opaque composite resin for the CR group and an opaquer powder for the M4M group might improve the esthetical result and hide the metal frame or the prosthetic screw in the access-hole [36, 37].

Some studies analyzed the effectiveness of a ceramic inlay to restore an access hole [38]. Above the screw, a channel of 3 to 4 mm is needed to achieve this technique and in some clinical situations, there is less than 2 mm. Despite the excellent aesthetical results, with ceramic inlay technique, crown or bridge retrieval is harder and generates an additional cost. The poor clinical result reported with the composite resin filling (control group) might be the fact that a ceramic primer and a bonding agent were not used.

Conclusions

Within the limitation of the study, it was concluded that:

The null-hypothesis "superficial and marginal deterioration of M4M and CR would not be significantly different" was accepted.
The M4M (modified 4-META/MMA-TBB resin) and CR (composite resin) combined with a ceramic primer showed comparable characteristics (marginal integrity and wear behavior) in an access hole filling.
The esthetical evaluation (VAS scale) showed that there were no significant differences between group M4M and CR.
After 12 months, the pattern of marginal wear showed a difference, but both materials clinically worked out successfully.

Further long-term investigation is necessary to confirm these findings.

Acknowledgements
The authors thank Sun Medical Corporation for their material supply.

Authors' contributions
RT and SS carried out the clinical data and their analysis. RT and SS have been involved in drafting the manuscript and approved the final version to be published.

Competing interests
The authors, Rémy Tanimura and Shiro Suzuki, declare that they have no financial, commercial or any other competing interests.

Author details
[1]8, place du Général Catroux, 75017 Paris, France. [2]Department of Clinical Community and Sciences, University of Alabama at Birmingham School of Dentistry, 1919 7th Avenue South, Birmingham, AL 35294-0007, USA.

References
1. Millen C, Brägger U, Wittneben JG. Influence of prosthesis type and retention mechanism on complications with fixed implant-supported prostheses: a systematic review applying multivariate analyses. Int J Oral Maxillofac Implants. 2015;30(1):110–24.
2. Guichet DL, Caputo AA, Choi H, Sorensen JA. Passivity of fit and marginal opening in screw- or cement-retained implant fixed partial denture designs. Int J Oral Maxillofac Implants. 2000;15:239–46.
3. de França DG, Morais MH, dasNeves FD, Carreiro AF, Barbosa GA. Precision fit of screw-retained implant-supported fixed dental prostheses fabricated by CAD/CAM, copy-milling, and conventional methods. Int J Oral Maxillofac Implants. 2016. doi:10.11607/jomi.5023.
4. Cho SC, Small PN, Elian N, Tarnow D. Screw loosening for standard and wide diameter implants in partially edentulous cases: 3- to 7-year longitudinal data. Implant Dent. 2004;13:245–50.
5. Korsch M, Obst U, Walter W. Cement-associated per-implantitis: a retrospective clinical observational study of fixed implant-supported restorations using a methacrylate cement. Clin Oral Implants Res. 2014;25(7):797–802.
6. Linkevicius T, Puisys A, Vindasiute E, Linkeviciene L, Apse P. Does residual cement around implant-supported restorations cause peri-implant disease? A retrospective case analysis. Clin Oral Implants Res. 2013;24(11):1179–84.
7. Hebel KS, Gajjar RC. Cement-retained versus screw-retained implant restorations: achieving optimal occlusion and esthetics in implant dentistry. J Prothet Dent. 1997;77:28–35.
8. Torrado E, Ercoli C, Al M, Graser GN, Tallents RH, Cordaro L. A comparison of the porcelain fracture resistance of screw-retained and cement-retained implant-supported metal-ceramic crowns. J Prosthet Dent. 2004;91:532–7.
9. Derafshi R, Farzin M, Taghva M, Heidary H, Atashkar B. The effects of new design of access hole on porcelain fracture resistance of implant-supported crowns. J Dent (Shiraz). 2015;16(1 Suppl):61–7.
10. Taylor RC, Ghoneim AS, McGlumphy EA. An esthetic technique to fill screw-retained fixed prostheses. J Oral Implantol. 2004;30(6):384–5.
11. Weininger B, McGlumphy E, Beck M. Esthetic evaluation of materials used to fill access holes of screw-retained implant crowns. J Oral Implantol. 2008;34(3):145–9.
12. Tanimura R, Suzuki S. In vitro evaluation of a modified 4-META/MMA-TBB resin for filling access holes of screw-retained implant prostheses. J Biomed Mater Res B ApplBiomater. 2015;103(5):1030–6.
13. Korsch M, Walther W. Peri-implantitis associated with type of cement: a retrospective analysis of different types of cement and their clinical correlation to the peri-implant tissue. Clin Implant Dent Relat Res. 2015;17(Suppl 2):e434–43.
14. Linkevicius T, Vindasiute E, Puisys A, Linkeviciene L, Maslova N, Puriene A. The influence of the cementation margin position on the amount of undetected cement. A prospective clinical study. Clin Oral Implants Res. 2013;24(1):71–6.
15. Vindasiute E, Puisys A, Maslova N, Linkeviciene L, Peciuliene V, Linkevicius T. Clinical factors influencing removal of the cement excess in implant-supported restorations. Clin Implant Dent Relat Res. 2015;17(4):771–8.
16. Thalji G, Bryington M, De Kok IJ, Cooper LF. Prosthodontic management of implant therapy. Dent Clin North Am. 2014;58(1):207–25.
17. Dittmer MP, Nensa M, Stiesch M, Kohorst P. Load-bearing capacity of screw-retained CAD/CAM-produced titanium implant frameworks (I-Bridge®2) before and after cyclic mechanical loading. J Appl Oral Sci. 2013;21(4):307–13.
18. Turkylmaz I, Patel NS, McGlumphy EA. Oral rehabilitation of a severely resorbed edentoulous maxilla with screw-retained hybrid denture using Cresco system: a case report. Eur J Dent. 2008;2(3):220–3.
19. Balshi SF, Wolfinger GJ, Balshi TJ. A protocol for immediate placement of a prefabricated screw-retained provisional prosthesis using computed tomography and guided surgery and incorporating planned alveoplasty. Int J Periodontics Restorative Dent. 2011;31(1):49–55.
20. Meloni SM, De Riu G, Pisano M, Tullio A. Full arch restoration with computer-assisted implant surgery and immediate loading in edentulous ridges with dental fresh extraction sockets. One year results of 10 consecutively treated patients: guided implant surgery and extraction sockets. J Maxillofac Oral Surg. 2013;12(3):321–5.
21. Lee A, Okayasu K, Wang HL. Screw-versus cement-retained implant restorations: current concepts. Implant Dent. 2010;19(1):8–15.
22. Cicciù M, Beretta M, Risitano G, Maiorana C. Cemented-retained vs screw-retained implant restorations: an investigation on 1939 dental implants. Minerva Stomatol. 2008;57(4):167–79.
23. Michalakis KX, Hirayama H, Garefis PD. Cement-retained versus screw-retained implant restorations: a critical review. Int J Oral Maxillofac Implants. 2003;18(5):719–28.
24. Taira Y, Sakai M, Sawase T. Effects of primer containing silane and thiophosphate monomers on bonding resin to a leucite-reinforced ceramic. J Dent. 2012;40(5):353–8.
25. Kato H, Matsumura H, Tanaka T, Atsuta M. Bond strength and durability of porcelain bonding systems. J Prosthet Dent. 1996;75(2):163–8.
26. Queiroz JR, Souza RO, Nogueira Junior Jr L, Ozcan M, Bottino MA. Influence of acid-etching and ceramic primers on the repair of a glass ceramic. Gen Dent. 2012;60(2):e79–85.
27. Bottino MA, Snellaert A, Bergoli CD, Özcan M, Bottino MC, Valandro LF. Effect of ceramic etching protocols on resin bond strength to a felspar ceramic. Oper Dent. 2015;40(2):E40–6.
28. Ozcan M, Allahbeickaraghi A, Dündar M. Possible hazardous effects of hydrofluoric acid and recommendations for treatment approach: a review. Clin Oral Investig. 2012;16(1):15–23.
29. Magne P, Cascione D. Influence of post-etching cleaning and connecting porcelain on the microtensile bond strength of composite resin to feldspatic porcelain. J Prothet Dent. 2006;96(5):354–61.
30. Leinfelder KF, Suzuki S. In vitro wear device for determining posterior composite wear. J Am Dent Assoc. 1999;130(9):1347–53.
31. Sumino N, Tsubota K, Takamizawa T, Shiratsuchi K, Miyazawa M, Latta MA. Comparison of the wear and flexural characteristics of flowable resin composites for posterior lesions. Acta Odontol Scand. 2013;71:820–7.
32. Ikeda T, Wakabayashi N, Ona M, Ohyama T. Effects of polymerization shrinkage on the interfacial stress at resin-metal joint in denture-base: a non-linear FE stress analysis. Dent Mater. 2006;22:413–9.
33. Kawai K, Leinfelder KF. Effect of resin composite adhesion on marginal degradation. Dent Mater J. 1995;14(2):211–20.
34. Naito K. Bonding and wear characteristics of a tri-n-butylborane initiated adhesive resin filled with pre-polymerized composite particles. J Oral Sci. 2011;53(1):109–16.
35. Wimmer T, Huffmann AM, Eichberger M, Schmidlin PR, Stawarczyk B. Two-body wear rate of PEEK, CAD/CAM resin composite and PMMA: effect of specimen geometries, antagonist materials and test set-up configuration. Dent Mater. 2016;32(6):e127–36.
36. Kurt M, Ural C, Kulunk T, Sanal AF, Erkoçak A. The effect of screw color and technique to fill access hole on the final color of screw-retained implants crowns. J Oral Implantol. 2011;37(6):673–9.
37. de Pereira R P, Rocha CO, Reis JM, Arioli-Filho JN. Influence of sealing of the screw access hole on the fracture resistance of implant-supported restorations. Braz Dent J. 2016;27(2):148–52.
38. Mihali S, Canjau S, Bratu E, Wang HL. Utilization of ceramic inlays for sealing implant prostheses screw access holes: a case-control study. Int J Oral Maxillofac Implants. 2016;31(5):1142–9.

19

The influence of systemically or locally administered mesenchymal stem cells on tissue repair in a rat oral implantation model

Miya Kanazawa[1†], Ikiru Atsuta[1*†] (iD), Yasunori Ayukawa[1], Takayoshi Yamaza[2], Ryosuke Kondo[1], Yuri Matsuura[1] and Kiyoshi Koyano[1]

Abstract

Background: Multipotent mesenchymal stem cells (MSCs) are used clinically in regenerative medicine. Our previous report showed systemically injected MSCs improved peri-implant sealing and accelerated tissue healing. However, the risks of systemic MSC administration, including lung embolism, must be considered; therefore, their local application must be assessed for clinical safety and efficacy. We investigated differences in treatment effect between local and systemic MSC application using a rat oral implantation model.

Methods: Rat bone marrow-derived MSCs were isolated and culture-expanded. The rat's right maxillary first molars were extracted and replaced with experimental titanium implants. After 24 h, MSCs (1×10^6/ml) were systemically or locally injected into recipient rats via the tail vein (systemic group) or buccal subcutaneous tissue (local group), respectively. Rats treated in the absence of MSCs were included as a control (control group). The maxillary epithelium was assessed histologically after 4 weeks to evaluate laminin-332 (Ln-332) distribution and horseradish peroxidase invasion, as indicators of peri-implant epithelium (PIE) formation and PIE sealing to the implant surface, respectively. The effect of MSCs on rat oral epithelial cell (OEC) morphology was determined by coculture.

Results: Systemic group MSCs accumulated early at the peri-implant mucosa, while local group MSCs were observed in various organs prior to later accumulation around the implant surface. PIE formation and Ln-332-positive staining at the implant interface were enhanced in the systemic group compared with the local and control groups. Furthermore, OEC adherence on implants was reduced in high-density compared with low-density MSC cocultures.

Conclusions: Local MSC injection was more ineffective than systemic MSC injection at enhancing PIE sealing around titanium implants. Thus, although local MSC administration has a wide range of applications, further investigations are needed to understand the exact cellular and molecular mechanisms of this approach prior to clinical use.

Keywords: Mesenchymal stem cell, Dental implant, Epithelial cell, Systemic and local administration

* Correspondence: atyuta@dent.kyushu-u.ac.jp
†Equal contributors
[1]Section of Implant and Rehabilitative Dentistry, Division of Oral Rehabilitation, Faculty of Dental Science, Kyushu University, 3-1-1 Maidashi, Higashi-ku, Fukuoka 812-8582, Japan
Full list of author information is available at the end of the article

Background

Mesenchymal stem cell (MSC)-based approaches can be broadly divided into two categories: cell therapy and regenerative medicine. Cell therapy is focused on the anti-inflammatory, immune-regulatory, and homeostasis-regulatory actions of MSCs to treat disorders like malignant lymphoma, angina pectoris, and atopic dermatitis. Conversely, regenerative medicine is focused on MSCs playing a tissue engineering role, to enhance tissue regeneration using growth factors and scaffolds; for example, to generate tissue-engineered skin or cartilage, which have been assessed in clinical trials.

Our previous study showed that systemically injected MSCs improved attachment of the peri-implant epithelium (PIE) to the titanium (Ti) implant surface and accelerated tissue healing around the implant. Because the systemically injected MSCs accumulated around the experimental implant, we believe they acted through both regenerative medicine and cell therapy modes [1]. Indeed, the peri-implant tissue is always exposed to the possibility of inflammation because the Ti implant penetrates through the oral mucosa. However, many studies have shown that the PIE has a low sealing ability within the oral environment [2–4], meaning bacteria can more readily accumulate around the implant and induce inflammatory destruction more easily than around the natural tooth [5, 6]. Additionally, it is important to prevent epithelial down-growth by promoting epithelial cell adherence and stabilizing the epithelial soft tissue seal [7]. Therefore, improving local defense within the mucosa is indispensable to enabling successful implantation.

Some studies report that epithelial healing after implant replacement is similar to mucosa wound healing [8]. Wound healing goes through a genetically programmed repair process involving inflammation, cell proliferation, re-epithelialization, formation of granulation tissue, angiogenesis, interactions between various cell types, and matrix/tissue remodeling [9]. Therefore, the aim of MSC treatment is to regulate many cells to restore the structure, function, and physiology of damaged tissues around the implant [10].

Accumulation of MSCs adjacent to the damaged tissue following their administration into an implant model can be determined following "systemic" or "local" transplantation. Although systemic MSC administration has proven efficacious and has a large advantage as our above previous studies [11, 12], possible risks, including pulmonary embolism, pose a serious issue [13, 14]. It is therefore important to provide an alternative low-risk method that avoids MSCs becoming trapped within healthy organs. Despite this, cell regulation following local cell administration is not well-documented with respect to peri-implant tissue regeneration.

The purpose of this study was to verify the effects and mechanisms of bone marrow-derived MSCs following their local administration using an oral implantation rat model, to deepen our understanding of this approach for effective utilization of MSCs.

Methods

MSC isolation

Bone marrow cells were flushed out of the femurs and tibias of 4-week-old green fluorescent protein-transgenic Wistar rats. Cells were treated with a 0.85% NH_4Cl solution for 10 min to lyse the red blood cells and were passed through a 70-μm cell strainer to obtain a single cell suspension. Cells were seeded into 100-mm plastic culture dishes (1×10^6 cells/dish), washed with phosphate buffered saline (PBS), and cultured in growth medium consisting of alpha minimum essential medium (α-MEM; Invitrogen, Grand Island, NY, USA), 20% fetal bovine serum (Equitech-Bio, Kerrville, TX), 2 mM L-glutamine (Invitrogen), 55 μm 2-mercaptoethanol (Invitrogen), 100 U/ml penicillin, and 100 μg/ml streptomycin (Invitrogen). Passage 3 (P3) cells were used experimentally in this study.

Immunofluorescent staining

MSCs (5×10^4 cells/ml) were seeded into 35-mm dishes and incubated for 12 h at 37 °C in 5% CO_2. The slides were then fixed in 4% paraformaldehyde (PFA) for 5 min and blocked with secondary antibody-matched normal serum for 1 h, followed by incubation with mouse anti-rat CD44, CD90, and CD105 antibodies (1:100, Sigma-Aldrich, St. Louis, MO,) overnight at 4 °C. The slides were then treated with fluorescein isothiocyanate (FITC)-conjugated secondary antibodies (1:200, Jackson Immuno Research, West Grove, PA) for 1 h at room temperature and mounted using VECTASHIELD® Mounting Medium containing 4′6-diamidino-2-phenylindole (DAPI) (Vector Laboratories, Burlingame, CA).

Experimental implants

Single piece, screw-type pure Ti (Japan Industrial Standards Class 1; equivalent to ASTM Grade 1) experimental implants with a machine-polished surface (Sky blue, Fukuoka, Japan) were used in accordance to our previous study [15] (Fig. 1a). Implant surface roughness was measured using a laser scanning microscope (VK-9710, Keyence, Osaka, Japan), and the arithmetic mean roughness (Ra) was found to be 0.16 μm. The implants were treated with 100% acetone and autoclave sterilized before use.

Oral implantation

All experimental procedures were approved by the Ethics Committee on Animal Experimentation at Kyushu University (Approval Number: A25-133-0), Japan, in accordance with the ARRIVE guidelines and the Guidelines of the

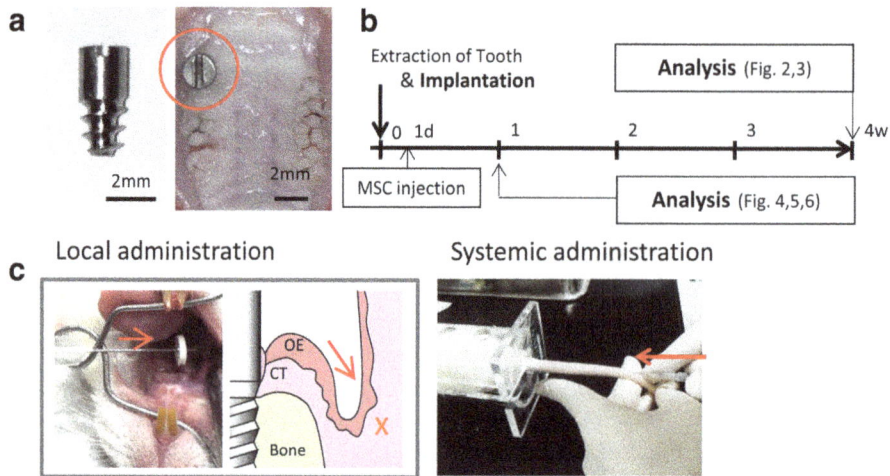

Fig. 1 In vivo experimental design. **a** Photographs of the experimental implant (left panel) and implant in the rat oral cavity (right panel). **b** Experimental protocol of in vivo study: Implantation was performed at the same time as tooth extraction, then 1 day after implantation, mesenchymal stem cells (MSCs) were injected via the tail vein or into the gingivobuccal fold around the dental implant. Epithelial tissue structure around the implant was observed after 4 weeks. MSC accumulation into various tissues was observed 1, 3, 5, and 7 days after MSCs injection. **c** Photograph of MSC administration into the model rat with the experimental implant

Japanese Physiological Society. Surgical implantation was performed in accordance with previously published protocols [4, 16]. Briefly, 6-week-old Wistar rats (27 males, 120–150 g) underwent immediate implant placement as follows: the maxillary right first molars were removed and an experimental implant was screwed into the socket under systemic chloral hydrate under systemic anesthesia.

MSC administration

Twenty-four hours after implantation, rats were lightly anesthetized with chloral hydrate and lidocaine hydrochloride, and ex vivo expanded P3 green fluorescent protein (GFP)-MSCs (1×10^6 cells) were administered via one of the following modes: (1) systemic injection via the tail vein (systemic group), (2) local injection into the gingivobuccal fold around the dental implant (local group), and (3) no MSC injection (control group).

Smear staining

Peripheral blood was collected from the retro-orbital plexus of the model rats. Samples were spread onto slides, dried for 30 min, and fixed in 4% PFA for 10 min. For fluorescence staining, samples were incubated with FITC-conjugated rat anti-GFP antibodies for 2 h at 37 °C. Imaging was performed using an Axiotech Microscope (Carl Zeiss, Göttingen, Germany).

Enzyme-linked immunosorbent assay for inflammatory markers

Peripheral blood was centrifuged to obtain the blood serum, corrected 24 h after the MSC administration. The supernatants from the blood were extracted using

M-PER® (Thermo Fisher Scientific, Waltham, MA) mammalian protein extraction reagent. The samples were centrifuged and used in an enzyme-linked immunosorbent assay (ELISA) for detection of interleukin (IL)-2, IL-4, and IL-10 (R&D Systems).

Instillation of horseradish peroxidase

The procedure for topical application of horseradish peroxidase (HRP) was similar to that reported previously [16, 17]. Four weeks after implantation, rats were placed under deep anesthesia, and 50 mg/ml of HRP (type 11, molecular weight 40,000 Da, Sigma-Aldrich) was instilled into the oral mucosa surrounding the implant for 60 min. The optimal length of HRP penetration was estimated using peroxidase 3,3′-diaminobenzidine (DAB, Nacalai tesque, Kyoto, Japan) and hematoxylin staining.

Tissue preparation and immunohistochemistry for immunofluorescence

Tissues were prepared in accordance to the methods described in our previous studies [8, 15]. After each experimental period, the rats were deeply anesthetized and perfused intracardially with heparinized PBS followed by 4% PFA (pH 7.4). Tissue samples (lung, liver, heart, and maxilla) were collected at each experimental period, dissected, and immersed in 4% PFA for 48 h at 4 °C. The oral mucosa surrounding the implant and tooth site was carefully removed from the bone, implant, or tooth, and cut into 10-μm bucco-palatal sections using a cryostat at − 20 °C. The sections were then stained immunohistochemically using mouse anti-rat GFP (1:100, Sigma-Aldrich), CD90 (1:100, Sigma-Aldrich), and Ln-332 (1:100, Santa Cruz

Biotechnology, Santa Cruz, CA) antibodies (1:100, Sigma-Aldrich) overnight at 4 °C. Samples were then treated with FITC-conjugated secondary antibody (1:200, Jackson Immuno Research, West Grove, PA, USA) for 1 h at room temperature and mounted with DAPI (Vector Laboratories), as described previously [17, 18].

Detection of cell apoptosis

For apoptosis detection, the 10-μm bucco-palatal sections from around the experimental implant were incubated overnight with FITC-conjugated anti-rat GFP (1:100, Sigma-Aldrich) and 7-amino actinomycin D (7-AAD, Apoptosis Detection Kit; BD Biosciences, Franklin Lakes, NJ) at 4 °C. Apoptotic cells were then counted and calculated as a percentage of the total cells.

Osteogenic differentiation assay

MSCs were cultured in osteogenic culture medium containing 1.8 mM KH_2PO_4 and 10 nM dexamethasone (Sigma-Aldrich). After 28 days of osteogenic induction, an expression of the osteogenic marker runt-related transcription factor 2 (Runx2, 1:100, Santa Cruz Biotechnology) was determined by immunofluorescent staining.

Adipogenic differentiation assay

MSCs were cultured in adipogenic culture medium containing 0.5 mM isobutylmethylxanthine, 60 μM indomethacin, 0.5 μM hydrocortisone, and 10 μg/ml insulin (all Sigma-Aldrich). After 14 days of adipogenic induction, expression of the adipogenic marker, peroxisome proliferator-activated receptor gamma (PPARγ, 1:100, Santa Cruz Biotechnology), was determined by immunofluorescent staining.

Isolation of oral mucosa epithelial cells

Oral mucosa epithelial cell (OEC) cultures were performed based on a previous report [19]. Briefly, oral mucosa derived from 4-day-old Wistar rats was incubated with dispase (1×10^3 IU/ml) in Mg^{2+} and Ca^{2+}-free PBS for 12 h at 4 °C. The oral epithelium was then peeled from the connective tissue using tweezers. The epithelium was dispersed by pipetting ten times and seeded onto dishes or Ti plates placed on the bottom of dishes. OECs were cultured in defined keratinocyte serum-free medium (DK-SFM; Invitrogen, Grand Island, NY) and gentamicin (50 μg/ml) on plastic in a humidified atmosphere of 95% air and 5% CO_2 at 37 °C.

OEC coculture with MSCs

OECs were cocultured indirectly with MSCs using Transwell® insert as a separator between the two cell types. Briefly, OECs were cultured at a density of 5×10^5 cells/mL on mirror-surfaced pure Ti plates [15 mm diameter by 1 mm thickness, 0.19 μm roughness (Ra),

Japan Industrial Standards Class 1 (equivalent for ASTM Grade I)] (KS40, Kobelco, Kobe, Japan). Transwell inserts without MSCs in the upper chamber served as controls (Fig. 7a). As shown in Fig. 7c, the upper chamber contained either 5×10^2, 5×10^3, 5×10^4, or 5×10^5 MSCs (in 0.5 ml of culture medium), while the bottom chamber contained 5×10^4 OECs (in 1.5 ml of medium) for the various assays described below.

Cell adhesion assays

OEC adhesion assays were conducted according to previously published methods [16, 20]. Non-adherent or weakly attached cells were removed by shaking (3 × 5 min at 75 rpm) using a rotary shaker (NX-20, Nissin, Tokyo, Japan). Adherent cells were then counted and calculated as a percentage of the initial count, which was used to define adhesive strength of the cells.

Scratch assays

Scratch assays were performed on Ti plates to model wounding using various numbers of MSCs in the upper Transwell chamber. The techniques were conducted as described previously [16, 20]. Briefly, confluent OEC monolayers were scratched with a cell scraper and cultured for 48 h. OECs at the edge of the wound were visualized immunofluorescently using antibodies against actin to observe cell migration, and then the migrating cells were counted on the wound area.

Statistical analysis

Data are presented as means ± standard deviation (SD). One-way analysis of variance (ANOVA) with Fisher's least significant difference test was performed. Significance was established when $p < 0.05$. Experiments were performed with triplicate samples and were repeated three or four times to verify reproducibility.

Results and discussion

Because MSC treatment is being introduced more widely as a clinically available therapy, the method of administration must be considered to better mitigate risk. Although for a number of other factors also need consideration, including cell source, cell donor condition, cell population, and timing of MSC administration, this study only focused on comparison between systemic and local injection of MSCs into a rat oral implant model.

Sealing and defense at the PIE–implant interface are very important because dental implants in the oral mucosa are at high risk of inflammation. However, sealing between the PIE and implant is much weaker than that between the junctional epithelium (JE) and teeth [3], possibly owing to an inferiority of adhesion structures at the PIE-implant interface [15]. We therefore aimed to

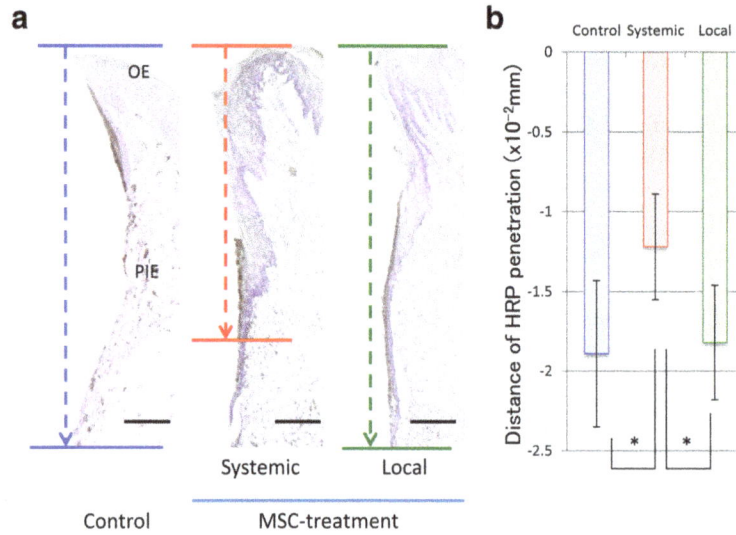

Fig. 2 HRP penetration on implant surface. **a** Light micrographs of the epithelial structure around the control, local, and systemic group implants after HRP penetration. Bar = 200 μm. **b** Median distance of HRP penetration. Each bar represents the mean ± SD of the three independent experiments. *$p < 0.05$ vs. Cont

assess the influence of MSCs during implant treatment. Our previous report showed a positive effect of systemically injected MSCs for the improvement of peri-implant tissue sealing and acceleration of tissue healing [11].

HRP penetration on implant surface

In the systemic group, a strong HRP reaction was seen only in the coronal portion of the PIE on the implant surface (Fig. 2a). In the control and local groups, HRP reaction was not only found in the coronal PIE region on the surface of the PIE but also in the connective tissue. Furthermore, in the middle and apical PIE regions of these latter groups, the deep layers of PIE cells exhibited the strongest HRP reaction. This result meant that the PIE with these groups had only a weak epithelial sealing, and had been penetration of the external factors to the surrounding tissue of implant.

The systemic group exhibited a significant improvement in blocking HRP penetration (Fig. 2b) compared

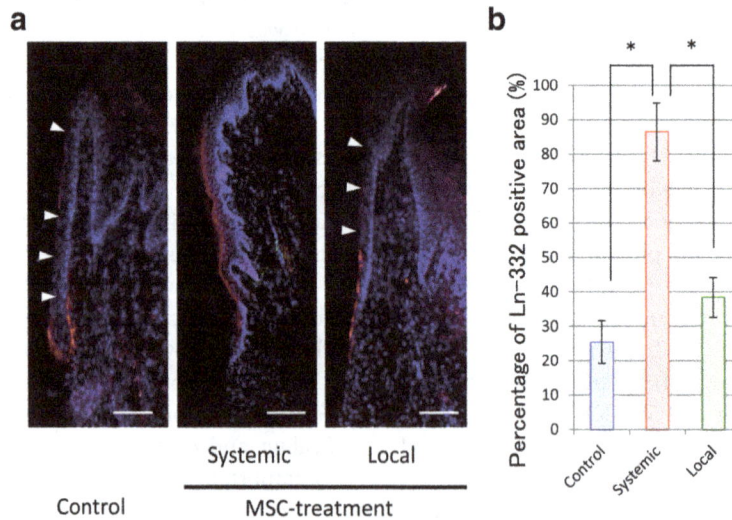

Fig. 3 Ln-332 distribution on peri-implant epithelium (PIE) after MSC injection. **a** Light micrographs of Ln-332 distribution (red staining) in the gingiva around the control, local, and systemic group implants after 4 weeks. White arrowheads indicated lack of positive reaction. Blue staining: DAPI (bar = 200 μm) (**b**). Quantitation of Ln-332 presence in the PIE. Images were analyzed to quantify Ln-332 expression in the PIE around the implants. Each data point represents the mean ± SD of the three independent experiments. *$p < 0.05$

with both the local and control groups, which were comparable.

Distribution of Ln-332 in the peri-implant oral mucosa

In the systemic group, immunohistochemical staining of Ln-332 showed a positive reaction along the whole implant-PIE interface at 4 weeks (Fig. 3a). In the local group, the Ln-332 deposition pattern in the PIE was comparable to that of the control group. In the oral mucosa around both local and control group implants, Ln-332-positive staining was apparent at the apical portion of the implant-PIE interface, but the upper portion of the interface did not exhibit Ln-332 detection. Only in the control group was the PIE-connective tissue interface intensely stained at the end of the PIE. Absence of Ln-332 staining was noted in the buccal mucosa underlying the OSE or OE in all groups.

As shown in Fig. 3b, expression of adhesion proteins on the interface between PIE-implant was significantly lower in the control and local groups compared with the systemic group.

Ln-332 is the major adhesive ligand for integrin α6β4, which interacts with the cytoskeletal elements, and is a component of the hemidesmosomes, epithelial adhesion plaques that tack the plasma membrane of the epithelial cells [21–23]. Moreover, Ln is expressed at the interface between the JE and natural tooth [24, 25] and is thought to be critical for the attachment of gingival epithelial cells to substrates [26, 27]. In our previous study, Ln was implicated in the adhesion of the PIE to the dental implant [20, 28]. Therefore, we observed the distribution of Ln during PIE formation around the implant to eliminate the influence of transplanted MSCs on the OE.

Connecting Ln and α6β4 integrin activates intracellular signaling pathways, such as the mitogen-activated protein kinase (MAPK) and phosphoinositide 3-kinase (PI3K) signaling pathways, which control cell migration, adhesion, and survival [29–31]. Our previous study showed that insulin-like growth factor-1 (IGF-1)-activated PI3K signaling promoted epithelial adhesion via HD activation of PI3K signaling and improved epithelial sealing around the implant [32]. Some studies indicate that MSCs activate intrinsic MSCs or various other cells through paracrine expression of IGF-1, epidermal growth factor (EGF), or platelet-derived growth factor (PDGF). Therefore, we

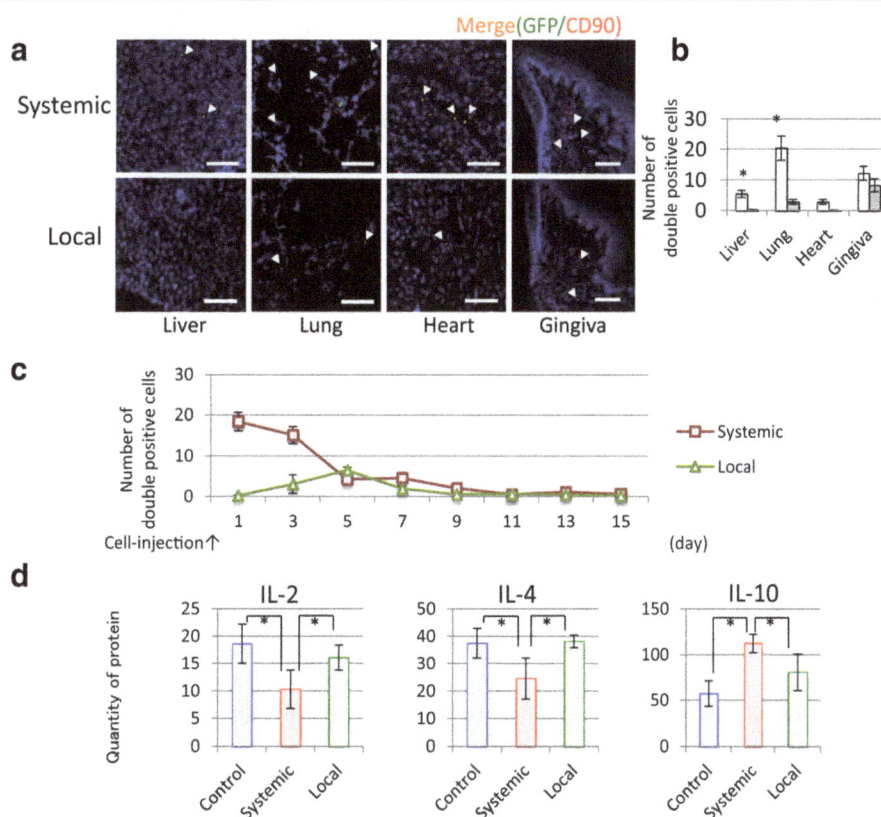

Fig. 4 Whole body accumulation of MSCs. **a** CD-90/GFP-FITC double-positive cell (white arrowhead) visualization at day 1. (Bar = 200 μm) (**b**) CD-90/GFP-FITC double-positive cell counts in various organs in the control, systemic (white), and local (gray) groups at day 1. **c** Change of intravascular MSCs number up to 14 days after systemic or local MSC injection. **d** Levels of serum inflammatory cytokines, IL-2, IL-4, and IL-10 in control, local, and systemic groups

highlight the importance of direct contact between MSCs and epithelial cells in order to change cell characteristics or activate cell differentiation.

Whole body MSC accumulation

GFP/CD-90 double-positive cells were detected and counted in various tissues, including the mucosa around the experimental implants (Fig. 4a, b). Although few double-positive MSCs were observed in the liver and heart 1 day after MSC injection, double-positive MSCs were observed in the lung and peri-implant tissue after both systemic and local injection. Figure 4c shows changes in MSC numbers in the rat blood over time. In the local group, intravascular MSC number peaked at day 5, while in the systemic group, MSC number declined quickly at the early time points 3 days after the administration.

Subcutaneously administrated cells or drugs are reported to take a few days to be delivered into the body through vessel bloods [33, 34]. This may be owed to difficulty of the cells in securing vascular accesses to the target site because of a lack of blood vessels at the buccinators, while systemic MSC homing occurs more readily through the bloodstream [35].

The effects of MSC treatment on levels of serum inflammatory cytokines IL-2, IL-4, and IL-10 in the implant model rat are shown (Fig. 4d). Systemic MSC injection resulted in lower IL-2 and IL-4 levels and higher IL-10 levels compared with local MSC injection and the control.

Accumulation of MSCs at the peri-implant tissue

An interesting study disclosed that intraperitoneal MSCs migrated and engrafted at the inflamed colon and passed through the whole intestinal wall reaching the luminal side [36]. Although we were unable to trace the exact migration of our locally administrated MSCs by observed fragmentary, in vivo imaging or tracking with superparamagnetic iron oxide might enable this using a series of flow [14, 37].

In this study, GFP-MSCs took several days to be observed at the target organ after local injection (Fig. 5B (b, c)). Some cells were observed in the mass of the injected area (Fig. 5B(a)), while others were observed indirectly circulating within the whole body or were slightly accumulating at the wound area (Fig. 5B (d)). Specially, these results showed that the most of injected MSCs in the local group got delayed to accumulate around the implant. In the systemic group, GFP/CD-90 double-positive cells were observed around the apical portion of the PIE-like epithelial structure at days 3 and 5 (Fig. 5B (b, c)), after which positive staining declined over time. In the local group, MSC location was limited to the buccal mucosa near the experimental implant at

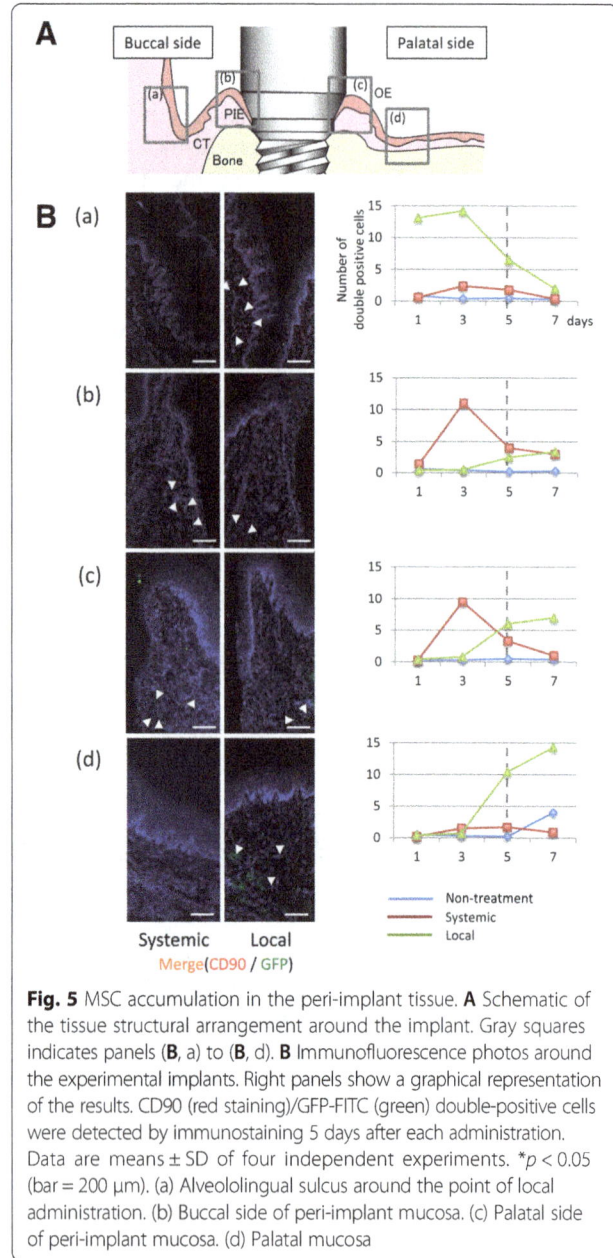

Fig. 5 MSC accumulation in the peri-implant tissue. **A** Schematic of the tissue structural arrangement around the implant. Gray squares indicates panels (**B**, a) to (**B**, d). **B** Immunofluorescence photos around the experimental implants. Right panels show a graphical representation of the results. CD90 (red staining)/GFP-FITC (green) double-positive cells were detected by immunostaining 5 days after each administration. Data are means ± SD of four independent experiments. *$p < 0.05$ (bar = 200 μm). (a) Alveololingual sulcus around the point of local administration. (b) Buccal side of peri-implant mucosa. (c) Palatal side of peri-implant mucosa. (d) Palatal mucosa

early stage; however, MSC accumulation was observed at the mucosa around the implant from day 5 onwards (Fig 5B). On the contrary, the MSCs did not accumulate on the implant surface, unlike in the systemic group, and they remained around the implantation site for approximately 1 week.

Detection of apoptotic GFP-MSCs

Due to the existence of muscles, connective tissue, dermal layer, and basement membrane, cells within the mass of the injected area encounter these barriers, inhibiting the distance of migration between the application region and inflammatory site, which has an estimated diameter of

20–30 μm (Fig. 6). High-density cell injection at the topical region is also an obstacle for homing, thus using a vasodilator like heparin, culturing the cells under hypoxic condition, maintaining a lower confluence, or the addition of IL-3, IL-6, IGF-1, tumor necrosis factor alpha (TNF-α), or interferon-gamma (IFN-γ), can be used to increase C-X-C chemokine receptor type 4 (CXCR-4) [38], which is a specific receptor for stromal-derived-factor-1 (SDF-1, also called CXCL12), an MSC chemotactic factor that could improve homing efficiency [39].

Locally injected MSCs decreased sharply in number from the buccal site within a week (Fig. 6a). One day after injection, some 7-AAD-positive cells were detected within the MSC mass at the subcutaneous tissue. From days 3 and 5, MSCs began to undergo apoptosis within the local administration region. At day 7 after injection, the level of MSC apoptosis was approximately 90% (Fig. 6b).

Relationship between cell density and differentiation

Isolated MSCs were seeded at four concentrations (5×10^2, 5×10^3, 5×10^4, 5×10^5 MSCs/ml) in adipogenic and osteogenic induction conditions. When the medium was switched to adipogenic and osteogenic differentiation medium, the MSC concentrations were approximately 30, 60, 80, and 100%, respectively. MSCs differentiation into adipocytes and osteoblasts was determined by PPARγ and Runx2 immunofluorescence staining, respectively (Fig. 7 A, B). At a density of 5×10^4 MSCs/ml, adipogenic and osteogenic differentiation were confirmed by increased expression of specific adipogenic markers and Runx2, respectively, using western blotting. Therefore, cells at a suitable cell density within the MSC mass were induced to undergo osteogenic or adipogenic differentiation. However, 3 days after injection, the MSCs began to undergo apoptosis over time in the local administration region. A high ratio of apoptosis occurred

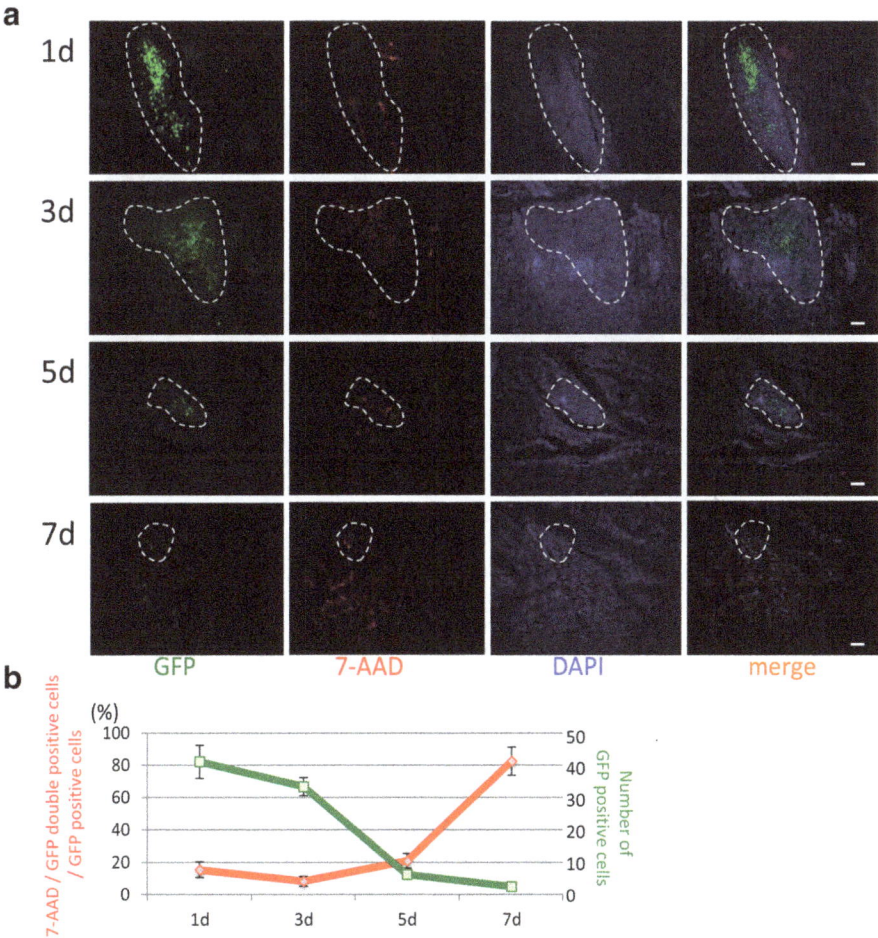

Fig. 6 MSC apoptosis after local administration. **a** GFP-conjugated MSCs (green) were stained by 7-AAD (red) as an apoptosis marker and nuclear DAPI (blue). (Bar = 80 μm) **b** Quantitation of 7-AAD/GFP double-positive or GFP-positive cell numbers in the mass (bound area by white dotted line) after local MSC administration

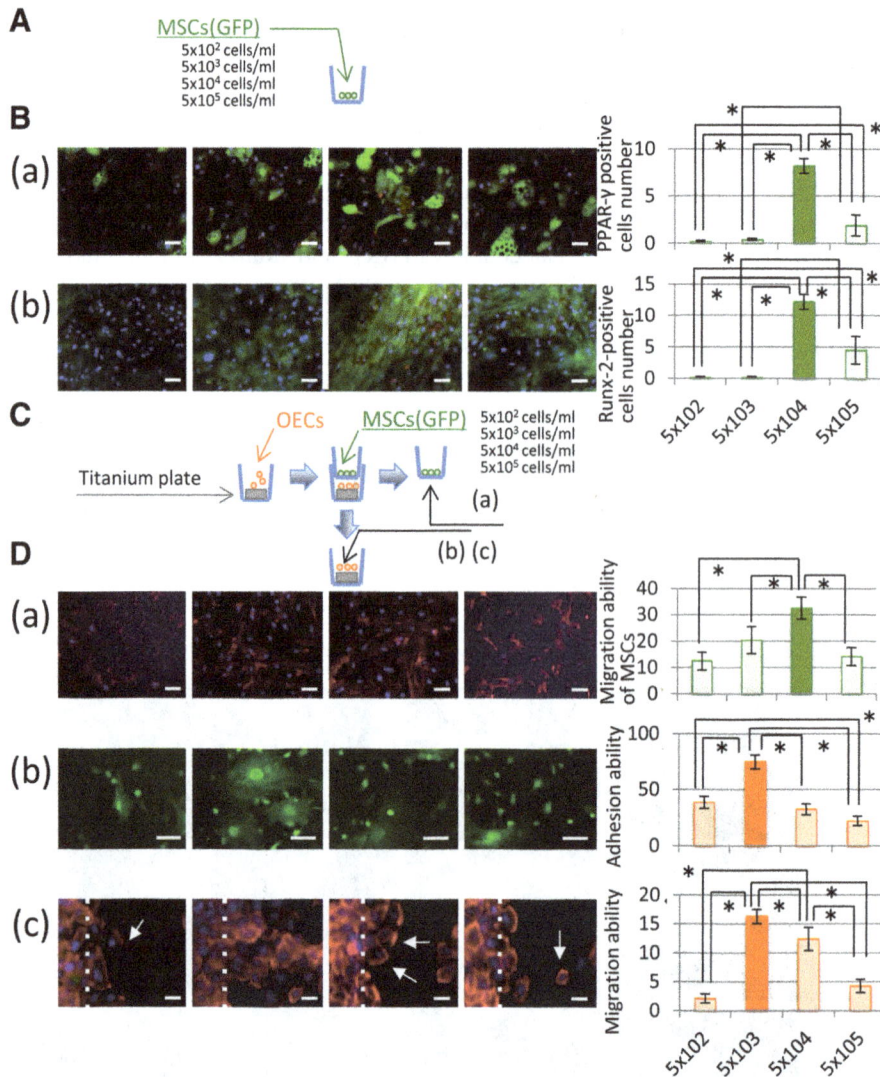

Fig. 7 Relationship between cell density and differentiation. **A** MSCs were seeded at four concentrations (5×10^2, 5×10^3, 5×10^4, 5×10^5 MSCs/ml) into culture wells. **B** Multipotent differentiation of MSCs related to cell density. (a) Adipogenic differentiation of MSCs. The graph shows quantification of PPAR-γ-positive cell numbers as differentiated adipocytes from independent experiments (means ± SD). (Bar = 40 μm) (b) osteogenic differentiation of MSCs. The graph shows quantification of Runx-2-positive cell numbers as differentiated osteoblasts from four independent experiments (means ± SD). (Bar = 50 μm) **C** schematic of in vitro coculture study. **D** Relationship between MSCs and OECs in coculture. (a) Quantification of MSCs number in the upper Transwell insert chamber to determine MSC migration through the 8-μm pores. (Bar = 20 μm) (b) OEC adhesion assay. Data show the percentage of OECs under MSC coculture. Bars represent the means ± SD of four independent experiments. *$p < 0.05$ (c) scratch assay. OECs were cultured for 3 days then observed by immunofluorescence staining for actin filaments (red). The white dotted line shows the limit of the wound area into which the cells migrated, while the white arrow indicates migrating cells. (Bar = 20 μm) the right panel graphically shows the number of migrating cells under each condition. Bars represent the means ± SD of four parallel experiments. *$p < 0.05$

immediately after local administration of MSCs, which reduced the amount of viable cells at early stage.

MSC migration from the local mass

Figure 7C and D showed the suitable amount of MSCs had much better positive effect for the migration and adhesion of OECs to titanium surface. MSC attachment within the upper Transwell chamber was determined 24 h after seeding by fluorescence microscopy, as shown in Fig. 7D (a). The majority of MSCs appeared flattened with numerous

cytoplasmic extensions and lamellipodia. The majority of MSCs passed through the transwell pores when seeded at a density of 5×104. However, at a density of 5×104 the MSCs more readily passed through the 8 μm pores compared with cells at other densities.

OEC and MSC coculture at various seeding densities.

MSCs were seeded at a range of densities (5×10^2, 5×10^3, 5×10^4, 5×10^5 cells/ml) within the upper Transwell chamber, and OECs were cultured on titanium plates like as titanium implant surface, as shown in Fig. 7D (b, c). Only at a density of 5×10^3 did the MSCs activate OEC migration and adhesion.

Furthermore, ELISA indicated that this may not have regulated inflammation because there was no significant difference in expression of IL-10 detected at 24-hour post injection compared with the control (data not shown). The blood stream is thought to be a suitable environment for MSCs, since their survival is higher in this source than within inflamed tissues [37]. To therefore ensure a constant number of viable cells, repeat doses with smaller cell numbers or scatter injection points may benefit local MSC administration. This may permit more cells to be intravasated into the blood vessels, and offer an antiphlogistic effect to the inflammation sites. In terms of MSC administration timing, an earlier response is believed to be more effective to clinical outcomes [36, 40], although similar results have been obtained following delayed administration in some studies. Above all, investing research efforts in identifying the most efficacious route for MSC delivery is a critical matter because there is currently no consensus.

Conclusions

Our study supports systemic administration of MSCs to enable accelerated soft tissue sealing of the Ti surface in our rat oral implantation model. Although local MSC administration had little positive effect in our model, the MSCs accumulated around the peri-implant oral mucosa and were identified in various organs, indicating a wide range of possible applications. This study highlights that clinical cases should be considered individually prior to practical application of MSCs, and that further investigations are needed to understand the exact cellular and molecular mechanisms of MSCs following their local administration.

Acknowledgements
This work was supported by JSPS KAKENHI Grant Numbers JP 15H05029 and 15H02573 to Y. Ayukawa.

Authors' contributions
MK, IA, YA, TY, RK, and YM were involved in the practical achievement of these experiments. MK, IA, RK, and YM collected, analyzed, and interpreted the data. IA, AY, and KK designed the study and provided financial and administrative support. IA, YA, TY, and KK wrote the manuscript. KK, YA, and IA revised the manuscript for publication. Each author participated sufficiently in the work to take public responsibility for appropriate portions of the content, and all authors read and approved the manuscript.

Competing interests
Miya Kanazawa, Ikiru Atsuta, Yasunori Ayukawa, Takayoshi Yamaza, Ryosuke Kondo, Yuri Matsuura, and Kiyoshi Koyano declare that they have no competing interests.

Author details
[1]Section of Implant and Rehabilitative Dentistry, Division of Oral Rehabilitation, Faculty of Dental Science, Kyushu University, 3-1-1 Maidashi, Higashi-ku, Fukuoka 812-8582, Japan. [2]Department of Molecular Cell and Oral Anatomy, Faculty of Dental Science, Kyushu University, Fukuoka, Japan.

References
1. Egusa H, Sonoyama W, Nishimura M, Atsuta I, Akiyama K. Stem cells in dentistry—part I: stem cell sources. J Prosthodont Res. 2012;56:151–65.
2. Lindhe J, Berglundh T. The interface between the mucosa and the implant. Periodontol. 1998;17:47–54.
3. Ikeda H, Shiraiwa M, Yamaza T, Yoshinari M, Kido MA, Ayukawa Y, Inoue T, Koyano K, Tanaka T. Difference in penetration of horseradish peroxidase tracer as a foreign substance into the peri-implant or junctional epithelium of rat gingivae. Clin Oral Implants Res. 2002;13:243–51.
4. Ikeda H, Yamaza T, Yoshinari M, Ohsaki Y, Ayukawa Y, Kido MA, Inoue T, Shimono M, Koyano K, Tanaka T. Ultrastructural and immunoelectron microscopic studies of the peri-implant epithelium-implant (Ti-6Al-4V) interface of rat maxilla. J Periodontol. 2000;71:961–73.
5. Ericsson I, Persson LG, Berglundh T, Marinello CP, Lindhe J, Klinge B. Different types of inflammatory reactions in peri-implant soft tissues. J Clin Periodontol. 1995;22:255–61.
6. Schou S, Holmstrup P, Stoltze K, Hjorting-Hansen E, Kornman KS. Ligature-induced marginal inflammation around osseointegrated implants and ankylosed teeth. Clin Oral Implants Res. 1993;4:12–22.
7. Atsuta I, Ayukawa Y, Kondo R, Oshiro W, Matsuura Y, Furuhashi A, Tsukiyama Y, Koyano K. Soft tissue sealing around dental implants based on histological interpretation. J Prosthodont Res. 2016;60:3–11.
8. Atsuta I, Yamaza T, Yoshinari M, Mino S, Goto T, Kido MA, Terada Y, Tanaka T. Changes in the distribution of laminin-5 during peri-implant epithelium formation after immediate titanium implantation in rats. Biomaterials. 2005;26:1751–60.
9. Tarnawski AS. Cellular and molecular mechanisms of gastrointestinal ulcer healing. Dig Dis Sci 50 Suppl. 2005;1:S24–33.
10. Knight DA, Rossi FM, Hackett TL. Mesenchymal stem cells for repair of the airway epithelium in asthma. Expert Rev Respir Med. 2010;4:747–58.
11. Kondo R, Atsuta I, Ayukawa Y, Yamaza T, Matsuura Y, Furuhashi A, Tsukiyama Y, Koyano K. Therapeutic interaction of systemically-administered mesenchymal stem cells with peri-implant mucosa. PLoS One. 2014;9:e90681.
12. Zhang R, Liu Y, Yan K, Chen L, Chen XR, Li P, Chen FF, Jiang XD. Anti-inflammatory and immunomodulatory mechanisms of mesenchymal stem cell transplantation in experimental traumatic brain injury. J Neuroinflammation. 2013;10:106.
13. Zhang L, Li K, Liu X, Li D, Luo C, Fu B, Cui S, Zhu F, Zhao RC, Chen X. Repeated systemic administration of human adipose-derived stem cells attenuates overt diabetic nephropathy in rats. Stem Cells Dev. 2013;22:3074–86.
14. Zheng B, von See MP, Yu E, Gunel B, Lu K, Vazin T, Schaffer DV, Goodwill PW, Conolly SM. Quantitative magnetic particle imaging monitors the transplantation, biodistribution, and clearance of stem cells in vivo. Theranostics. 2016;6:291–301.
15. Atsuta I, Yamaza T, Yoshinari M, Goto T, Kido MA, Terada Y, Tanaka T. Ultrastructural localization of laminin-5 (gamma2 chain) in the rat peri-implant oral mucosa around a titanium-dental implant by immuno-electron microscopy. Biomaterials. 2005;26:6280–7.
16. Oshiro W, Ayukawa Y, Atsuta I, Furuhashi A, Yamazoe J, Kondo R, Sakaguchi M, Matsuura Y, Tsukiyama Y, Koyano K. Effects of CaCl2 hydrothermal treatment of titanium implant surfaces on early epithelial sealing. Colloids Surf B Biointerfaces. 2015;131:141–7.
17. Atsuta I, Ayukawa Y, Ogino Y, Moriyama Y, Jinno Y, Koyano K. Evaluations of epithelial sealing and peri-implant epithelial down-growth around "step-type" implants. Clin Oral Implants Res. 2012;23:459–66.
18. Furuhashi A, Ayukawa Y, Atsuta I, Okawachi H, Koyano K. The difference of fibroblast behavior on titanium substrata with different surface characteristics. Odontology. 2012;100:199–205.
19. Shiraiwa M, Goto T, Yoshinari M, Koyano K, Tanaka TA. Study of the initial attachment and subsequent behavior of rat oral epithelial cells cultured on titanium. J Periodontol. 2002;73:852–60.
20. Atsuta I, Ayukawa Y, Furuhashi A, Ogino Y, Moriyama Y, Tsukiyama Y, Koyano K. Vivo and in vitro studies of epithelial cell behavior around titanium implants with machined and rough surfaces. Clin Implant Dent Relat Res. 2014;16:772–81.
21. Borradori L, Sonnenberg A. Structure and function of hemidesmosomes:

more than simple adhesion complexes. J Invest Dermatol. 1999;112:411–8.

22. Rabinovitz I, Mercurio AM. The integrin alpha6beta4 functions in carcinoma cell migration on laminin-1 by mediating the formation and stabilization of actin-containing motility structures. J Cell Biol. 1997;139:1873–84.

23. Stepp MA, Spurr-Michaud S, Tisdale A, Elwell J, Gipson IK. Alpha 6 beta 4 integrin heterodimer is a component of hemidesmosomes. Proc Natl Acad Sci U S A. 1990;87:8970–4.

24. Schroeder A, van der Zypen E, Stich H, Sutter F. The reactions of bone, connective tissue, and epithelium to endosteal implants with titanium-sprayed surfaces. J Maxillofac Surg. 1981;9:15–25.

25. Schroeder HE, Listgarten MA. Fine structure of the developing epithelial attachment of human teeth. 2d rev. ed. Basel. New York: S. Karger; 1977.

26. Shimono M, Ishikawa T, Enokiya Y, Muramatsu T, Matsuzaka K, Inoue T, Abiko Y, Yamaza T, Kido MA, Tanaka T, Hashimoto S. Biological characteristics of the junctional epithelium. J Electron Microsc. 2003;52:627–39.

27. Tamura RN, Oda D, Quaranta V, Plopper G, Lambert R, Glaser S, Jones JC. Coating of titanium alloy with soluble laminin-5 promotes cell attachment and hemidesmosome assembly in gingival epithelial cells: potential application to dental implants. J Periodontal Res. 1997;32:287–94.

28. Okawachi H, Ayukawa Y, Atsuta I, Furuhashi A, Sakaguchi M, Yamane K, Koyano K. Effect of titanium surface calcium and magnesium on adhesive activity of epithelial-like cells and fibroblasts. Biointerphases. 2012;7:27.

29. O'Connor KL, Nguyen BK, Mercurio AM. RhoA function in lamellae formation and migration is regulated by the alpha6beta4 integrin and cAMP metabolism. J Cell Biol. 2000;148:253–8.

30. Shaw LM, Rabinovitz I, Wang HH, Toker A, Mercurio AM. Activation of phosphoinositide 3-OH kinase by the alpha6beta4 integrin promotes carcinoma invasion. Cell. 1997;91:949–60.

31. Tang K, Nie D, Cai Y, Honn KV. The beta4 integrin subunit rescues A431 cells from apoptosis through a PI3K/Akt kinase signaling pathway. Biochem Biophys Res Commun. 1999;264:127–32.

32. Atsuta I, Ayukawa Y, Furuhashi A, Yamaza T, Tsukiyama Y, Koyano K. Promotive effect of insulin-like growth factor-1 for epithelial sealing to titanium implants. J Biomed Mater Res A. 2013;10:2896–904.

33. Spriet M, Buerchler S, Trela JM, Hembrooke TA, Padgett KA, Rick MC, Vidal MA, Galuppo LD. Scintigraphic tracking of mesenchymal stem cells after intravenous regional limb perfusion and subcutaneous administration in the standing horse. Vet Surg. 2015;44:273–80.

34. Bazhanov N, Ylostalo JH, Bartosh TJ, Tiblow A, Mohammadipoor A, Foskett A, Prockop DJ. Intraperitoneally infused human mesenchymal stem cells form aggregates with mouse immune cells and attach to peritoneal organs. Stem Cell Res Ther. 2016;7:27.

35. Goldmacher GV, Nasser R, Lee DY, Yigit S, Rosenwasser R, Iacovitti L. Tracking transplanted bone marrow stem cells and their effects in the rat MCAO stroke model. PLoS One. 2013;8:e60049.

36. Wang M, Liang C, Hu H, Zhou L, Xu B, Wang X, Han Y, Nie Y, Jia S, Liang J, Wu K. Intraperitoneal injection (IP), intravenous injection (IV) or anal injection (AI)? Best way for mesenchymal stem cells transplantation for colitis. Sci Rep. 2016;6:30696.

37. Strohschein K, Radojewski P, Winkler T, Duda GN, Perka C, von Roth P. In vivo bioluminescence imaging—a suitable method to track mesenchymal stromal cells in a skeletal muscle trauma. Open Orthop J. 2015;9:262–9.

38. De Becker A, Riet IV. Homing and migration of mesenchymal stromal cells: how to improve the efficacy of cell therapy? World J Stem Cells. 2016;8:73–87.

39. Luo Q, Zhang B, Kuang D, Song G. Role of stromal-derived factor-1 in mesenchymal stem cell paracrine-mediated tissue repair. Curr Stem Cell Res Ther. 2016;11:585–92.

40. Park WS, Sung SI, Ahn SY, Sung DK, Im GH, Yoo HS, Choi SJ, Chang YS. Optimal timing of mesenchymal stem cell therapy for neonatal intraventricular hemorrhage. Cell Transplant. 2016;25:1131–44.

β-TCP/HA with or without enamel matrix proteins for maxillary sinus floor augmentation: a histomorphometric analysis of human biopsies

James Carlos Nery[1,6*], Luís Antônio Violin Dias Pereira[2], George Furtado Guimarães[1], Cassio Rocha Scardueli[3,4], Fabiana Mantovani Gomes França[1], Rubens Spin-Neto[4] and Andreas Stavropoulos[5]

Abstract

Background: It is still unclear whether enamel matrix proteins (EMD) as adjunct to bone grafting enhance bone healing. This study compared histomorphometrically maxillary sinus floor augmentation (MSFA) with β-TCP/HA in combination with or without EMD in humans.

Methods: In ten systemically healthy patients needing bilateral MSFA, one side was randomly treated using β-TCP/HA mixed with EMD (BC + EMD) and the other side using only β-TCP/HA (BC). After 6 months, biopsies were harvested from grafted areas during implant installation, being histologically and histomorphometrically analyzed. Differences between the groups considering new bone formation, soft tissues, and remaining BC were statistically evaluated.

Results: All patients showed uneventful healing after MSFA, and dental implant installation was possible in all patients after 6 months. Histological analysis showed newly formed bone that was primarily woven in nature; it was organized in thin trabeculae, and it was occasionally in contact with residual bone substitute particles, which appeared in various forms and sizes and in advanced stage of degradation. Mean bone area was 43.4% (CI95 38.9; 47.8) for the BC group and 43.0% (CI95 36.6; 49.5) for the BC + EMD group. Mean soft tissue area was 21.3% (CI95 16.5; 26.2) for BC group and 21.5% (CI95 17.7; 25.3) for BC + EMD group, while the remaining biomaterial was 35.3% (CI95 36.6; 49.5) and 35.5% (CI95 29.6; 41.3) for BC and BC + EMD group, respectively.

Conclusions: MSFA with BC resulted in adequate amounts of new bone formation allowing successful implant installation; adding EMD did not have a significant effect.

Keywords: Bone substitute, Maxillary sinus floor, Enamel matrix proteins, Histomorphometry, Human

Background

Reconstruction of the edentulous and severely atrophied posterior maxilla is often performed by means of maxillary sinus floor augmentation in combination with dental implants [1, 2]. Various bone graft materials are typically used for enhancing bone formation within the sinus cavity; autogenous bone (AB) is considered as the gold standard due to its osteogenic, osteoinductive, and osteoconductive properties [3–5]. However, harvesting AB from intraoral sites is associated with a number of pitfalls such as donor site morbidity, surgical complications, and extra time, while in some occasions there is limited availability in intraoral bone [6]. Furthermore, the available scientific evidence neither supports nor refutes the superiority of AB over other graft materials for maxillary sinus augmentation with regard to implant survival or complications at the recipient site [7].

Various bone substitute materials, that attempt to incorporate several features of AB, have been evaluated

* Correspondence: jamescnery@gmail.com
[1]Department of Implantology, São Leopoldo Mandic Research Center, Brasília, DF, Brazil
[6]Implant Center, SEPS 710/910, Lotes CD, Office 226, CEP: 70390-108 Brasília, DF, Brazil
Full list of author information is available at the end of the article

with the aim to replace AB grafting [1]. Biphasic calcium phosphate has been widely used as a bone substitute in orthopedics, periodontology, and maxillofacial and oral surgery. It has been shown to be a safe biocompatible scaffold supporting new bone formation, used either alone or in combination with growth factors [8, 9]. Bone Ceramic® (BC; Straumann, Basel, Switzerland) is among the biphasic calcium phosphates currently available in the market. It is a fully synthetic bone graft substitute of medical grade purity in particulate form (particle size 500–1000 μm), consisting of 60% hydroxyapatite (HA) and 40% beta tri-calcium phosphate. Studies have shown that BC acts as osteoconductive material when used for maxillary sinus floor augmentation [4, 10].

An enamel matrix protein derivative (EMD; Emdogain, Straumann, Basel, Switzerland) has been used in periodontal regenerative procedures for over 20 years, and it has been shown to efficiently enhance the outcome of healing [11, 12]. Although the few available preclinical studies have not shown any clear benefit when EMD was used for bone regeneration, emerging evidence shows that EMD upregulates the expression of several chemokines and growth factors relevant for bone wound healing [13]. In this context, clinical testing on the possible potential of EMD to enhance bone formation in other types of bone defects (i.e., non-periodontal) is sparse and the results are unclear [14].

The aim of the present study was to compare histomorphometrically the outcome of maxillary sinus floor augmentation with β-TCP/HA with or without enamel matrix proteins (BC + EMD and EMD, respectively) in humans.

Methods

This research project was approved by the Ethics Committee of the School of Dentistry and Dental Research Center São Leopoldo Mandic, Brazil, under the protocol 2010/0360.

Sample definition

Ten consecutive patients (age range 35–75 years) with the need of bilateral maxillary sinus floor augmentation prior to the placement of four dental implants (two in each side of posterior maxilla) were selected for the study. The main inclusion criterion was a vertical dimension of the residual alveolar bone between 3 and 5 mm in the sites selected for implant placement in the posterior maxilla, as assessed on a cone beam CT. Only patients with no need for additional bone augmentation (i.e., lateral or vertical) were included. The patients did not suffer from any systemic disease that might interfere with bone healing (e.g., uncontrollable diabetes; osteoporosis) and did not smoke more than 10 cigarettes per day. Sample size calculation was based on the statistical

mean and standard deviation of percent new bone formation within the augmented maxillary sinus, reported previously in a similar study including histomorphometric evaluation [15].

Maxillary sinus floor augmentation, biopsy harvesting, and dental implant placement

All patients received systemic antibiotics (amoxicillin 500 mg, every 8 h for 7 days) and anti-inflammatory drugs (nimesulide 100 mg twice daily for 5 days), starting all the medication 1 h before surgery. Patients were also prescribed analgesics (paracetamol 750 mg, max. four times a day) if there was pain. Chlorexidine digluconate 0.12% mouth rinses, four times daily, were also prescribed for 14 days post-operatively.

Surgery was planned using cone beam CT images (i-CAT, Image Sciences International, USA) with 0.25 mm voxel size, in 1-mm-thick sections, generated every 1 mm in the region of interest (posterior maxilla). After extra and intraoral disinfection of the operating field, local anesthesia was administered using lidocaine hydrochloride 2% with epinephrine 1:100.000 (DFL Industry and Trade, Rio de Janeiro, Brazil). Maxillary sinus floor augmentation with a lateral window technique was performed, and each of the sinuses received either β-TCP/HA (Straumann® BoneCeramic, Basel, Switzerland – BC group) or β-TCP/HA manually mixed using a periosteal elevator with EMD (Straumann® Emdogain, Basel, Switzerland), in a proportion of 1 g of BC for 0.3 ml of EMD (BC + EMD group), in a random fashion (by tossing a coin) and using a split-mouth design. In both groups, a very limited amount of sterile ;physiological saline solution (NaCl 0.9%) was added to the graft material mixture, insufficient amount to provide the consistency needed to ease handling and transferring into the sinus. No membrane or other material was used for closing the lateral window. After flap repositioning, closure was performed using simple interrupted nylon sutures (4-0, Ethicon, Johnson & Johnson). No radiographic examination immediately after sinus augmentation procedure was undertaken.

Six months after grafting, another CBCT examination was carried out for implant planning. In the sequence, following the previously described antiseptic and anesthetic procedures, two implants with a sand-blasted and acid etching surface were installed in each of the grafted sinuses, i.e., 40 implants in total (32—Neoporous, Neodent, Curitiba, Paraná, Brazil; 8—SLA, Straumann, Basel, Switzerland). A 10-mm-long cylindrical bone biopsy was harvested using a 2-mm internal diameter trephine bur during preparation for the most anterior implant site (i.e., two biopsies were retrieved from each patient). Six months later, the prosthetic rehabilitation of the patient was performed.

Biopsy handling and evaluation

Immediately after retrieval, the apical aspect of the harvested biopsies was marked using India ink, to be used as a guide during histological evaluation. The biopsies were routinely processed (maintained in formaldehyde during 2 days, washed, and decalcified using EDTA solution, under continuous shaking, for 2 months) and embedded in paraffin. Six 6-μm-thick sections representing the central aspect of the cylindrical biopsy were obtained from each biopsy. These sections were stained using hematoxylin-eosin and were used for histological and histomorphometric analyses. Images were acquired using a DIASTAR light microscope (Leica Reichert & Jung products, Germany) connected to a Leica Microsystems DFC-300-FX digital camera (Leica Microsystems, Germany). Additional sections were stained using picrosirius-hematoxylin for microscopic examination under polarized light.

From the entire biopsy, only the 6 mm towards the apical aspect was considered as the region of interest (ROI), in order to allow visualization of approximately 80% of grafted bone and 20% of resident bone. Histological evaluation assessed morphological characteristics of the newly formed bone, remaining grafted material, integration of the grafted material with the newly formed bone, soft tissues, and local inflammation. Also, the newly formed bone was assessed regarding the aggregation and organization of the collagen bundles, reflected in the variation in birefringence intensity. The relative amounts (%) of bone, soft tissues, and "other material" (i.e., remaining grafting material or empty spaces due removal of the grafting material during histological processing, artifacts, and debris), within the ROI were planimetrically estimated using ImageJ (NIH, Bethesda, MD, USA) (Fig. 1).

Data analysis

The data for each tissue component from the three histological sections were averaged to represent the biopsy. Commercially available software (GraphPad Prism 5.0 for Windows, GraphPad Software Inc., USA) was utilized for statistical comparisons between groups and for drawing the graphics. The assumption of normality was checked using D'Agostino & Pearson omnibus test. The data for each evaluated tissue, for BC and BC + EMD groups were analyzed as two paired samples from normal distributions based on a paired t test. Estimates were given with 95% confidence intervals, and statistical significance was set at 5% ($p < 0.05$).

Results

Clinical evaluation

All ten patients showed uneventful healing after the sinus floor augmentation procedure as well as after dental implant placement, with no overt postoperative

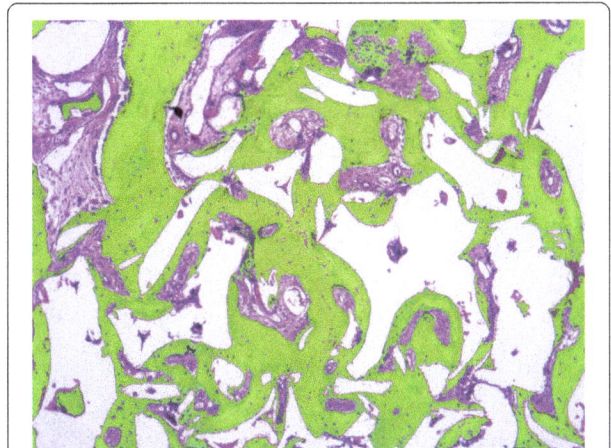

Fig. 1 Histomicrograph illustrating the various tissue areas measured on the sections: newly formed bone (*green mask*), soft tissues (*purple mask*), and "others", including residual bone substitute particles and empty spaces either due to removal of the bone substitute particles during to the decalcification processing or due to artifacts (*white mask*)

inflammation or infection. Consistently, in all ten patients, no significant jiggling of the drill was noticed during biopsy harvesting, while subjective drilling resistance during implant placement was similar in both groups and all implants had appropriate primary stability as judged clinically. Further, even though bone substitute particles could still be recognized in the retrieved biopsy, all particles appeared well integrated in the biopsy tissue.

Histological evaluation

The histological evaluation showed various amounts of newly formed bone, soft tissue, and remaining grafted material particles in all biopsies, with no apparent difference between groups (Figs. 2 and 3). In all samples, most part of the grafted material was removed due to decalcification during the histological processing. From the ghost images of the grafted material, the particles appeared in various forms and sizes, and in advanced stage of degradation. Evaluation under polarized light showed both areas of high birefringence in the newly formed bone, indicative of the high aggregation and organization of collagen bundles of mature lamellar bone, as well as areas of low birefringence, indicative of the disorganized collagen bundles of immature bone. No apparent differences in bone maturation were observed between the groups (Figs. 4 and 5). The new bone was in contact with the remaining graft particles at a variable extend within each biopsy, but again there were no apparent differences between the two groups. In all samples, only few inflammatory cells, mostly macrophages, were observed.

Histomorphometric analysis

Within the ROI, mean bone area was 43.4% (SD 6.1; CI95 38.9–47.8) for the BC group and 43.0% (SD 9.0;

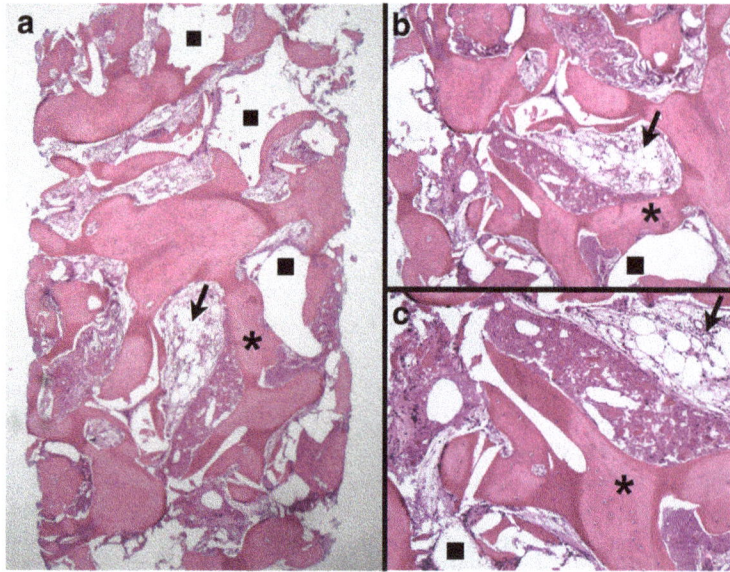

Fig. 2 Histomicrograph of a biopsy from the BC group. **a** Overview—×25 magnification; **b** ×30 magnification; **c** ×60 magnification. Areas corresponding to BC removed during histological processing (*square*) in direct contact with newly formed bone (*asterisk*), containing a large number of osteocytes, and with soft tissue (*arrow*) can be observed (hematoxylin-eosin stain)

CI95 36.6–49.5) for the BC + EMD group. The mean soft tissue area was 21.3% (SD 6.8; CI95 16.5–26.2) for BC group and 21.5% (SD 5.3; CI95 17.7–25.3) for BC + EMD group. The mean area of "other material" was 35.3% (SD 9.0; CI95 36.6–49.5) for BC group, and 35.5% (SD 8.2; CI95 29.6–41.3) for BC + EMD group. The data is graphically presented in Fig. 6. No differences between the groups were found for any of the three parameters

evaluated (p value was 0.94 for bone, 0.96 for soft tissue, and 0.97 for other materials).

Discussion

The present study compared the histological and histomorphometrical outcome of healing after maxillary sinus floor augmentation with BC with or without EMD, based on human biopsies. The results showed that

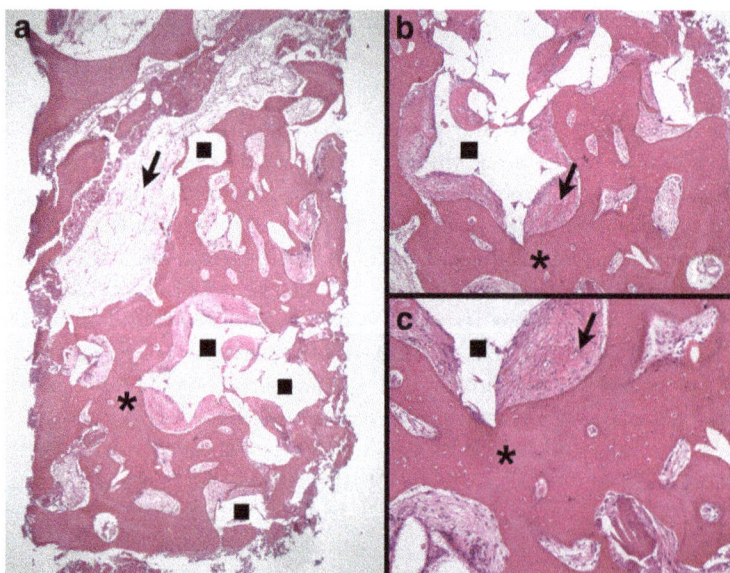

Fig. 3 Histomicrograph of a biopsy from the BC + EMD group. Overview—×25 magnification; **b** ×30 magnification; **c** ×60 magnification. Areas corresponding to BC + EMD removed during histological processing (*square*) surrounded by newly formed bone (*asterisk*), with large numbers of osteocytes and soft tissue (*arrow*) can be observed. There is direct contact between the BC reminiscent, soft tissues, and vital bone (hematoxylin-eosin stain)

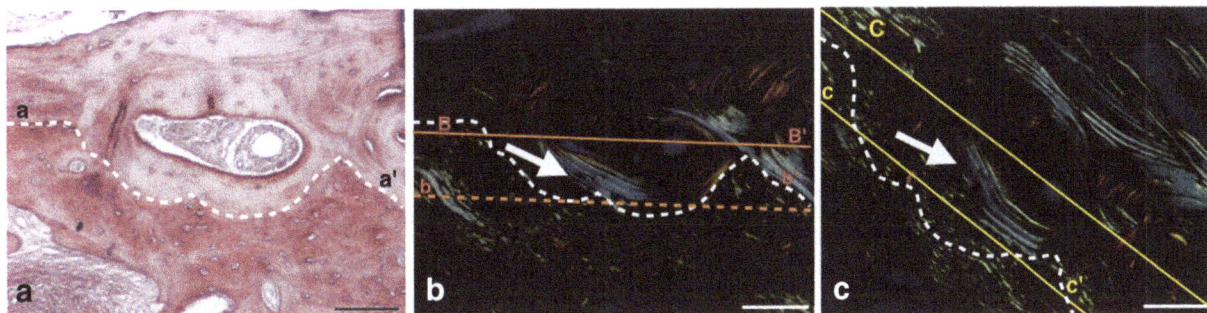

Fig. 4 Histomicrograph of a biopsy from the BC group, showing an aspect of newly formed bone. Section stained with picrosirius-hematoxylin and digitalized with bright-field (**a**) and linearly polarized light (**b** and **c**). **b, c** Results of near 45° section rotation (between axes *B–B'* and *C–C'*) to compensate some of the orientation-related effects associated with linearly polarized light. In **a**, typical Haversian systems are showed (area observed above *dotted line*, *a* to *a'*). In **b** and **c**, the *arrows* indicate thin birefringent collagen bundle (appearing as *bright lines*) arranged around Haversian canals, suggestive of mature lamellar bone. The area observed below the *dotted line* is suggestive of immature (non-lamellar) bone, where collagen fibers undulations can be observed. The dark area corresponds to complete disorganization of the collagen fibers. *Bar* = 100 μm

addition of EMD did not enhance the outcome of healing, neither in terms of quality nor quantity of new bone. Nevertheless, the amount of bone generated after maxillary sinus floor augmentation with BC or BC + EMD was adequate to support successful implant placement and osseointegration of implants.

EMD is used for almost 20 years for enhancing tissue regeneration in periodontal defects, and it has been shown to exert anabolic action on several types of cells and factors relevant for bone regeneration [11, 12]. Nevertheless, there is still only sparse information from the clinic on the possible beneficial effect of adding EMD on a bone substitute material in terms of enhancing bone tissue regeneration in non-periodontal sites. In particular, a single study has previously evaluated the BC + EMD combination vs. BC in sinus lift, but due to the fact that only radiographic analysis was performed, the results were unclear [14]; thus, the present study, including histological evaluation, was performed. After 6 months of healing, about 43% of the evaluated part of

the biopsy consisted of newly formed mineralized bone and about 35% consisted of grafting material; no differences between the groups were observed also in regard to bone tissue organization and maturation, as revealed by analysis of birefringence. Herein, only the 6 mm towards the apical aspect of the 10-mm-long biopsies was considered as the region of interest (ROI), in order to minimize any influence on the results from counting aspects of the alveolar ridge present before surgery.

Aiming to enhance bone formation and bone quality when bone substitute materials such as BC are used, biologics have often been added and positive results have occasionally been observed [16, 17]. The possibility that absence of any beneficial effect of EMD on bone regeneration herein was due to the sterile physiological saline solution added to the graft material mixture to facilitate its handling and transferring into the sinus, cannot be excluded. Indeed, the saline solution may have either diluted the concentration of EMD necessary to exert a beneficial effect or it may have interfered with adequate

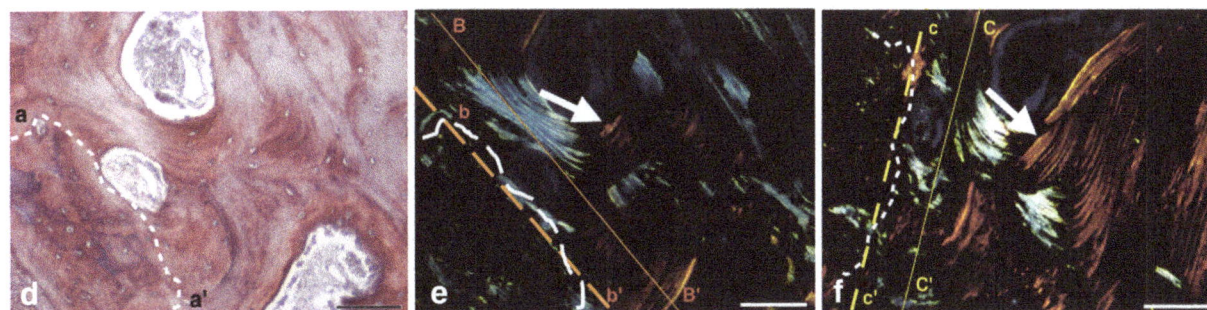

Fig. 5 Histomicrograph of a biopsy from the BC + EMD group, showing an aspect of newly formed bone. Section stained with picrosirius-hematoxylin and digitalized with bright-field (**d**) and linearly polarized light (**e** and **f**). **e, f** Results of near 45° section rotation (between axes *B–B'* and *C–C'*) to compensate some of the orientation-related effects associated with linearly polarized light. In **d**, typical Haversian systems are showed (area observed above *dotted line*, *a* to *a'*). In **e** and **f**, the *arrows* indicate thin birefringents (appears visually as brilliance) collagen arrangement around Haversian canals suggestive of lamellar mature bone. Areas observed below *dotted lines* are suggestive of immature (non-lamellar) bone where collagen fiber undulations can be observed. The dark area corresponds to complete disorganization of the collagen fibers. *Bar* = 100 μm

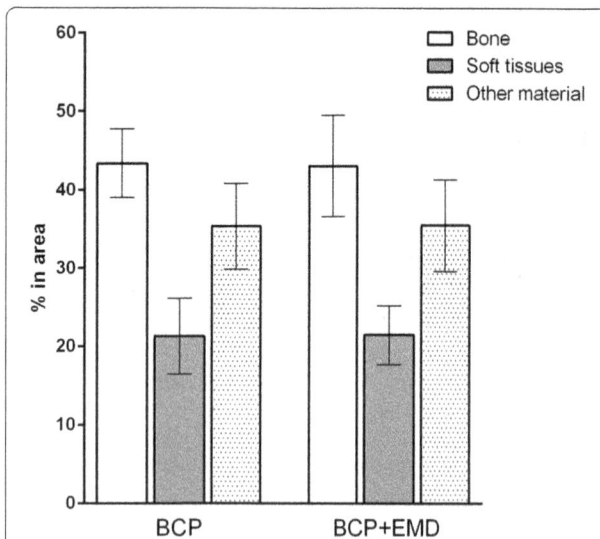

Fig. 6 Histomorphometric evaluation results (considering six sections for each biopsy), for newly formed bone, soft tissues, and others

adsorption of EMD on the BC particles, resulting in altered (reduced) presence of EMD on the site during healing. In fact, in an in vitro study, published after the clinical procedures of the present study were concluded, it was shown that best adsorption of EMD on bone substitute particles is achieved when particles are dry and EMD is allowed to adsorb for at least 5 min. Further, in that study it was shown that inadequate adsorption of EMD on the bone substitute particles had negative influences in osteoblast proliferation and differentiation [14, 15, 18].

Nevertheless, the amount of bone generated with BC or BC + EMD herein was adequate to support successful implant placement and osseointegration of implants. In fact, more or less similar amounts of bone formation have been reported in studies evaluating human sinus biopsies after grafting with a variety of biomaterials (bone formation ranging approximately from 30 to 50%) [19]. On the other hand, an ideal situation would be that BC becomes gradually resorbed and completely substituted by vital bone tissue [8]. A few studies have indeed showed that biologics accelerate the degradation of biomaterials and consequently lead to larger bone formation at the grafted region [20, 21]. However, in the present study, EMD did not seem to influence graft remodeling in that manner. The possible biological and biomechanical long-term challenges of a loaded implant inserted in largely non-vital BC-grafted bone sites remain unknown. Recent studies, in fact, indicate high failure rates of implants inserted in sites augmented laterally and/or vertically with fresh-frozen allogeneic bone blocks [22], a material that remains largely necrotic for several months, despite good clinical graft incorporation [22–24]. In perspective, high long-term implant survival rates are reported after sinus augmentation with a variety of bone substitute materials [25].

Conclusions

The present study showed that maxillary sinus floor augmentation with BC resulted in adequate amounts of new bone formation allowing successful implant installation, while adding EMD did not have a significant effect.

Authors' contributions

JCN, LAVDP, GFG, and RSN performed the experiments and data analysis. CRS, FMGF, RSN, and AS conceived and designed the study, performed the experiments, and wrote the manuscript. CRS, RSN, and AS participated in the manuscript preparation. All authors read and approved the final version of the manuscript.

Competing interests

James Carlos Nery, Luís Antônio Violin Dias Pereira, George Furtado Guimarães, Cassio Rocha Scardueli, Fabiana Mantovani Gomes França, Rubens Spin-Neto, and Andreas Stavropoulos declare that they have no competing interests.

Author details

[1]Department of Implantology, São Leopoldo Mandic Research Center, Brasília, DF, Brazil. [2]Department of Biochemistry and Tissue Biology, UNICAMP – State University of Campinas, Institute of Biology, Campinas, São Paulo, Brazil. [3]Department of Periodontology, UNESP – Univ. Estadual Paulista, Araraquara Dental School, Araraquara, São Paulo, Brazil. [4]Department of Dentistry and Oral Health – Oral Radiology, Aarhus University, Aarhus, Denmark. [5]Department Periodontology – Faculty of Odontology, Malmö University, Malmö, Sweden. [6]Implant Center, SEPS 710/910, Lotes CD, Office 226, CEP: 70390-108 Brasília, DF, Brazil.

References

1. Esposito M, Felice P, Worthington HV. Interventions for replacing missing teeth: augmentation procedures of the maxillary sinus. Cochrane Database Syst Rev. 2014;17:CD008397.
2. Jungner M, Cricchio G, Salata LA, Sennerby L, Lundqvist C, Hultcrantz M, et al. On the early mechanisms of bone formation after maxillary sinus membrane elevation: an experimental histological and immunohistochemical study. Clin Implant Dent Relat Res. 2015;17:1092–102.
3. Boyne PJ, James RA. Grafting of the maxillary sinus floor with autogenous marrow and bone. J Oral Surg. 1980;38:613–6.
4. Frenken JW, Bouwman WF, Bravenboer N, Zijderveld SA, Schulten EA, ten Bruggenkate CM. The use of Straumann bone ceramic in a maxillary sinus floor elevation procedure: a clinical, radiological, histological and histomorphometric evaluation with a 6-month healing period. Clin Oral Implants Res. 2010;21:201–8.
5. Wallace SS, Froum SJ. Effect of maxillary sinus augmentation on the survival of endosseous dental implants. A systematic review. Ann Periodontol. 2003;8:328–43.
6. Galindo-Moreno P, Padial-Molina M, Fernandez-Barbero JE, Mesa F, Rodriguez-Martinez D, O'Valle F. Optimal microvessel density from composite graft of autogenous maxillary cortical bone and anorganic bovine bone in sinus augmentation: influence of clinical variables. Clin Oral Implants Res. 2010;21:221–7.
7. Nkenke E, Stelzle F. Clinical outcomes of sinus floor augmentation for implant placement using autogenous bone or bone substitutes: a systematic review. Clin Oral Implants Res. 2009;20 Suppl 4:124–33.
8. Stavropoulos A, Becker J, Capsius B, Acil Y, Wagner W, Terheyden H. Histological evaluation of maxillary sinus floor augmentation with recombinant human growth and differentiation factor-5-coated beta-tricalcium phosphate: results of a multicenter randomized clinical trial. J Clin Periodontol. 2011;38:966–74.
9. Stavropoulos A, Windisch P, Gera I, Capsius B, Sculean A, Wikesjo UM. A phase IIa randomized controlled clinical and histological pilot study evaluating rhGDF-5/beta-TCP for periodontal regeneration. J Clin Periodontol. 2011;38:1044–54.

10. Schmitt CM, Doering H, Schmidt T, Lutz R, Neukam FW, Schlegel KA. Histological results after maxillary sinus augmentation with Straumann(R) BoneCeramic, Bio-Oss(R), Puros(R), and autologous bone. A randomized controlled clinical trial. Clin Oral Implants Res. 2013;24:576–85.

11. Miron RJ, Sculean A, Cochran DL, Froum S, Zucchelli G, Nemcovsky C, et al. Twenty years of enamel matrix derivative: the past, the present and the future. J Clin Periodontol. 2016;43:668–83.

12. Sculean A, Nikolidakis D, Nikou G, Ivanovic A, Chapple IL, Stavropoulos A. Biomaterials for promoting periodontal regeneration in human intrabony defects: a systematic review. Periodontol 2000. 2015;68:182–216.

13. Wyganowska-Swiatkowska M, Urbaniak P, Nohawica MM, Kotwicka M, Jankun J. Enamel matrix proteins exhibit growth factor activity: a review of evidence at the cellular and molecular levels. Exp Ther Med. 2015;9:2025–33.

14. Favato MN, Vidigal BC, Cosso MG, Manzi FR, Shibli JA, Zenobio EG. Impact of human maxillary sinus volume on grafts dimensional changes used in maxillary sinus augmentation: a multislice tomographic study. Clin Oral Implants Res. 2015;26:1450–5.

15. Boeck-Neto RJ, Gabrielli M, Lia R, Marcantonio E, Shibli JA, Marcantonio Jr E. Histomorphometrical analysis of bone formed after maxillary sinus floor augmentation by grafting with a combination of autogenous bone and demineralized freeze-dried bone allograft or hydroxyapatite. J Periodontol. 2002;73:266–70.

16. Alam I, Asahina I, Ohmamiuda K, Enomoto S. Comparative study of biphasic calcium phosphate ceramics impregnated with rhBMP-2 as bone substitutes. J Biomed Mater Res. 2001;54:129–38.

17. Alam MI, Asahina I, Ohmamiuda K, Takahashi K, Yokota S, Enomoto S. Evaluation of ceramics composed of different hydroxyapatite to tricalcium phosphate ratios as carriers for rhBMP-2. Biomaterials. 2001;22:1643–51.

18. Miron RJ, Bosshardt DD, Hedbom E, Zhang Y, Haenni B, Buser D, et al. Adsorption of enamel matrix proteins to a bovine-derived bone grafting material and its regulation of cell adhesion, proliferation, and differentiation. J Periodontol. 2012;83:936–47.

19. Friedmann A, Dard M, Kleber BM, Bernimoulin JP, Bosshardt DD. Ridge augmentation and maxillary sinus grafting with a biphasic calcium phosphate: histologic and histomorphometric observations. Clin Oral Implants Res. 2009;20:708–14.

20. Koo KT, Susin C, Wikesjo UM, Choi SH, Kim CK. Transforming growth factor-beta1 accelerates resorption of a calcium carbonate biomaterial in periodontal defects. J Periodontol. 2007;78:723–9.

21. Wikesjo UM, Sorensen RG, Kinoshita A, Wozney JM. RhBMP-2/alphaBSM induces significant vertical alveolar ridge augmentation and dental implant osseointegration. Clin Implant Dent Relat Res. 2002;4:174–82.

22. Carinci F, Brunelli G, Franco M, Viscioni A, Rigo L, Guidi R, et al. A retrospective study on 287 implants installed in resorbed maxillae grafted with fresh frozen allogenous bone. Clin Implant Dent Relat Res. 2010;12:91–8.

23. Spin-Neto R, Stavropoulos A, Coletti FL, Faeda RS, Pereira LA, Marcantonio Jr E. Graft incorporation and implant osseointegration following the use of autologous and fresh-frozen allogeneic block bone grafts for lateral ridge augmentation. Clin Oral Implants Res. 2014;25:226–33.

24. Spin-Neto R, Stavropoulos A, Coletti FL, Pereira LA, Marcantonio Jr E, Wenzel A. Remodeling of cortical and corticocancellous fresh-frozen allogeneic block bone grafts–a radiographic and histomorphometric comparison to autologous bone grafts. Clin Oral Implants Res. 2015;26:747–52.

25. Corbella S, Taschieri S, Del Fabbro M. Long-term outcomes for the treatment of atrophic posterior maxilla: a systematic review of literature. Clin Implant Dent Relat Res. 2015;17:120–32.

21

Evaluation of symptomatic maxillary sinus pathologies using panoramic radiography and cone beam computed tomography—influence of professional training

Michael Dau[1]*[iD], Paul Marciak[2], Bial Al-Nawas[2], Henning Staedt[3], Abdulmonem Alshiri[4], Bernhard Frerich[1] and Peer Wolfgang Kämmerer[1]

Abstract

Background: A comparison of panoramic radiography (PAN) alone and PAN together with small field of view cone beam computed tomography (sFOV-CBCT) for diagnosis of symptomatic pathologies of the maxillary sinus was carried out by clinicians of different experience.

Methods: Corresponding radiographic images (PAN/sFOV-CBCT) of 28 patients with symptomatic maxillary sinus pathologies were chosen and analyzed by two general practitioners (GP), two junior maxillofacial surgeons (MS1), and three senior maxillofacial surgeons (MS2) via questionnaire.

Results: Visibility of maxillary pathologies in PAN was significantly different between the groups (GP 39%, MS1 48%, MS2 61%; $p < 0.05$). The number of incidental findings varied within examiner groups in PAN with a significant increase in MS2 ($p = 0.027$). The majority of examiners rated an additional sFOV-CBCT as "reasonable"/ "required" with a significant influence of the examining groups (GP 98.2%, MS1 94.6%, MS2 80.9%; $p = 0.008$). In 58% of cases, an additional sFOV-CBCT was seen as "affecting therapy" with significant differences between the groups (GP 68%, MS1 50%, MS2 55%; $p < 0.001$).

Conclusions: PAN alone is not sufficient for the evaluation of pathologies of the maxillary sinus. But, depending on the examiners' clinical experience, it remains a useful diagnostic tool. Along with the observers' training, significant benefits of an additional sFOV-CBCT for evaluation of symptomatic maxillary sinus pathologies were detected.

Keywords: Panoramic radiography, Cone beam computed tomography, Maxillary sinus site, Subjective rating, Incidental radiographic findings, Education

Background

Non-symptomatic abnormalities of the maxillary sinus such as mucosal thickening, retention cysts, and opacification are reported to occur in up to 74% of all cases [1–6]. For diagnosis of symptomatic pathologies of the maxillary sinus like retention cysts, polyps, and tumors, panoramic radiographies (PAN) are commonly used and widely available. In PAN, not every area of interest is accurately detected and allocated. Furthermore, small maxillary sinus lesions with diameter less than 3 mm show poor detection rates [7]. Three-dimensional imaging is useful in the maxilla for a wide range of clinical settings, such as trauma, bone pathology, and neoplastic diseases, as well as in dental implantology and sinus augmentation [8–12].

Computed tomography (CT) is an excellent tool for maxillary sinus examination and diagnosis [13, 14]. A survey among 331 otolaryngologists showed that the majority (75%) did not obtain confirmatory CT scan before initial

* Correspondence: michael.dau@med.uni-rostock.de
[1]Department of Oral, Maxillofacial and Plastic Surgery, University Medical Center, Schillingallee 35, 18057 Rostock, Germany
Full list of author information is available at the end of the article

non-surgical therapy. Though, prior proceeding with sinus surgery, an average of one (59%) or even two (37%) CT scans was reported [15]. Cone beam computed tomography (CBCT) is mostly used for dental implant planning [6, 10, 16] and offers diagnostic options similar to CT scans but without contrast agents and with about 10–50% less radiation exposure [17, 18]. Especially if small fields of view are used for CBCT, radiation exposure is significantly reduced. However, this exposure to radiation as well as the costs are still significantly higher when compared to those of conventional dental imaging [19–22]. For diagnosis and general preoperative planning, both PAN and CBCT are described to be useful and important diagnostic tools [11, 23, 24]. Nonetheless, there are only few studies [7, 12, 14, 25] and some case reports [26–28] that showed an additional clinical benefit of CBCT for evaluation of maxillary sinus when compared to PAN. In most studies, non-symptomatic sites were visualized in order to exclude pathologic findings prior to dental implant surgery [1, 7, 23, 24, 29, 30].

In order to justify CBCT use for clinical examination and diagnosis of the maxillary sinus, the aim of this study was to compare the subjective quality rating of PAN and PAN together with a small field of view (sFOV) CBCT to evaluate symptomatic maxillary sinus by clinicians with different training and clinical experience.

Methods

Patients and examiners

In an experimental diagnostic comparison, radiographic images of 15 female and 13 male patients were assessed. Patients' radiographs were selected from the Department of Oral, Maxillofacial and Facial Plastic Surgery of the University Medical Centre of Mainz and Rostock, Germany. All patients have had referrals to the hospitals with symptomatic maxillary sinus pathologies and received PAN (Orthophos XG Plus (Sirona Dental Systems GmbH, Bensheim, Germany)) as well as CBCT (KaVo 3D eXam, KaVo Dental GmbH, Biberach/Riß, Germany or Accuitomo Morita, J. MORITA Mfg. Corp., Kyoto, Japan) for radiographic analysis and diagnosis. All CBCT images contained a limited field of view (size of FOV 60×60 mm) for the pathological site only (sFOV-CBCT). Clinical information were given to all examiners before rating. Patients with incomplete medical records were excluded. Seven examiners with a different professional training and experience in using PAN and CBCT were participating. They were two general practitioners with 2–3 years of clinical experience (GP), two junior maxillofacial surgeons with 2–3 years of clinical experience (MS1), and three senior maxillofacial surgeons with 6–7 years of clinical experience (MS2). A standardized questionnaire for PAN (three questions) and CBCT (two questions) was given to each individual separately to

answer. The participant examined only PAN in the first part of the project. Afterwards, he/she filled out the respective questionnaire. At the next step, he/she examined the CBCT scans and answered its related questions. All examiners had undergone a structured postgraduate curriculum for usage of CBCT before, and they used CBCT on daily basis. This curriculum, as demanded by German authorities for using CBCT, consisted of at least two classroom-based trainings (each for 1 day) together with 25 documented CBCT cases and a written examination. Besides, there was no further training for this study. In each case, the same reading environment using a beamer (Epson® EB G5450WU, Epson® Germany, Meerbusch, Germany; data sheet: resolution 1920×1200, brightness 4000 lumens, contrast ratio 1000:1) and a 2×3 m screen was provided. This study on anonymous radiographic images was performed in accordance to the current version of the Declaration of Helsinki [31].

Questionnaire

The first question for PAN addressed the imaging quality in the clinical relevant area of interest (clinical data were given). Three answers were possible: 1 = good visibility and can be evaluated, 2 = visible but cannot be evaluated, and 3 = not visible. The second question asked for an additional need for CBCT scans. Three answers were possible: 1 = required, 2 = reasonable, and 3 = not required. The third question was referring to the number of additional incidental findings in PAN not related to the sinus disease that led to the radiographic examination.

For CBCT, the first question was referring to a possible additional value in the area of interest. The examiners had to choose between three possible answers (1 = showed no additional information, 2 = was useful, 3 = was affecting therapy). The second question targeted the number of incidental findings in CBCT in addition to PAN not related to the sinus disease that led to the radiographic examination.

Statistics

Due to the experimental design, no prior power analysis was conducted. All results in this study were expressed as number of cases, incidence value (percentage), or as arithmetic means ± standard deviation (SD). For comparison of groups, one-way analyses of variance (ANOVA) with Tukey B simultaneous post hoc tests as well as chi-square tests were performed and descriptive p values of the tests are reported. A p value ≤ 0.05 was termed significant. All statistical analyses were performed with SPSS version 20.0 (SPSS Inc., Chicago, IL, USA).

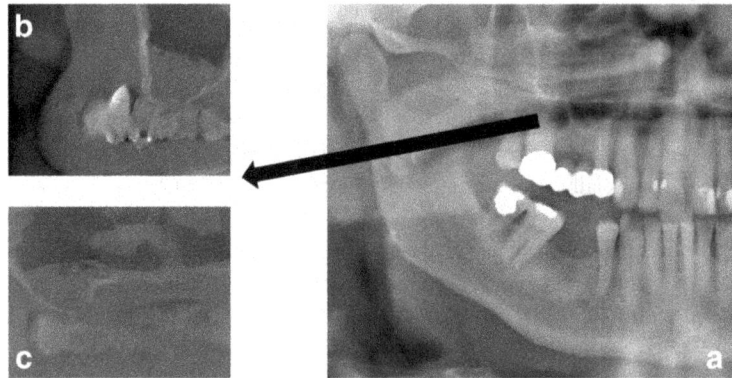

Fig. 1 a Panoramic radiography with area of interest (maxillary sinus) and **b, c** examples of corresponding images in cone beam computed tomography

Results

This study focused on three different aspects in our analysis—PAN, PAN and CBCT, as well as the influence of the different clinical and radiological experience (examples in Figs. 1 and 2).

(a) Panoramic radiography (PAN)

When assessing PAN, the ratings were significantly lower at "good visible and can be evaluated" (9.9%) compared to "visible but cannot be evaluated" (39.5%; $p < 0.001$) and compared to "not visible" (50.6%; $p < 0.001$) ratings (Table 1). An additional CBCT was needed in most cases ("required" (28%) and "reasonable" (63.3%) versus "not required" (8.7%; Table 2)). All examiners found an average number of 1.7 ± 1.3 additional findings in PAN (Table 3). The three most common findings were retained third molars with putative follicular cysts (22% of all findings), followed by radiological insufficient root filling (21%) and caries/insufficient filling of teeth (19%; Table 4).

(b) Cone beam computed tomography (CBCT)

The majority of the answers indicated the usefulness of an additional sFOV-CBCT. Whereas it only "showed no additional information" in 10.1% and was "useful" in 32.4% of cases, an additional CBCT was rated as "affecting therapy" in 57.5% of cases (Table 5).

Overall, the examiners observed an average number of 0.6 ± 0.6 additional incidental findings (Table 3). The findings were radiological caries/insufficient filling of teeth (88%) as well as insufficient root filling (22%).

(c) Influence of examiners' clinical background

In PAN, MS1 (51.8%) and MS2 (39.3%) rated significantly less for "not visible" when compared to GPs (60.7%; $p < 0.001$). The difference was significant between MS1 and MS2 as well ($p < 0.05$). Significantly more "good visibility" ratings were obtained for MS2 (15.5%) when compared to MS1 (8.9%; $p = 0.021$) and GP (5.4%; $p < 0.001$; Table 1). A significant higher number of additional incidental findings in PAN was seen in MS2 (mean = 2.1 ± 1.5) versus GP (mean = 1.5 ± 1.3; $p = 0.021$) as well as in MS2 versus MS1 (mean = 1.6 ± 1.1; $p = 0.048$; Table 3).

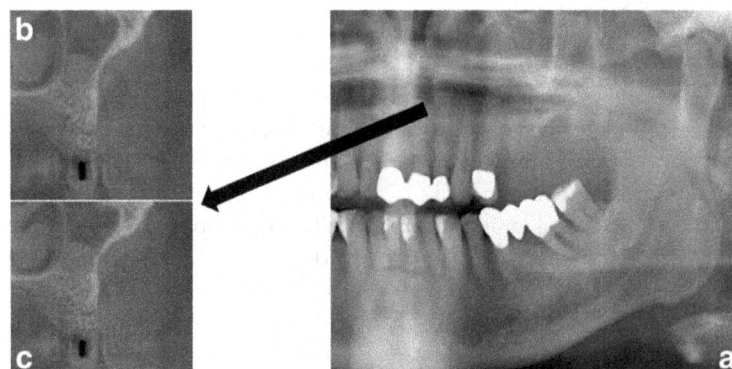

Fig. 2 a Panoramic radiography with area of interest (maxillary sinus) and **b, c** examples of corresponding images in cone beam computed tomography

Table 1 Results of the question "Based on PAN, the clinical area of interest, is..."

Question	General practitioner (n = 2)	Junior maxillofacial surgeon (n = 2)	Senior maxillofacial surgeon (n = 3)	p value*
1 = good visibility and can be evaluated	3 (5.4%)	5 (8.9%)	13 (15.5%)	p < 0.002
2 = visible but cannot be evaluated	19 (33.9%)	22 (39.3%)	38 (45.2%)	
3 = not visible	34 (60.7%)	29 (51.8%)	33 (39.3%)	

*One-way ANOVA test with post hoc Tukey B: GP versus MS1 p = 0.034, MS1 versus MS2 p = 0.211, and GP versus MS2 p = 0.001

GPs rated an additional CBCT significantly less often to be "not required" (1.8%) when compared to MS1 (5.4%; p = 0.038) and to MS2 (19%; p = 0.006). Moreover, GPs rated significantly more for a CBCT to be "reasonable" or "required" (98.2%) when compared to MS1 (94.6%; p = 0.002) and compared to MS2 (80.9%; p = 0.001; Table 2). Also, in the GP group, the additional CBCT was seen significantly more often to be "affecting therapy" (67.8%) when compared to MS1 (50%) and to MS2 (53.8%; all p < 0.001; Table 5). Between the groups, there was no difference in the average number of additional incidental diagnoses in sFOV-CBCT scans (GD, average = 0.7 ± 0.5; MS1, average = 0.6 ± 0.5; MS2, average = 0.7 ± 0.7; p = 0.912, Table 3).

Discussion

In dentistry, PAN is a widely available, useful, and important diagnostic tool for diagnosis and general preoperative planning [32] with less radiation exposure then CBCT [21]. While most dentists have used it routinely successful for years and gained significant experience in doing so [33], there are certain limitations in dependence of the region to be examined [10]. The high number of "not visible" ratings of the area of interest in the study at hand underlines this conclusion. Nevertheless, PAN showed several additional incidental findings showing its important value being a basic diagnostic tool, also in preventive dentistry [32, 33]. It is noticeable that most of these incidental findings were described by senior surgeons. This demonstrates the impact of clinical experience of evaluation of PAN [12, 34]. A lack of experience in 2D

Table 2 Results of the question "An additional sFOV-CBCT of the clinical area of interest is..."

Question	General practitioner (n = 2)	Junior maxillofacial surgeon (n = 2)	Senior maxillofacial surgeon (n = 3)	p value*
1 = required	14 (25.0%)	21 (37.5%)	18 (21.4%)	p = 0.008
2 = reasonable	41 (73.2%)	32 (57.1%)	50 (59.5%)	
3 = not required	1 (1.8%)	3 (5.4%)	16 (19.0%)	

*One-way ANOVA test with post hoc Tukey B: GP versus MS1 p = 0.369, MS1 versus MS2 p = 0.006, and GP versus MS2 p = 0.038

Table 3 Number of additional incidental findings in PAN and sFOV-CBCT not related to the sinus disease that led to the radiographic examination

Number of cases	General practitioner (n = 2)	Junior maxillofacial surgeon (n = 2)	Senior maxillofacial surgeon (n = 3)	p value*
	Number of incidental findings in PAN			
(n = 28)	1.5 ± 1.3	1.6 ± 1.1	2.1 ± 1.5	p = 0.027
	Number of additional, incidental findings in sFOV-CBCT			
(n = 28)	0.7 ± 0.5	0.6 ± 0.5	0.7 ± 0.7	p = 0.912

*One-way ANOVA test

imaging might even result in unnecessary additional 3D diagnostics (such as additional CBCTs) [12].

For the diagnosis of symptomatic pathologies in the maxillary sinus, PAN alone is not sufficient. Benefits (in dependence of clinical and radiological experience) offered from additional sFOV-CBCT imaging were proven in the presented study. The high number of "therapy affecting" ratings when adding CBCT supports such statement. Wolf et al. reported the general demand for three-dimensional imaging of maxillary sinus in order to minimize intra- and postoperative complications and to localize any foreign body in relation to other anatomical structures [35]. Similarly, various studies reported an average of one or more CT scans prior proceeding with sinus surgery [15]. Sharma et al. recommended CT scans prior sinus surgery in order to guide the surgeon [36]. Other researcher found the same diagnostic accuracy of CBCT scans of maxillary sinus pathologies when compared to sinus endoscopy [37] which underlines the importance of CBCT within this field. As shown by others as well [2, 38–43], a better evaluation of anatomical structures was found when using CBCT. CBCT scans offer an extremely valuable diagnostic and clinical tool for maxillary sinus pathologies in general [36, 44, 45] for vital findings like posterior superior alveolar arteries in the lateral sinus wall [46] as well as for anatomical variations [47]. Especially in cases with symptomatic

Table 4 Description of incidental findings in PAN not related to the sinus disease that led to the radiographic examination

Additional incidental findings in panoramic radiography	Relative incidence (%) in relation to total number of therapy affecting findings
Retained third molar/follicular cyst	22
Insufficient root filling	21
Caries/insufficient filling of teeth	19
Apical ostitis	17
Remaining root remnants	9
Periodontal bone loss	8
Anatomic particularities (enlargement of the mental foramen/retromolar foramen/bifid nerve)	4

Table 5 Results of the question "Is there an additional clinical value of sFOV-CBCT?"

Question	General practitioner ($n = 2$)	Junior maxillofacial surgeon ($n = 2$)	Senior maxillofacial surgeon ($n = 3$)	p value*
1 = it showed no additional information	2 (3.6%)	5 (8.9%)	15 (17.9%)	$p < 0.001$
2 = it was useful	16 (28.6%)	23 (41.1%)	23 (27.4%)	
3 = it was affecting therapy	38 (67.8%)	28 (50.0%)	46 (54.8%)	

*One-way ANOVA test with post hoc Tukey B: GP versus MS1 $p = 0.002$, MS1 versus MS2 $p = 0.890$, and GP versus MS2 $p = 0.001$

maxillary sinus pathologies, three-dimensional diagnostic is helpful [13, 36, 48] and a sFOV-CBCT offers limited radiation exposure as well.

The influence of clinical experience of evaluation of PAN [34] as well as the clinical experience and routine analysis of 3D radiographs (as assumed for maxillofacial surgeons when compared to those for general practitioners) strongly influence the diagnostic value of additional three-dimensional imaging. The number of incidental findings in CBCT in addition to those seen in PAN was not of major difference and did not correlate to the examiners' experience. This difference can be explained by using sFOV-CBCTs for evaluation of symptomatic maxillary sinus pathologies only. The smaller field of view shows less incidental findings, but the radiation exposure will be kept lower as well. Nonetheless, sFOV-CBCT is not meant to be a replacement for PAN especially for patients' screening. It seems that advanced diagnostic tools such as CBCT offer an effective solution with more precise diagnosis of the maxillary sinus when compared to PAN together with a lower radiation dose compared to a CT.

There are some limitations of the study and potential bias caused by the experimental design, the subjective evaluation, and the low number of patients. Nevertheless, the additional value of CBCT strongly depends on the level on medical and radiographic knowledge of the anatomy of sites of interest [16, 38] and the surrounding structures [2]. Based on the findings of this study and the literature, an adjunct sFOV-CBCT is a valuable diagnostic tool for cases of symptomatic maxillary sinus pathologies.

Conclusions

Depending on the observers' clinical and radiological experience, PAN alone may not be sufficient for evaluation of pathologies of the maxillary sinus. On the contrary, significant benefits of sFOV-CBCT for diagnosing symptomatic maxillary sinus pathologies were reported. Having sFOV-CBCT seems to have added additional information and confidence in comparison to PAN alone. Nonetheless, also with the examiners' increased clinical experience, PAN remains a valuable diagnostic tool.

Authors' contributions
The organization of data acquisition as well as preparation and evaluation of questionnaires were conducted by PM, BA, HS, and PWK. MD, BA, AA, BF, and PWK did the statistical evaluation together with the preparation, drafting, and finalization of the manuscript. All authors read and approved the final manuscript.

Competing interests
Michael Dau, Paul Marciak, Bial Al-Nawas, Henning Staedt, Abdulmonem Alshiri, Bernhard Frerich, and Peer Wolfgang Kämmerer declare that they have no competing interests.

Informed consent
This experimental diagnostic comparison was performed without any further consequences for the patient. According to this and the hospital laws of the individual states (see *Krankenhausgesetz RLP and MV*), no formal consent was required.

Author details
[1]Department of Oral, Maxillofacial and Plastic Surgery, University Medical Center, Schillingallee 35, 18057 Rostock, Germany. [2]Department of Oral and Maxillofacial Surgery, Plastic Surgery, University Medical Centre, Mainz, Germany. [3]Private Dental Praxis Dr. Rossa, Ludwigshafen, Germany. [4]Department of Biomaterial and Prosthetic Sciences, King Saud University, Riyadh, Saudi Arabia.

References
1. Dragan E, et al. Maxillary sinus anatomic and pathologic CT findings in edentulous patients scheduled for sinus augmentation. Rev Med Chir Soc Med Nat Iasi. 2014;118(4):1114–21.
2. Raghav M, et al. Prevalence of incidental maxillary sinus pathologies in dental patients on cone-beam computed tomographic images. Contemp Clin Dent. 2014;5(3):361–5.
3. Lyros I, et al. An incidental finding on a diagnostic CBCT: a case report. Aust Orthod J. 2014;30(1):67–71.
4. Steier L, et al. Maxillary sinus unilateral aplasia as an incidental finding following cone-beam computed (volumetric) tomography. Aust Endod J. 2014;40(1):26–31.
5. Vogiatzi T, et al. Incidence of anatomical variations and disease of the maxillary sinuses as identified by cone beam computed tomography: a systematic review. Int J Oral Maxillofac Implants. 2014;29(6):1301–14.
6. Warhekar S, et al. Incidental findings on cone beam computed tomography and reasons for referral by dental practitioners in Indore City (m.p). J Clin Diagn Res. 2015;9(2):ZC21–4.
7. Shiki K, et al. The significance of cone beam computed tomography for the visualization of anatomical variations and lesions in the maxillary sinus for patients hoping to have dental implant-supported maxillary restorations in a private dental office in Japan. Head Face Med. 2014;10:20.
8. Dammann F, et al. Diagnostic imaging modalities in head and neck disease. Dtsch Arztebl Int. 2014;111(23-24):417–23.
9. Kuhnel TS, Reichert TE. Trauma of the midface. Laryngorhinootologie. 2015; 94 Suppl 1:S206–47.
10. Dau M, et al. Presurgical evaluation of bony implant sites using panoramic radiography and cone beam computed tomography-influence of medical education. Dentomaxillofac Radiol. 2017;46(2):20160081.
11. Kammerer PW, et al. Surgical evaluation of panoramic radiography and cone beam computed tomography for therapy planning of bisphosphonate-related osteonecrosis of the jaws. Oral Surg Oral Med Oral Pathol Oral Radiol. 2016;121(4):419–24.
12. Malina-Altzinger J, et al. Evaluation of the maxillary sinus in panoramic radiography—a comparative study. Int J Implant Dent. 2015;1(1):17.
13. Guerra-Pereira I, et al. Ct maxillary sinus evaluation—a retrospective cohort study. Med Oral Patol Oral Cir Bucal. 2015;20(4):e419–26.
14. Gang TI, et al. The effect of radiographic imaging modalities and the observer's experience on postoperative maxillary cyst assessment. Imaging Sci Dent. 2014;44(4):301–5.
15. Batra PS, et al. Computed tomography imaging practice patterns in adult chronic rhinosinusitis: survey of the American Academy of Otolaryngology-

Head and Neck Surgery and American Rhinologic Society Membership. Int Forum Allergy Rhinol. 2015;5(6):506–12.

16. Whitesides LM, Aslam-Pervez N, Warburton G. Cone-beam computed tomography education and exposure in oral and maxillofacial surgery training programs in the United States. J Oral Maxillofac Surg. 2015;73(3):522–8.

17. Shah N, Bansal N, Logani A. Recent advances in imaging technologies in dentistry. World J Radiol. 2014;6(10):794–807.

18. De Cock J, et al. A comparative study for image quality and radiation dose of a cone beam computed tomography scanner and a multislice computed tomography scanner for paranasal sinus imaging. Eur Radiol. 2015;25(7):1891–900.

19. Roberts JA, et al. Effective dose from cone beam CT examinations in dentistry. Br J Radiol. 2009;82(973):35–40.

20. Deman P, et al. Dose measurements for dental cone-beam CT: a comparison with MSCT and panoramic imaging. Phys Med Biol. 2014;59(12):3201–22.

21. Shin HS, et al. Effective doses from panoramic radiography and CBCT (cone beam CT) using dose area product (DAP) in dentistry. Dentomaxillofac Radiol. 2014;43(5):20130439.

22. Al-Okshi A, et al. Using GafChromic film to estimate the effective dose from dental cone beam CT and panoramic radiography. Dentomaxillofac Radiol. 2013;42(7):20120343.

23. Poleti ML, et al. Anatomical variation of the maxillary sinus in cone beam computed tomography. Case Rep Dent. 2014;2014:707261.

24. Friedland B, Metson R. A guide to recognizing maxillary sinus pathology and for deciding on further preoperative assessment prior to maxillary sinus augmentation. Int J Periodontics Restorative Dent. 2014;34(6):807–15.

25. Agacayak KS, et al. Alterations in maxillary sinus volume among oral and nasal breathers. Med Sci Monit. 2015;21:18–26.

26. Jafari-Pozve N, et al. Aplasia and hypoplasia of the maxillary sinus: a case series. Dent Res J (Isfahan). 2014;11(5):615–7.

27. Rivis M, Valeanu AN. Giant maxillary cyst with intrasinusal evolution. Rom J Morphol Embryol. 2013;54(3 Suppl):889–92.

28. Yilmaz SY, Misirlioglu M, Adisen MZ. A diagnosis of maxillary sinus fracture with cone-beam CT: case report and literature review. Craniomaxillofac Trauma Reconstr. 2014;7(2):85–91.

29. Lana JP, et al. Anatomic variations and lesions of the maxillary sinus detected in cone beam computed tomography for dental implants. Clin Oral Implants Res. 2012;23(12):1398–403.

30. Jadhav AB, Lurie AG, Tadinada A. Chronic osteitic rhinosinusitis as a manifestation of cystic fibrosis: a case report. Imaging Sci Dent. 2014;44(3):243–7.

31. World Medical A. World Medical Association Declaration of Helsinki: ethical principles for medical research involving human subjects. JAMA. 2013;310(20):2191–4.

32. Kammerer PW, et al. Clinical parameter of odontoma with special emphasis on treatment of impacted teeth—a retrospective multicentre study and literature review. Clin Oral Investig. 2016;20(7):1827–35.

33. Schafer T, et al. Incidental finding of a foreign object on a panoramic radiograph. Pediatr Dent. 2015;37(5):453–4.

34. Turgeon DP, Lam EW. Influence of experience and training on dental students' examination performance regarding panoramic images. J Dent Educ. 2016;80(2):156–64.

35. Wolf MK, et al. Preoperative 3D imaging in maxillary sinus: brief review of the literature and case report. Quintessence Int. 2015;46(7):627–31.

36. Sharma BN, et al. Computed tomography in the evaluation of pathological lesions of paranasal sinuses. J Nepal Health Res Counc. 2015;13(30):116–20.

37. Zojaji R, et al. Diagnostic accuracy of cone-beam computed tomography in the evaluation of chronic rhinosinusitis. ORL J Otorhinolaryngol Relat Spec. 2015;77(1):55–60.

38. Noar JH, Pabari S. Cone beam computed tomography—current understanding and evidence for its orthodontic applications? J Orthod. 2013;40(1):5–13.

39. Guerrero ME, Noriega J, Jacobs R. Preoperative implant planning considering alveolar bone grafting needs and complication prediction using panoramic versus CBCT images. Imaging Sci Dent. 2014;44(3):213–20.

40. Machtei EE, Oettinger-Barak O, Horwitz J. Axial relationship between dental implants and teeth/implants: a radiographic study. J Oral Implantol. 2014;40(4):425–31.

41. Stratemann SA, et al. Evaluating the mandible with cone-beam computed tomography. Am J Orthod Dentofacial Orthop. 2010;137(4 Suppl):S58–70.

42. Quintero JC, et al. Craniofacial imaging in orthodontics: historical perspective, current status, and future developments. Angle Orthod. 1999;69(6):491–506.

43. Tadinada A, et al. Radiographic evaluation of the maxillary sinus prior to dental implant therapy: a comparison between two-dimensional and three-dimensional radiographic imaging. Imaging Sci Dent. 2015;45(3):169–74.

44. Ritter L, et al. Prevalence of pathologic findings in the maxillary sinus in cone-beam computerized tomography. Oral Surg Oral Med Oral Pathol Oral Radiol Endod. 2011;111(5):634–40.

45. Maillet M, et al. Cone-beam computed tomography evaluation of maxillary sinusitis. J Endod. 2011;37(6):753–7.

46. Varela-Centelles P, et al. Detection of the posterior superior alveolar artery in the lateral sinus wall using computed tomography/cone beam computed tomography: a prevalence meta-analysis study and systematic review. Int J Oral Maxillofac Surg. 2015;44(11):1405–10.

47. Shahidi S, et al. Evaluation of anatomic variations in maxillary sinus with the aid of cone beam computed tomography (CBCT) in a population in south of Iran. J Dent (Shiraz). 2016;17(1):7–15.

48. Hssaine K, et al. Paranasal sinus mucoceles: about 32 cases. Rev Stomatol Chir Maxillofac Chir Orale. 2016;117(1):11–4.

22

Investigation of peri-implant tissue conditions and peri-implant tissue stability in implants placed with simultaneous augmentation procedure: a 3-year retrospective follow-up analysis of a newly developed bone level implant system

Jonas Lorenz[1], Henriette Lerner[2], Robert A. Sader[1] and Shahram Ghanaati[1*]

Abstract

Background: Guided bone regeneration (GBR) has been proven to be a reliable therapy to regenerate missing bone in cases of atrophy of the alveolar crest. The aim of the present retrospective analysis was to assess peri-implant tissue conditions and document peri-implant tissue stability in C-Tech implants when placed simultaneously with a GBR augmentation procedure.

Methods: A total of 47 implants, which were placed simultaneously with a GBR procedure with a synthetic bone substitute material in 20 patients, were investigated clinically and radiologically at least 3 years after loading. Implant survival, the width and thickness of peri-implant keratinized gingiva, probing depth, bleeding on probing (BOP), the Pink Esthetic Score (PES), peri-implant bone loss, and the presence of peri-implant osteolysis were determined.

Results: The follow-up investigation revealed a survival rate of 100% and only low median rates for probing depths (2.7 mm) and BOP (30%). The mean PES was 10.1 from the maximum value of 14. No osseous peri-implant defects were obvious, and the mean bone loss was 0.55 mm.

Conclusions: In conclusion, implants placed in combination with a GBR procedure can achieve long-term stable functionally and esthetically satisfying results for replacing missing teeth in cases of atrophy of the alveolar crest.

Keywords: C-Tech implants, Guided bone regeneration, Oral implantology, Peri-implantitis

Background

The prevalence of peri-implantitis has grown in the past few years and has become a major issue in implant dentistry. Long-term stable and healthy soft- and hard-tissue conditions should be achieved in combination with esthetically and functionally satisfying results. However, the rising number of placed implants in the past decades has come with an increase in the prevalence of peri-implantitis [1].

Peri-implantitis is defined as a pathological inflammation of the peri-implant soft and hard tissue leading to peri-implant bone loss. For pathogenesis, many different factors are discussed in the literature. Reviews have shown that oral hygiene, implant surgery factors such as implant position, soft- and hard-tissue amount and quality, prosthetic concepts and design, general medical history, and other factors have an impact on the establishment and progression of peri-implantitis [2].

Peri-implant soft tissue forms the first border of the peri-implant tissue to the oral cavity and therefore to the migration of microorganisms that can cause and accelerate peri-implant infections. Dental implants, unlike the

---

* Correspondence: shahram.ghanaati@kgu.de

[1]Department for Oral, FORM-Lab, Cranio-Maxillofacial, and Facial Plastic Surgery, Medical Center of the Goethe University Frankfurt, Frankfurt am Main, Germany

Full list of author information is available at the end of the article

natural teeth, do not possess a compact barrier against penetration properties of the oral cavity. Peri-implant soft tissue acts as a cuff-like barrier [3]. In contrast to the periodontal attachment, there is no connective tissue fiber insertion into the implant surface. The peri-implant soft tissue possesses a lower number of blood vessels [4, 5] and cells but a higher amount of collagen [3, 6]. As a consequence of these anatomical differences, the peri-implant soft tissue has a decreased defending mechanism against microorganisms that in a pathological amount causes peri-implant infections.

A major etiological factor for peri-implantitis is the position of the implant in the surrounding bone [2]. In addition to bone quality and vascularization, a sufficient amount of peri-implant bone is important for the long-term stability of the implant and a sufficient underlining to the peri-implant soft tissue [2]. However, in most patients, the local bone amount is reduced due to atrophy, inflammatory processes, or resectional defects. Therefore, in the past few years, different techniques have been described to enlarge the local bone amount in prospective implant sites [7]. Besides methods such as GBR or the sinus augmentation technique, different augmentation materials have been investigated and established in the daily clinical routine. Autologous bone in the context of hard tissue augmentations is still the gold standard due to its osteogenic capacity [8]. To avoid the disadvantages that come with autologous bone transfer, such as a second surgical site and an increase in postoperative pain, biomaterial research has focused on the development of bone substitute materials that serve as scaffolds for the ingrowth of bone and its progenitor cells from the surrounding tissue [9].

The ability of bone substitute materials to form a sufficient and stable implantation bed has been proven in numerous clinical trials; however, it is still to a certain degree unclear if the different tissue reactions have an impact on the establishment of a peri-implant infection, especially when these biomaterials are used for augmentations around the implant shoulder. Due to the two-stage design of the implant, the implant shoulder presents a potential micro-gap between the abutment and the implant and a port of entry for microorganisms and peri-implant infections leading to a manifestation of peri-implantitis [10].

Regarding the stability of peri-implant hard and soft tissue, biological or anatomical factors are not the only elements that could be proven to have an impact. Technical factors such as the implant-abutment connection are also known to be key factors for long-term stable hard- and soft-tissue health [11]. Regarding the implant-abutment connection, which seems to be the key issue, located on the interface between the implant, the peri-implant bone, the peri-implant soft tissue, and

the oral cavity, different studies have shown that a Morse-tapered conical connection reduces the micromovement and therefore the micro-motions, which results in a pump effect of sulcus fluid and microorganisms in the fragile peri-implant soft tissue [10, 12]. The conical connection leads to a kind of "cold welding" type of connection that seems to prevent bone loss compared to external implant-abutment connections [10, 12].

A further factor, which has been detected to improve peri-implant hard- and soft-tissue health and is related to a conical implant-abutment connection, is a "platform switching" design. By switching the platform between the implant and the abutment from the outside surface of the implant to the inside region and therefore in larger distance to the peri-implant hard and soft tissue, the colonization of microorganisms seems to be reduced. Furthermore, the conical connection in combination with a platform switching design decreases stress transferred onto the peri-implant bone. As a result, peri-implant bone loss is prevented and the peri-implant soft- and hard-tissue health can be preserved [11, 13].

The aim of the present retrospective investigation was to assess clinically and radiologically peri-implant tissue conditions and document peri-implant tissue stability in C-Tech implants when placed simultaneously with a GBR augmentation procedure after at least 3 years of loading.

Methods

Patient population

In the present retrospective study, 47 dental implants (C-Tech Esthetic Line implants) from 20 patients (11 female, 9 male) with a mean age of 58.5 years (45–75 years) were analyzed clinically and radiologically. Implant placement and follow-up investigation was performed at the HL Dentclinic in Baden-Baden, Germany. The study was approved by the ethics commission of the medical department of Goethe University in Frankfurt am Main, Germany (378/16). All participating patients gave written informed consent to participate in the study and for publication of the obtained data. All patients from the private practice from one of the authors (H.L) that received C-Tech Esthetic Line implants in combination with a GBR augmentation procedure over a period of 1 year that have been available for follow-up investigation have been included in the present study. Furthermore, implants had to be loaded for at least 3 years. Patients with incomplete data collection or refusing to participate in the study have been excluded. Implants were placed in combination with simultaneous augmentation procedures on the implant shoulder (lateral augmentation, GBR) with synthetic (alloplastic) biomaterials. Hydroxyapatite (HA)-based bone substitute materials and bone substitute materials consisting of HA and beta-tricalcium phosphate (β-TCP) were used. Maxresorb° (Botiss Biomaterials, Berlin, Germany) is a synthetic derived bone substitute material made of biphasic calcium phosphate. It is composed of 60% HA and 40% β-TCP and has been applied for augmentation in 26 implants, while in 21 implants, Osbone° (Curasan, Frankfurt, Germany), a synthetic bone substitute material made of pure HA, has been used.

Implants were placed in native alveolar bone and augmentation around the implant shoulder due to horizontal and vertical bone defects that led to dehiscences of the implant surface. Twenty-three implants were placed in the upper jaw and 24 implants in the lower jaw. All implant placements were delayed at least 3 months after the extraction of teeth not worth preserving, and loading was done after a mean osseointegration period of 4 months. Prosthetic rehabilitation consisted of fixed prosthetics in 43 implants and removable prosthetics in 4 implants. The clinical and radiological follow-up investigation was performed after a loading period of at least 3 years (36–48 months after incorporation of prosthetics, mean 42.6 months). Implant survival and peri-implant hard- and soft-tissue health were analyzed to determine the manifestations of peri-mucositis by analysis of bleeding on probing (BOP) or peri-implantitis by analysis of marginal bone loss. Table 1 gives an overview of retrospectively investigated implants with patient information, implant localization, and implant data.

C-Tech implant system

In the present retrospective study, bone level implants (C-Tech Esthetic Line implants) were investigated clinically and radiologically. The bone level implant system has a Morse-locking conical implant-abutment connection with platform switching and an indexing hex that allows subcrestal implant placement and aims to prevent peri-implant bone loss. The surface of the implant system is manufactured by grit-blasting and acid-etching. The macrostructure of the implant consists of a beveled shoulder and three different threading profiles changing along the length of the implant.

Figure 1 gives a representation of the technical characteristics of the investigated C-Tech Esthetic Line implant system.

Clinical and radiological follow-up investigation

After a mean period of 3 years after loading, the implants were investigated clinically and radiologically according to previously published methods [14, 15]. To determine the stability of the peri-implant hard and soft tissue, the following parameters were analyzed: implant survival, that is, the implants being in situ; the width

and thickness of the peri-implant keratinized gingiva (in millimeters); the probing depth (in millimeters); BOP; peri-implant bone loss (in millimeters); and the presence of peri-implant osteolysis. The probing depth was measured with a blunt periodontal probe at four sites (mesio-buccal, distal-buccal, mesio-oral, and disto-oral). Simultaneously to the measurement of the probing depths, the implant was checked to see if probing provoked bleeding (BOP).

To analyze the esthetic appearance of the implant-retained prosthetics, the PES was determined. Digital photographs including the neighboring and opposite teeth were recorded and evaluated by two independent experienced blinded investigators familiar with the PES scoring method. The PES score is generated using seven items (mesial papilla, distal papilla, soft-tissue level, soft-tissue contour, alveolar process deficiency, soft-tissue color, and texture) and an evaluation with a point score from 0 = very bad to 2 = excellent. Thus, a maximum score of 14 can be achieved. For determination of peri-implant bone loss, digitally recorded panoramic radiographies taken routinely after implant insertion and upon reexamination were analyzed with appropriate radiological software. Bone loss was measured mesially and distally, and a mean bone loss value was calculated.

Investigation parameters:

- Implant being in situ
- Width and thickness of peri-implant keratinized gingiva
- Pink Esthetic Score (PES)
- Probing depth
- BOP
- Peri-implant bone loss
- Presence of peri-implant osteolysis

Results

Altogether, 47 implants were placed in the upper and lower jaws of a total of 20 patients. In all implants, lateral augmentation in a GBR process was performed simultaneously with implant placement due to reduced horizontal or vertical height of the alveolar crest. A total of 23 implants were placed in the upper jaw and 24 implants in the lower jaw. The implant diameter varied between 3.5 mm (32 implants) and 4.3 mm (15 implants). The implant length varied between 11 mm (37 implants) and 13 mm (10 implants). Prosthetic restoration consisted of fixed prosthetics (43 implants) and removable prosthetics (r.p.) (4 implants) (Table 1).

The bone substitute materials applied for the horizontal and vertical GBR procedures were of synthetic (HA and β-TCP) origin.

Table 1 Participating patients and the number and site of the inserted implants

Patient	Gender (m/f)	Age (years)	Implant localization (region)	Implant diameter (mm)	Implant length (mm)	Augmentation material	Prosthetic rehabilitation
1	f	50	32	3.5	13	HA + β-TCP	r.p
			34	4.3	11	HA + β-TCP	r.p
			42	3.5	13	HA + β-TCP	r.p
			44	4.3	11	HA + β-TCP	r.p
2	m	61	36	3.5	11	HA + β-TCP	f.p.
			37	3.5	11	HA + β-TCP	f.p.
			46	3.5	11	HA + β-TCP	f.p.
			47	3.5	11	HA + β-TCP	f.p.
3	m	48	26	4.3	11	HA + β-TCP	f.p.
4	f	54	21	4.3	11	HA + β-TCP	f.p.
5	f	45	23	3.5	13	HA	f.p.
			26	4.3	11	HA	f.p.
			27	4.3	11	HA	f.p.
6	m	56	32	3.5	13	HA + β-TCP	f.p.
			42	3.5	13	HA + β-TCP	f.p.
7	m	54	36	4.3	11	HA + β-TCP	f.p.
			46	3.5	11	HA + β-TCP	f.p.
			36	4.3	11	HA + β-TCP	f.p.
8	f	73	16	3.5	11	HA + β-TCP	f.p.
			26	3.5	11	HA + β-TCP	f.p.
9	m	64	27	4.3	11	HA + β-TCP	f.p.
10	f	62	15	3.5	11	HA + β-TCP	f.p.
			16	3.5	11	HA + β-TCP	f.p.
			17	3.5	11	HA + β-TCP	f.p.
			24	3.5	11	HA + β-TCP	f.p.
			36	4.3	11	HA + β-TCP	f.p.
			46	3.5	11	HA + β-TCP	f.p.
11	f	75	35	3.5	11	HA + β-TCP	f.p.
			36	3.5	11	HA + β-TCP	f.p.
12	f	52	16	4.3	11	HA + β-TCP	f.p.
13	m	46	24	3.5	11	HA + β-TCP	f.p.
			25	3.5	11	HA + β-TCP	f.p.
			26	3.5	11	HA + β-TCP	f.p.
			46	4.3	11	HA + β-TCP	f.p.
14	f	66	36	3.5	11	HA + β-TCP	f.p.
			37	3.5	11	HA + β-TCP	f.p.
15	f	63	11	3.5	13	HA	f.p.
16	f	53	36	3.5	11	HA + β-TCP	f.p.
			46	3.5	11	HA + β-TCP	f.p.
			47	3.5	11	HA + β-TCP	f.p.
17	f	51	14	3.5	13	HA + β-TCP	f.p.
			15	3.5	13	HA + β-TCP	f.p.
18	m	60	27	4.3	11	HA + β-TCP	f.p.
			47	4.3	11	HA + β-TCP	f.p.

Table 1 Participating patients and the number and site of the inserted implants *(Continued)*

19	m	75	22	3.5	13	HA + β-TCP	f.p.
			24	3.5	13	HA + β-TCP	f.p.
20	m	62	26	4.3	11	HA + β-TCP	f.p.
Total 20	Total 11*f; 9*m	Mean 58.5	Total 47; 23*u.j, 24*l.j.	Total 32*3.5 mm, 15*4.3 mm	Total 37*11 mm, 10*13 mm	Total 43*HA + β-TCP, 4*HA	Total 43*f.p., 4*r.p

f female, *m* male, *f.p.* fixed prosthetics, *r.p.* removable prosthetics, *u.j.* upper jaw, *l.j.* lower jaw, *HA + β-TCP* synthetic biphasic bone substitute material composed of 60% HA and 40% β-TCP, *HA* synthetic bone substitute material made of pure HA

At the follow-up investigation 3 years after implant loading, all of the 47 placed implants were in situ, leading to a survival rate of 100%. No prosthetic complications, major infections, or incompatibility reactions were observed.

Clinical analysis of the probing depths and the presence of BOP was performed to uncover an inflammatory reaction in the peri-implant soft tissue. The mean probing depth calculated from the probing depths at four sites per implant was 2.4 mm, varying from 1 to 4 mm. BOP was observed during probing in 14 of the 47 implants (30%). A distinct correlation between an accumulation of increased probing depth and BOP was obvious, as most implants with BOP presented increased probing depths.

The amount of peri-implant attached keratinized gingiva in the implants of the present study was analyzed to determine a potential correlation between keratinized peri-implant gingiva, a potential inflammatory response, and peri-implant bone loss and peri-implant osteolysis. All implants had a band of keratinized gingiva of at least 1 mm width and thickness. The mean width was 3.2 mm, ranging from 2 to 6 mm, and the mean thickness was 2.4 mm, ranging from 1 to 4 mm. No distinct and statistically significant correlation of the amount of keratinized gingiva and the evaluated soft-tissue parameters (probing depth and BOP) was observed.

Investigation of the esthetic appearance via PES revealed a mean point score of 10.1 (ranging from 7 to 13) from a maximum of 14. The highest values and therefore acceptance were found in the alveolar process deficiency and the soft-tissue level, which can be interpreted as a benefit of the augmentation procedure around the implant shoulder.

Peri-implant bone loss calculated using the average bone loss mesially and distally of each implant was

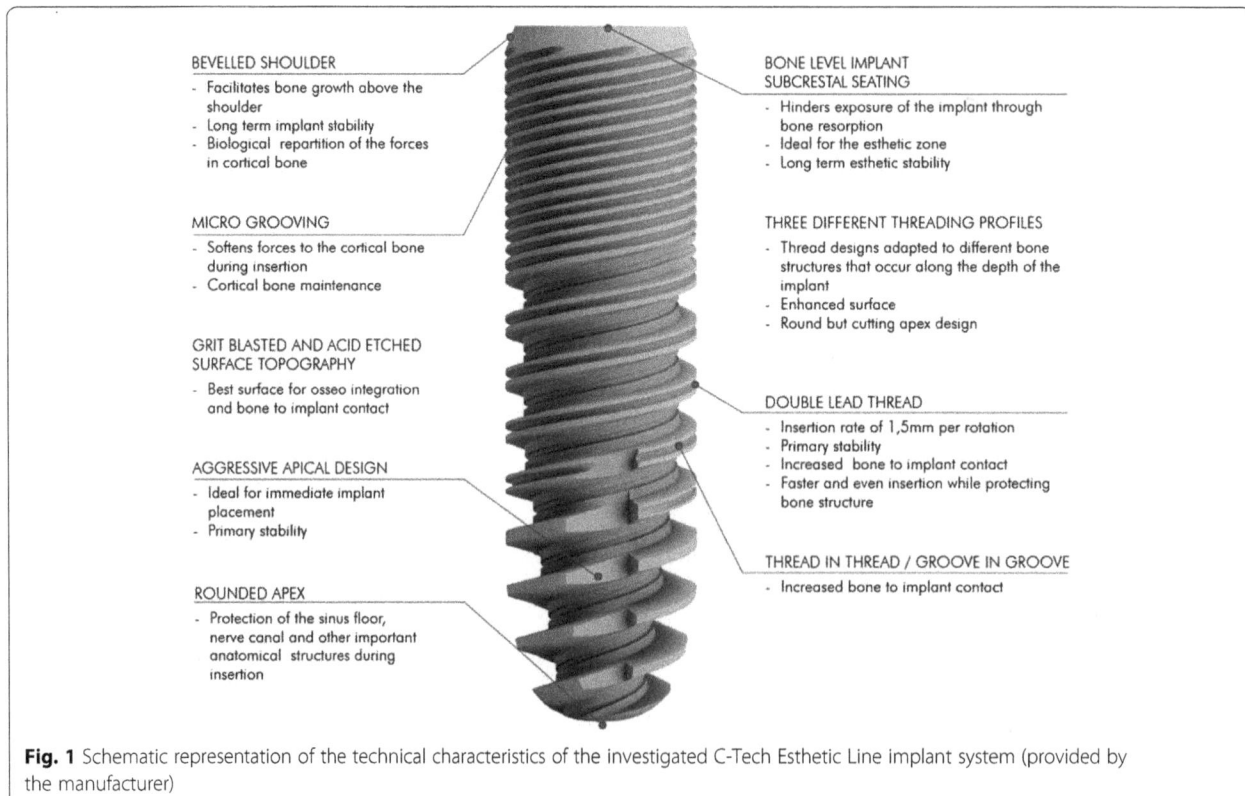

Fig. 1 Schematic representation of the technical characteristics of the investigated C-Tech Esthetic Line implant system (provided by the manufacturer)

0.55 mm (ranging from 0 to 3 mm) without any signs of acute infection or peri-implant osteolysis. Furthermore, the radiological analysis revealed a stable bone level in all implants 3 years after loading.

Table 2 gives an overview of the results of the clinical and radiological 3-year follow-up investigation. Figure 2a–d shows clinical images of the placed implant in patient 4.

Discussion

In the present retrospective study, C-Tech bone level implants placed simultaneously with a GBR procedure around the implant shoulder were investigated clinically and radiologically after at least 3 years of loading to assess peri-implant tissue conditions and document peri-implant tissue stability.

A total of 47 implants were placed in the upper (23 implants) and lower jaw (24 implants) of 20 patients. In all implants, lateral augmentation in a GBR process was performed simultaneously with implant placement due to a reduced horizontal or vertical height of the alveolar crest. The bone substitute materials applied to the horizontal and vertical GBR procedures were of synthetic origin. The clinical and radiological follow-up investigation revealed a survival rate of 100% and only low median rates for probing depths (2.7 mm) and BOP (30%). The mean PES was 10.1 from a maximum value of 14. No osseous peri-implant defects were obvious, and the mean bone loss calculated digitally was 0.55 mm, ranging from 0 to 3 mm.

The tissue reactions to bone substitute materials of different origins have been widely investigated by our research group [16–18]. It could be shown that the origin, the physico-chemical structure, and the processing techniques have an impact on the cellular tissue reaction within the augmentation bed. In a clinical study, the tissue reaction to a synthetic, HA-based and xenogeneic, bovine-based bone substitute material was compared histologically and histomorphometrically in a two-stage sinus augmentation procedure. It was shown that the synthetic bone substitute material induced a significantly higher expression of multinucleated giant cells (MNGCs) within the implantation bed compared to the xenogeneic bone substitute material. However, the induced MNGC-related tissue reaction came with a significantly higher vascularization within the implantation bed. Regarding the new bone formation within the implantation bed, it must be mentioned that the results of new bone formation after an integration period of 6 months did not differ between the synthetic and the xenogeneic bone substitute material [16].

The tissue reaction, however, did not only differ in bone substitute materials of different origin but also in bone substitute materials of the same origin. In an in vivo trial, two xenogeneic bone substitute materials processed with different techniques were implanted subcutaneously in CD-1 mice for up to 60 days. Both bone substitute materials showed good integration within the peri-implant tissue with no signs of adverse inflammatory effects. However, within the implantation bed of the bone substitute of low sintering temperature, few MNGCs were obvious on the surface of small bone substitute granules in the early integration period, while the tissue reaction to the larger granules at later stages consisted mainly of mononuclear cells. In contrast, the tissue reaction to the bone substitute material of high sintering temperature consisted mainly of biomaterial surface-associated MNGCs. Previous in vivo and clinical investigations indicated that MNGCs, which are widely known to be an expression of an ongoing foreign body reaction, are expressed especially on the surface of synthetic biomaterial granules, trying to degrade the biomaterial, but without really reducing the ratio of the biomaterial. In fact, multinucleated giant cells, which do not have the ability of degrading synthetic bone substitute materials, can be characterized more as foreign body giant cells than as osteoclastic cells [17–19].

Previously, our group performed another retrospective study with the same bone level implant system placed immediately after the extraction of teeth not worth preserving [14]. In a collective of 21 patients (11 female, 10 male), 50 dental implants were placed immediately in fresh extraction sockets in the upper (31 implants) and lower jaws (19 implants). The same clinical and radiological parameters were applied to investigate implants 2 years after loading. During the mean observation period of 2 years, none of the implants failed or presented an acute infection or peri-implantitis. All of the implants presented a sufficient amount of peri-implant keratinized soft tissue, low rates of probing depth (mean 2.25 mm), and presence of BOP (34%). The peri-implant bone level was stable, with a mean bone loss 2 years after loading of 0.83 mm [14].

Comparing the present results to the aforementioned study with the same implant system on immediately placed implants, it seems that the GBR augmentation procedure has no influence on the long-term stability of the implants. In both studies with different placement modalities and protocols, comparable clinical and radiological results were achieved. This leads to the assumption that the investigated C-Tech bone level implant system is able to achieve long-term stable function and to render esthetically satisfying results for replacing missing teeth in cases of atrophy of the alveolar crest, as well as in cases of immediate implant placement.

However, the biomaterial-related tissue reaction is still not clarified in detail and more studies need to be performed to investigate the interaction of biomaterials, such as bone substitute materials and dental implants.

Table 2 Results from the clinical and radiological 3-year follow-up investigation

Patient	Implant-localization (region)	Implant loss (+/−)	Buccal width of keratinized peri-implant gingiva (mm)	Buccal thickness of keratinized peri-implant gingiva (mm)	Pink Esthetic Score (PES)	Probing depth (mm) at four sites (mb, db, mo, do)	Bleeding on Probing (+/−) at four sites (mb, db, mo, do)	Peri-implant bone loss (mm)	Presence of peri-implant osteolysis (+/−)
1	32	−	2	2	−	3, 2, 2, 3	−, −, −, −	0	−
	34	−	3	3	−	2, 2, 2, 3	−, −, −, −	0	−
	42	−	3	2	−	3, 2, 3, 2	−, −, −, −	0	−
	44	−	2	3	−	3, 3, 2, 3	−, −, −, −	0	−
2	36	−	2	3	8	3, 3, 3, 4	−, −, −, +	0.5	−
	37	−	2	3	7	2, 3, 2, 3	−, −, −, −	0.5	−
	46	−	3	2	8	3, 3, 2, 3	−, −, −, −	0	−
	47	−	3	2	9	3, 4, 3, 4	−, +, −, +	0	−
3	26	−	4	3	8	2, 3, 3, 3	−, −, −, −	1	−
4	21	−	3	3	8	2, 2, 2, 3	−, −, −, −	0	−
5	23	−	4	2	9	3, 2, 2, 2	−, −, −, −	0	−
	26	−	3	2	9	3, 3, 3, 4	−, −, −, +	0.5	−
	27	−	3	3	8	3, 4, 4, 4	−, +, −, +	1	−
6	32	−	3	2	11	2, 3, 2, 3	−, −, −, −	1	−
	42	−	2	2	11	2, 1, 1, 2	−, −, −, −	0	−
7	36	−	3	2	10	3, 3, 3, 4	−, +, −, −	0.5	−
	46	−	2	3	9	4, 5, 3, 4	+, −, +, −	0.5	−
	36	−	3	3	10	3, 2, 2, 3	−, −, −, −	3	−
8	16	−	3	2	11	2, 2, 2, 3	−, −, −, −	0.5	−
	26	−	3	2	10	3, 2, 2, 2	−, −, −, −	1	−
9	27	−	3	2	9	3, 3, 3, 4	−, −, −, +	1	−
10	15	−	4	3	12	3, 2, 2, 2	−, −, −, −	0	−
	16	−	4	3	11	3, 3, 2, 2	−, −, −, −	0	−
	17	−	3	2	9	3, 3, 4, 3	−, −, +, −	0	−
	24	−	4	4	12	2, 3, 2, 3	−, −, −, −	0	−
	36	−	2	1	10	3, 4, 3, 3	−, +, −, −	0.5	−
	46	−	2	2	9	3, 3, 3, 3	−, −, −, −	1	−
11	35	−	3	2	11	2, 2, 3, 2	−, −, −, −	0.5	−
	36	−	3	2	11	3, 3, 2, 2	−, −, −, −	1	−
12	16	−	4	2	12	3, 2, 2, 2	−, −, −, −	0	−
13	24	−	5	3	12	1, 2, 2, 2	−, −, −, −	0	−
	25	−	5	2	11	2, 2, 1, 1	−, −, −, −	0	−
	26	−	4	2	9	2, 2, 3, 2	−, −,−, −	1	−
	46	−	3	2	8	3, 3, 4, 3	−, −, +, −	2	−
14	36	−	3	2	7	4, 3, 3, 2	+, −, −, −	0.5	−
	37	−	2	2	10	3, 4, 3, 3	−, −, −, −	1	−
15	11	−	4	3	13	2, 2, 3, 2	−, −, −, −	0	−
16	36	−	2	2	11	3, 3, 2, 2	−, −, −, −	0.5	−
	46	−	3	2	10	3, 4, 3, 3	−, +, −, −	1	−
	47	−	2	2	11	3, 3, 2, 3	−, −, −, −	1	−
17	14	−	5	2	12	2, 2, 1, 2	−, −, −, −	0	−
	15	−	4	3	13	2, 2, 2, 3	−, −, −, −	0	−

Table 2 Results from the clinical and radiological 3-year follow-up investigation *(Continued)*

18	27	–	3	2	11	3, 3, 4, 3	–, +, –, +	1	–
	47	–	2	2	9	4, 4, 3, 3	+, –, –, –	2	–
19	22	–	5	3	13	2, 2, 1, 2	–, –, –, –	0	–
	24	–	6	3	12	2, 3, 3, 2	–, –, –, –	1	–
20	26	–	4	2	11	3, 3, 2, 3	–, –, –, –	1	–
Total 20	Total 47; 23*u.j, 24*l.j.	Total 0	Mean 3.2 mm (2–6 mm)	Mean 2.4 mm (1–4 mm)	Mean 10.1 (7–13)	Mean 2.7 mm (1–5 mm)	Total 9.6% of the sites; 30% of the implants	Mean 0.55 mm (0–3 mm)	Total 0

mb mesio-buccal, *db* disto-buccal, *mo* mesio-oral, *do* disto-oral, + present, – absent, *f.p.* fixed prosthetics, *r.p.* removable prosthetics, *u.j.* upper jaw, *l.j.* lower jaw

Fig. 2 Clinical image of patient 4: **a** region 21 before implant placement. **b**, **c** Implant placement using the GBR procedure with a synthetic bone substitute material composed of HA + β-TCP

Conclusions

In the present study, the implant and peri-implant hard- and soft-tissue stability was analyzed in a bone level implant system placed simultaneously with a GBR procedure 3 years after prosthetic loading. Peri-implant hard- and soft-tissue parameters such as width and thickness of peri-implant keratinized gingiva, probing depth, BOP, PES, peri-implant bone loss, and the presence of peri-implant osteolysis were analyzed. The 3-year follow-up investigation revealed a survival rate of 100% and comparably low values for probing depth (2.7 mm) and BOP (30%). Furthermore, analysis of PES showed a favorable esthetic appearance of the implants and prosthetics. The synthetic HA and HA + β-tricalcium phosphate-based bone substitute materials used for the GBR seem to have had no negative influence on the peri-implant health, as all investigated parameters were in accordance with or better than the results presented in the international literature. In conclusion, the investigated bone level implant system seems to be suitable to achieve functionally and esthetically satisfying results in indications that require simultaneous augmentation procedures 3 years after loading.

Abbreviations
β-TCP: β-tricalcium phosphate; BOP: Bleeding on probing; F.P.: Fixed prosthetics; GBR: Guided bone regeneration; HA: Hydroxyapatite; MNGCs: Multinucleated giant cells; PES: Pink Esthetic Score; R.P.: Removable prosthetics

Funding
The authors declare no funds for the research.

Authors' contributions
JL and SG designed the study; HL and JL performed the patient treatment and data collection. SG and RS performed the data analysis. All authors read and approved the final version of the manuscript.

Competing interests
Jonas Lorenz, Henriette Lerner, Robert Sader, and Shahram Ghanaati declare that they have no competing interests.

Author details
[1]Department for Oral, FORM-Lab, Cranio-Maxillofacial, and Facial Plastic Surgery, Medical Center of the Goethe University Frankfurt, Frankfurt am Main, Germany. [2]HL-Dentclinic, Baden-Baden, Germany.

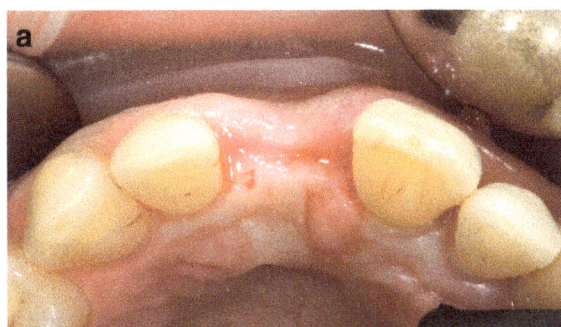

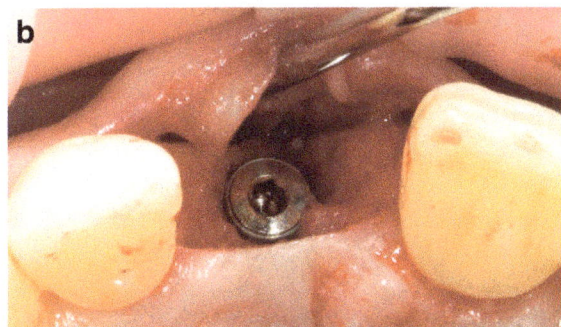

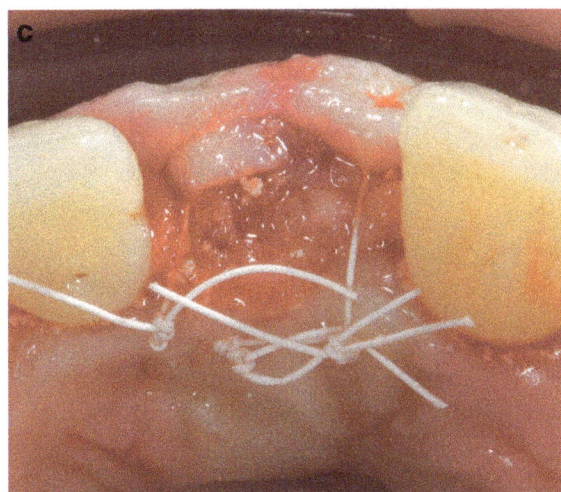

References

1. Gurgel BC, Montenegro SC, Dantas PM, Pascoal AL, Lima KC, Calderon PD. Frequency of peri-implant diseases and associated factors. Clin Oral Implants Res. 2016; doi: 10.1111/clr.12944

2. Qian J, Wennerberg A, Albrektsson T. Reasons for marginal bone loss around oral implants. Clin Implant Dent Relat Res. 2012;14(6):792–807.

3. Berglundh T, Lindhe J, Ericsson I, Marinello C, Liljenberg B, Thomsen P. The soft tissue barrier at implants and teeth. Clin Oral Implants Res. 1991;2:81–90.

4. Berglundh T, Lindhe J, Jonsson K, Ericsson I. The topography of the vascular systems in the periodontal and peri-implant tissues in the dog. J Clin Periodontol. 1999;21:189–93.

5. Moon I, Berglundh T, Abrahamsson I, Linder E, Lindhe J. The barrier between the keratinized mucosa and the dental implant. An experimental study in the dog. J Clin Periodontol. 1999;26:658–63.

6. Lindhe J, Berglundh T. The interface between the mucosa and the implant. Periodontol. 1998;17:47–54.

7. Masaki C, Nakamoto T, Mukaibo T, Kondo Y, Hosokawa R. Strategies for alveolar ridge reconstruction and preservation for implant therapy. J Prosthodont Res. 2015;59(4):220–8.

8. Damien CJ, Parsons JR. Bone graft and bone graft substitutes: a review of current technology and applications. J Appl Biomater. 1991;2:187–208.

9. Cordaro L, Torsello F, Miuccio MT, di Torresanto VM, Eliopoulos D. Mandibular bone harvesting for alveolar reconstruction and implant placement: subjective and objective cross-sectional evaluation of donor and recipient site up to 4 years. Clinical Oral Impl Res. 2011;22:1320–6.

10. Canullo L, Penarrocha-Oltra D, Soldini C, Mazzocco F, Penarrocha M, Covani U. Microbiological assessment of the implant-abutment interface in different connections: cross-sectional study after 5 years of functional loading. Clin Oral Implants Res. 2015;26(4):426–34.

11. Misch C. Implant design considerations for the posterior regions of the mouth. Implant Dent. 1999;8(4).

12. Steigenga J, al-Shammari K, Nociti F, Misch C, Wang H. Dental implant design and its relationship to long-term implant success. Implant Dent. 2001;12(4):306–17.

13. Canullo L, Pace F, Coelho P, Sciubba E, Vozza I. The influence of platform switching on the biomechanical aspects of the implant-abutment system. A three dimensional finite element study. Med Oral Patol Oral Cir Bucal. 2011;16(6):852–6.

14. Lerner H, Lorenz J, Sader R, Ghanaati S. Two-year retrospective study of periimplant health and periimplant bone stability after immediate implant placement of a newly developed bone level implant system—a first report. EDI Journal (European Association of Dental Implantologists, Teamwork Media); 2017; ahead of print.

15. Ghanaati S, Lorenz J, Obreja K, Choukroun J, Landes C, Sader R. Nanocrystalline hydroxyapatite-based material already contributes to implant stability after 3 months: a clinical and radiologic 3-year follow-up investigation. In: Journal of Oral Implantology. 2014;40(1):103–9.

16. Lorenz J, Kubesch A, Korzinskas T, Barbeck M, Landes C, Sader R, et al. TRAP-positive multinucleated giant cells are foreign body giant cells rather than osteoclasts: results from a split-mouth study in humans. J Oral Implantol. 2015;41(6):e257–66.

17. Barbeck M, Udeabor S, Lorenz J, Schlee M, Grosse Holthaus M, Raetscho N, et al. High-temperature sintering of xenogeneic bone substitutes leads to increased multinucleated giant cell formation: in vivo and preliminary clinical results. J Oral Implantol. 2015;41(5):e212–22.

18. Barbeck M, Udeabor S, Lorenz J, Kubesch A, Choukroun J, Sader R, et al. Induction of multinucleated giant cells in response to small sized bovine bone substitute (Bio-Oss TM) results in an enhanced early implantation bed vascularization. Ann Maxillofac Surg. 2014;4(2):150–7.

19. Lorenz J, Barbeck M, Sader R, Russe P, Choukroun J, Kirkpatrick CJ, et al. Foreign body giant cell related encapsulation of a synthetic material three years after augmentation. J Oral Implantol. 2016;42(3):273–7.

23

Histomorphometric and immunohistochemical evaluation of collagen containing xenogeneic bone blocks used for lateral bone augmentation in staged implant placement

Alberto Ortiz-Vigón, Sergio Martinez-Villa, Iñaki Suarez, Fabio Vignoletti and Mariano Sanz[*]

Abstract

Background: The osteoconductive properties of collagen containing xenogeneic bone blocks (CCXBB) remain unclear. The aim of this prospective single-arm clinical study was to assess the histological outcomes of CCXBB blocks used as bone replacement grafts for lateral bone augmentation procedures.

Methods: In 15 patients with severe horizontal alveolar ridge resorption, lateral augmentation procedures were performed using CCXBB as bone replacement grafts. Twenty-six weeks postoperatively, a re-entry procedure was performed to evaluate the bone width for adequate implant placement and two histological specimens were retrieved from each patient, one being processed for ground sectioning and the other for decalcified paraffin-included sections. In non-decalcified sections, the relative proportions occupied by bone, biomaterials, and connective tissue present in the biopsies were identified. In de-calcified sections, structures and cells positive for osteopontin (OPN), tartrate-resistant acid phosphatase activity (TRAP), osteocalcin (OSC), and alkaline phosphatase (ALP) were assessed.

Results: Soft tissue dehiscence occurred during the follow-up in 5 out of 15 patients (33.3%). The mean crest width at baseline was 2.78 mm (SD 0.57) and the mean crest width at re-entry was 6.90 mm (SD 1.22), with a mean ridge width increase of 4.12 mm (SD 1.32). Twenty-six bone biopsies were obtained from 13 patients. Histomorphometric analysis showed a mean of 26.90% (SD 12.21) of mineralized vital bone (MVB), 21.37% (SD 7.36) of residual CCXBB, 47.13% (SD 19.15) of non-mineralized tissue, and 0.92% of DBBM. The immunohistochemical analysis revealed a large number of OPN-positive cells 8.12% (SD 4.73), a lower proportion of TRAP positive multinuclear cells 5.09% (SD 4.91), OSC-positive cells 4.09% (SD 4.34), and a limited amount of ALP positive cells 1.63% (SD 2).

Conclusions: CCXBB achieved significant horizontal crestal width allowing for staged implant placement in most of the patients. In light of the histological outcomes and implant failures, special attention must be placed to prevent soft tissue dehiscence when CCXBB is used in severe atrophic alveolar crests.

Keywords: Clinical trial, Bone regeneration, Alveolar ridge augmentation, Xenogeneic bone substitutes, Heterografts, Histology, Immunohistochemistry, Dental implants

* Correspondence: marsan@ucm.es
ETEP Research Group, Facultad de Odontología, Universidad Complutense de Madrid, Plaza Ramón y Cajal, 28040 Madrid, Spain

Background

Different techniques and grafting materials have been used for the horizontal reconstruction of deficient alveolar processes before implant placement, resulting in different degrees of predictability and clinical outcomes [1]. Among the grafting materials, particulated xenogeneic materials have been extensively studied in both experimental and clinical studies and when combined with porcine-derived natural collagen membranes have resulted in predictable clinical and histological outcomes [2].This combined treatment has shown to be safe and efficacious in horizontal ridge augmentations resulting in regenerated bone with similar implant survival rates when compared to implants placed in pristine bone and demonstrating a low degree of morbidity and a low rate of post-operative complications [3, 4]. However, in clinical situations with severe bone resorption of the alveolar process, which results in non-self-containing bone defects, the use of particulate bone replacement grafts with its inherent weak volumetric stability may limit the predictability of the regenerative therapy [5, 6]. In these cases, dental implants are usually placed staged to the lateral bone augmentation procedure and autogenous bone blocks have been the state of the art procedure, resulting in superior results in mean horizontal bone gains when compared with guided bone regeneration with particulate bone grafts [4, 7, 8]. The use of bone blocks, however, has been associated with increased surgical time, morbidity [9, 10], and a higher frequency of post-operative complications [11, 12]. Moreover, the availability for harvesting intraoral bone blocks is limited [13, 14] and these autologous bone grafts may suffer a high degree of bone resorption during healing [15].

To overcome these limitations, the use of xenogeneic bone grafts as an alternative to autogenous bone blocks has been proposed [16]. Recently, a new equine-derived collagen containing xenogeneic bone block (CCXBB) was evaluated in preclinical studies [17, 18], demonstrating to be safe and adequate for ridge augmentation and better graft integration when compared to other xenogeneic bone blocks. Its performance in humans has been recently tested on 10 patients where these xenogeneic bone blocks were placed in single-tooth alveolar bone defects [19]. Clinically, a mean horizontal gains of 3.88 ± 1.75 mm was reported and the histological outcomes resulted in a homogeneous new bone formation within the CCXBB. These results were concordant with a recent histological study also reporting that equine bone grafts were biocompatible and underwent advanced remodelling at the time of implant placement [20]. Although this preliminary evidence on the performance and histological behaviour of equine bone blocks seems promising, there is still limited information when used in staged horizontal bone augmentation of large osseous defects. It was, therefore, the aim of this prospective study to evaluate the histological outcomes of CCXBB blocks used for lateral bone augmentation in large alveolar horizontal defects of at least two adjacent missing teeth.

Methods

Study design

The present manuscript reports the histological outcomes of a prospective single arm study evaluating the safety and clinical performance of CCXBB blocks when used as replacement bone grafts for lateral bone augmentation prior to staged implant placement. The results of the clinical and radiographic outcomes have been reported in a previous publication [21]. For correlation of the histological with the clinical outcome, respective data of the previous publication have been inserted.

Patient sample

Adults (≥18 years of age) were screened on the bases of having single or multiple teeth absences and a severe horizontal collapse of the alveolar ridge in need of one or more implants for implant supported fixed prosthetic rehabilitation.

Patients were selected on the bases of fulfillment of the following inclusion and exclusion criteria:

- Written informed consent
- Insufficient bone ridge width (<4 mm) for implant placement measured on a cone beam computed tomography (CBCT)
- Sufficient bone height for implant placement
- Healthy oral mucosa and ≥3 mm of attached keratinized mucosa

Patients were excluded if they had any of these conditions:

- General contraindications for dental and/or surgical treatments

Inflammatory and autoimmune disease of the oral cavity

- Allergy to collagen
- Diabetes
- History of myeloma, respiratory tract cancer, breast cancer, prostate cancer or kidney cancer requiring chemotherapy or radiotherapy within the past 5 years

Concurrent or previous radiotherapy of head area

- Concurrent or previous immunosuppressant, bisphosphonate, or high-dose corticosteroid therapy

- Smokers
- Pregnant or lactating women
- Women of child bearing age, who are not using a highly effective method of birth control
- Participation in an investigational device, drug, or biologics study within the last 24 weeks prior to the study start

Before final inclusion, patients received meticulous verbal and written descriptions of the interventions and conditions and were requested to sign an informed consent form (directive 95/46/EC on data protection, in accordance with current legal provisions by the European Community).

Experimental product information

CCXBB (Bio-Graft® Geistlich Pharma) is a bone substitute material in a natural block form. The dimensions of the Bio-Graft block are 10 mm in height, 10 mm in length and 5 mm in width. It consists of a natural cancellous bone structure of hydroxyapatite and endogenous collagen type I and III, equine origin and is a class III medical device according to the Medical Device Directive 93/42 EECs' definition (rule 8 implantable, resorbable device) and 17 (animal origin) in annex lX CE certificate G7 11 04 39446 050 for Geistlich Bio-Graft® was issued in June 2011.

The manufacture of Geistlich Bio-Graft is according to a standardized, controlled process and good manufacturing practices (GMPs). Each batch is manufactured and documented according to standard operating procedures, and the entire process has been validated.

Outcomes variables

The study design and follow-up visits have been summarized in Fig. 1. The primary outcome of this study was to assess the performance of the CCXBB by measuring the final crestal ridge width after 6 months of healing and evaluating its appropriateness for implant placement and the occurrence of adverse effects during healing.

Furthermore, the histological outcomes of this xenogeneic bone replacement graft were evaluated by harvesting a core biopsy of the regenerated area immediately before implant placement (after 6 months of healing), as well as the implant survival of those implants placed in the regenerated bone.

Surgical procedure and clinical measurements

The surgical placement of the CCXBB blocks and the clinical evaluation has been described in detail in a previous publication [21]. In brief, severe alveolar horizontal bone deficiencies were isolated after rising full-thickness mucoperiosteal flaps. Once the horizontal width of the alveolar crest was measured 2 mm below the crest with a bone calliper bone blocks were shaped, pre-drilled and pre-hydrated for 5 min with sterile physiological saline before placement and were fixed with titanium osteosynthesis screws allowing for a stable contact between the block graft and the underlying bone. The spaces between the bone block and the surrounding bone were filled with DBBM particles (Geistlich Bio-Oss®, Geistlich Pharma AG, Wolhusen, Switzerland) and covered with a native collagen membrane (CM) (Geistlich Bio-Gide®, Geistlich Pharma AG, Wolhusen, Switzerland) fixed to the underlying bone with titanium tacks (FRIOS Fixation-Set®, SYMBIOS, Mainz, Germany). The muco-periosteal flaps were then coronally advanced and sutured achieving a tension-free primary closure (Fig. 2).

Bone biopsies harvesting procedure

Twenty-six weeks after the regenerative procedure the patient returned for the re-entry intervention for placement of dental implants. After raising full-thickness flaps, the augmented area was exposed and horizontal crestal width measurements were performed. Then, the surgeon evaluated the bone availability and if implant placement was considered possible, a core bone biopsy was harvested with the use of a trephine, replacing the first drill of the implant bed preparation

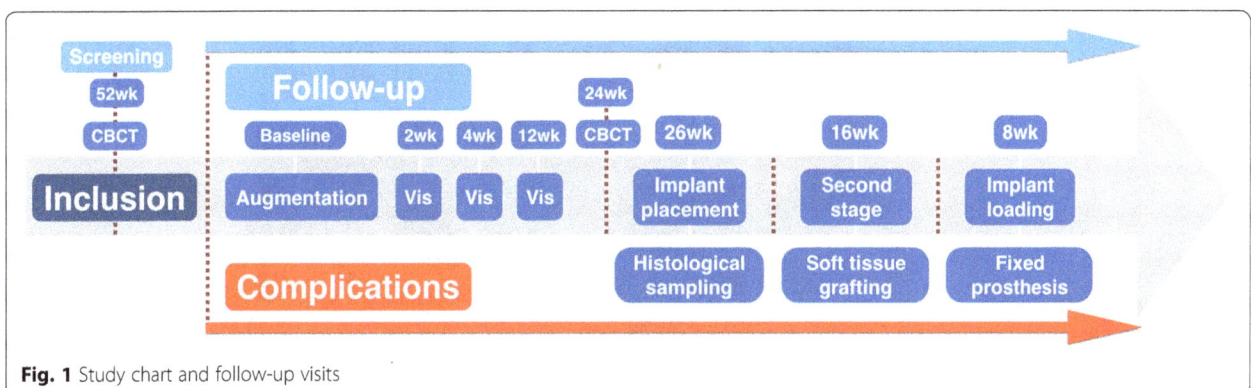

Fig. 1 Study chart and follow-up visits

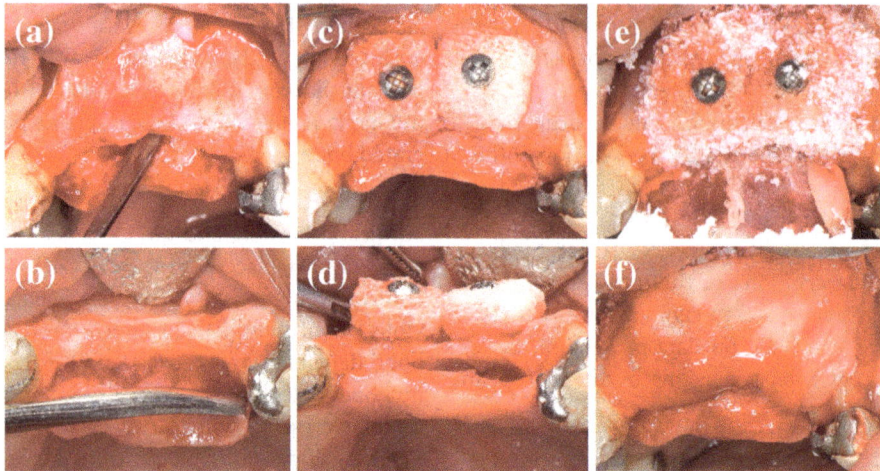

Fig. 2 Lateral bone augmentation of the alveolar crest (**a**) atrophic ridge. **b** Perforations and adaptation of the cortical layer. **c** Shaping, prewetting and fixation of CCXBB with titanium screws. **d** Horizontal contour and peripheral gap between CCXBB and bone layer. **e** Outlying DBBM filling. **f** CM stabilized with pins

(2 mm diameter and 10 mm length, Hager and Meisinger® Neuss, Germany).

The retrieved trephine containing the bone biopsy was irrigated with saline to remove the blood and was introduced in a tube containing 10% formalin solution, which was coded and stored until processing. Commercially available titanium dental implants were inserted in accordance with manufacturer guidelines and after 8 weeks of healing, fixed screwed-retained prosthetic restorations were placed (Fig. 3).

Histological processing

One biopsy per patient was processed for ground sectioning according to the method described by Donath and Breuner (1982). In brief, the specimens including the trephines were fixed in neutral-buffered formalin, stored in

compartment biopsy cassettes, and appropriately coded for identification. Once fixed, the blocks containing the trephines were dissected, dehydrated with ascending alcohol grades and embedded in a light-curing resin (Technovit 7200 VLC; Heraeus-Kulzer, Wehrheim, Germany). At least two longitudinal sections of each core biopsy were grounded and reduced to a thickness of approximately 40 microns using Exakt cutting and grinding equipment (Exakt Apparatebau, Norderstedt, Germany). All the sections were stained using the Levai-Laczkó technique [22].

The second biopsies were processed for decalcification, included in paraffin, stained with hematoxyline-eosine (H-E) and further processed for immune-histochemical analysis. The biopsies were fixed overnight in 4% neutral buffered formalin. Decalcification was achieved by immersing the specimens in 1 mM EDTA solution and

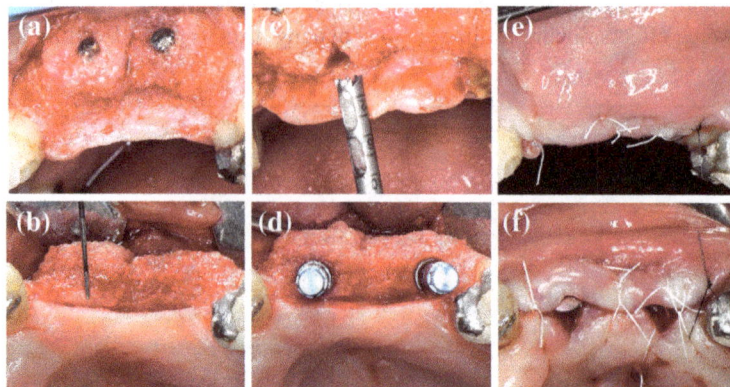

Fig. 3 Re-entry procedure of patient in Fig. 1. **a** Buccal aspect of the augmented region. **b** Horizontal bone augmentation. **c** Screws and pins removal and bone trephine sampling. **d** Implants placement and buccal bone width from the implant shoulder. **e** Primary flap closure. **f** Implants submerged healing

then embedded in paraffin following standard procedures. Semi-thin sections of 4-μm-thick were obtained and stained with hematoxyline-eosine (H-E).

For the immunohistochemical analysis, the semi-thin sections were incubated over night with primary antibodies at 4 °C (Santa Cruz Biotechnology Inc., Santa Cruz, Calif., USA). The antibody dilutions used were alkaline phosphatase (ALP) 1:100, osteopontin (OPN) 1:100, osteocalcin (OSC) 1:100, and tatrate resistant acid phosphatase (TRAP) 1:100.

Histological analysis
Qualitative analysis
The obtained semi-thin sections were evaluated with a motorized (Märzhäuser, Wetzlar-Steindorf, Germany) light microscope connected to a digital camera and a PC-based image-capture system (BX51, DP71, Olympus Corporation, Tokyo, Japan). Photographs were obtained at ×5 and ×20 magnifications (Fig. 4).

Histomorphometric analysis
From the obtained images, areas within the biopsies occupied by bone, biomaterial and connective tissue were identified using a pen computer (Cintiq companion, Wacom, Düsseldorf, Germany), coloured (Photoshop, Adobe, San José, CA, USA) and digitally measured using an automated image-analysis system (CellSens, Olympus Corporation) (Fig. 5).

Immunohistochemical analysis
The obtained histological sections were observed in a light microscope using 5x magnification. In the centre of each trephine biopsy, a rectangular region of interest (ROI) with a size of 30,000,000 to 32,000,000 pixels was defined and standardized photographs were obtained. The intensity of the antibody staining in the images was analysed using the software ImageJ, which by evaluating the antibody staining intensity in the area of interest allows for assessing quantitatively the specific marker (*ImageJ*®, *IHC Profiler plugin*). With this tool, the specimens were categorized into four groups: high positive (HP), positive (P), low positive (LP), and negative (N). To reduce false positives, only the HP and P values were considered for evaluating the percentage of positiveness for each immunohistochemical marker (Fig. 6).

Statistical analysis
Data were entered into an Excel (Microsoft Office 2011) database and proofed for entry errors. The software package (IBM SPSS Statistics 21.0; IBM Corporation, Armonk, NY, USA) was used for the analysis. A subject level analysis was performed for each outcome measurement reporting data as mean values, standard deviations, medians, 95% confidence intervals (CI), and frequencies. Shapiro–Wilk goodness-of-fit tests were used to assess the normality and distribution of data. Descriptive analysis of the histological and immunohistochemical outcomes was carried out by reporting means and standard deviations and comparisons between these histological outcomes between patients with subsequent implant loss versus patients with successful implant outcomes were evaluated using the paired sample t test or U Mann-Whitney if the distributions were non-normalized. Results were considered statistically significant at $p < 0.05$.

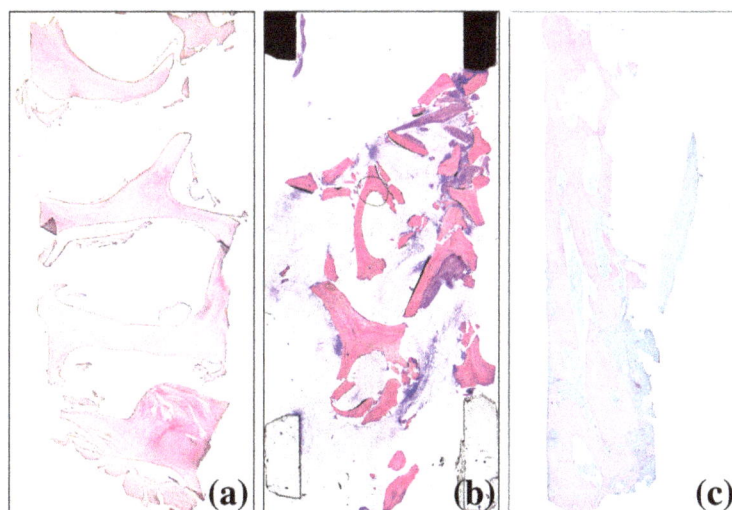

Fig. 4 Histological samples. **a** CCXBB control without implantation. **b** Histologic samples with acute inflammatory infiltration. **c** Histologic sample with limited remaining CCXBB and large bone ingrowth

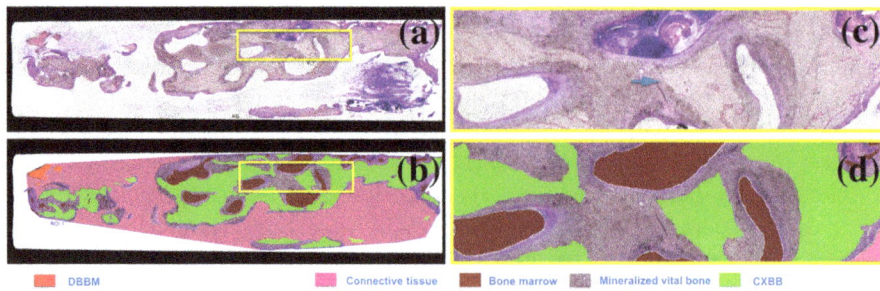

Fig. 5 Histomorphometric analysis of the same sample. **a** Ground section stained with Levai-Laczkó. **b** Tissue identification of the ROI. **c** Closer view **a** *arrow* pointing a cement line between new mineralized bone and CCXBB. **d** Closer view of **b**

Results

Twenty-eight CCXBB blocks were placed in 15 patients that fulfilled the selection criteria (12 women and 3 men) with a mean age of 54.5 (SD 8.34).

Clinical results

The detailed clinical and radiographical outcomes have been reported previously [21]. In brief, one patient experienced pain and soft tissue dehiscence leading to removal of the graft material 3 days after the regenerative procedure. Another patient refused to proceed to implant placement after suffering an early dehiscence also leading to a complete removal of the graft. From the remaining 13 patients completing the study, the alveolar ridge width augmented from a mean 2.78 mm (SD 0.55) at baseline to 6.90 mm (SD 1.22) at re-entry, resulting in a statistical significant mean alveolar crest width gain of 4.12 mm (SD 1.32) Sixteen weeks after implant placement a second stage procedure and a soft tissue augmentation was performed (Fig. 7).

Although soft tissue dehiscence, with different degrees of graft exposure, occurred at different time points in 5 out of 15 patients (33.3%) (Fig. 8), 24 implants were placed in 13 patients. Table 1 depicts the data on survival rates at the time of loading. Three implants were lost in three patients at the time of abutment connection, and one patient presenting very narrow ridge at baseline (<2 mm) lost all the implants. Nevertheless, all implants could be replaced without additional grafting procedure.

Histological observations

Histological biopsies from 13 patients were harvested and processed for histological analysis. The histomorphology of the healed CCXBB bone grafts evidenced in most of the samples newly formed mineralized vital woven bone, as well as residual graft material, bone marrow, and non-mineralized connective tissue (Fig. 5). Residual CCXBB appeared to be integrated with the new bone, which had grown within the graft trabeculae. CCXBB and DBBM were identified only by the presence of empty lacunae and cement lines separating the graft from the parent bone (Fig. 5c). In four of the specimens analyzed, minimal or no signs of new bone formation were appreciated, showing an inflammatory infiltrate with neutrophils and macrophages associated with tissue destruction (Fig. 4b).

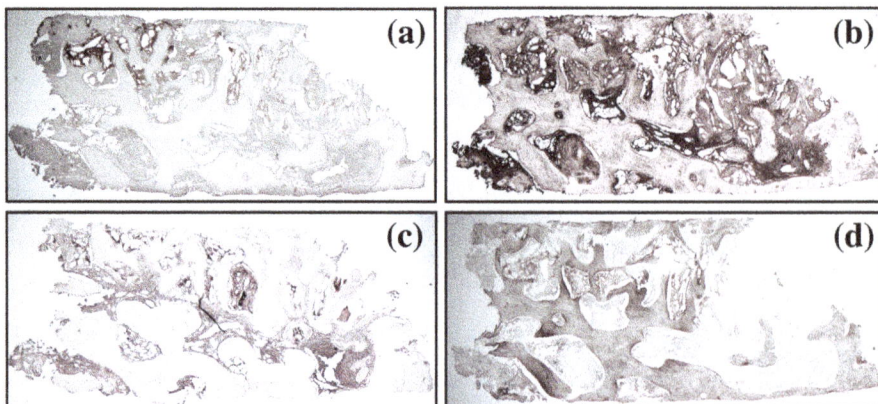

Fig. 6 Immunohistochemical analysis of slices from the same sample with four different markers. **a** TRAP. **b** OPN. **c** ALP. **d** OSC

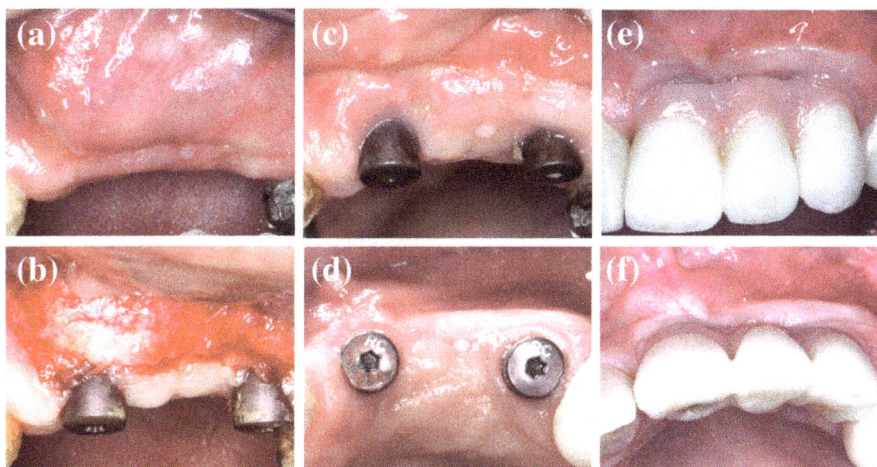

Fig. 7 Second stage surgery of patient in Fig. 1. **a** Vestibular depth reduction after augmentation and implant placement. **b** Partial thickness and apical repositioned flap. **c** CMX healing and soft tissue dehiscence with CCXBB exposure. **d** Dehiscence healing after re-contouring and buccal emergency profile. **e** Buccal aspect of the final restoration. **f** Buccal ridge contour

Histomorphometrical results

The results from the histomorphometric measurements are depicted in Table 2. Bone biopsies were composed by 21.37% (SD 7.36) of residual CCXBB, 26.90% (SD 12.21) of mineralized vital bone (MVB), 47.13% (SD 19.15) of non-mineralized tissue and 0.92% of DBBM (Fig. 5b). Biopsies from patients who lost their implants had a statistical significant lower amount of MVB ($p = 0.01^u$) and a statistical significant larger proportion of connective tissue ($p = 0.02^t$) (Table 4). Furthermore, although no statistically significant correlation was observed between presence of soft tissue dehiscence and specific histomorphological outcomes, a tendency towards a low amount of new bone was observed in the specimens from patients where the bone graft had been exposed ($p = 0.06$).

Immunohistochemical results

Results from the immune-histochemical analysis are presented in Table 3. A large number of OPN-positive cells (mesenchymal, hematopoietic cells and osteoblast) were observed in most of the tissue samples (Fig. 6a). Similarly, TRAP positive multinuclear cells (osteoclasts) were also observed mainly in contact with the residual CCXBB (Fig. 6b). More limited amounts of OSC-positive cells (mature osteoclast) were observed (Fig. 6c) whereas ALP-positive cells (osteoblast) were mainly detected on the surface of the newly formed woven bone and in proximity of vascular units (Fig. 6d). The newly formed bone in close contact with the CCXBB remnants showed signs of modelling and remodelling. When the correlation between the immunohistochemical results and implant loss was investigated, a statistically significant correlation between implant loss and number of OSC positive cells was observed (2 versus 8.78% $p = 0.02^u$) (Table 4).

Discussion

The purpose of this investigation was to evaluate histologically and immunohistochemically the behavior of CCXBB blocks when used for staged lateral bone

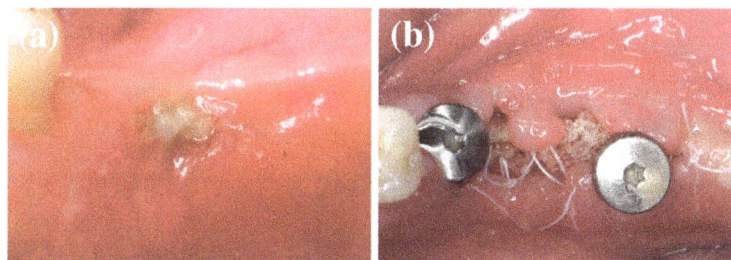

Fig. 8 Soft tissue dehiscence (**a**) CCXBB exposure 15 weeks after bone augmentation, the dehiscence healed 2 weeks later after reducing the graft exposure (**b**) after soft tissue augmentation and abutment connection leading to the loss of the mesial implant. After partial removal of the bone graft and place a connective tissue graft the area healed properly and a month later it was possible to replace the implant

Table 1 Clinical and histomorphometry assessments (i.e., dehiscences, mineralized bone, CCXBB, bone marrow, connective tissue, and implant lost)

Patient	Soft tissue dehiscence	Mineralized bone (%)	CCXBB (%)	Bone marrow (%)	Connective tissue (%)	Implant lost
1	No	22.56	25.26	15,443	36.03	No
2	Yes	0	28.49	0.000	71.50	Yes
3	No	30.39	21.10	14,248	33.24	No
4	No	31.59	21.79	13,982	32.62	No
5	No	41.44	11.90	17,259	25.88	Yes
6	Yes	39.41	5.88	54,461	0	No
7	No	24.31	13.21	32,813	26.84	No
8	Yes	26.19	21.09	52,714	0	No
9	No	23.39	30.18	39,455	6.96	No
10	No	17.73	15.79	26,590	39.88	Yes
11	Yes	12.95	27.09	10,104	48.83	Yes
12	No	37.45	21.37	35,035	3.89	No
13	No	42.31	28.35	29,129	0	No
%	Yes: 30.7 No: 69.2	26.90	20.89	26.24	25.05	Yes: 30.7 No: 69.2
Median		26.19	21.37	26.59	26.84	
SD		12.21	7.35	16.43	22.07	
IR		18.28	13.22	23.13	36.01	
95% CI		19.52;34.28	16.44;25.33	16.31;36.18	11.71;38.39	

Abbreviations: CCXBB Collagen containing xenogenic bovine bone, *SD* Standard deviation, *IR* Interquartile range, *CI* Confidence interval

augmentation in severe human horizontal residual bone defects. Six months after the regenerative intervention using the CCXBB blocks, the mean increase in bone width was 4.12 mm and hence, this outcome allowed for the placement of dental implants in 11 out of 15 patients (73.3%). These results were concordant with the reported weighted mean width increases (3.90 mm (SD 0.38)) from a recent systematic review evaluating intraoral autogenous bone blocks [4]. These results were also similar to those reported with the use of allogeneic bone blocks (4.50 mm (SD 1.3)) [23] or with those from a pilot study using the same CCXBB xenogeneic bone blocks for the staged regeneration of single tooth bone defects (Schwarz, et al. 2016). In this study, in eight patients, the mean crestal width gain was 3.88 mm (SD 1.75) and implant placement was feasible in eight out of ten (80%) patients at re-entry [19].

To the best of our knowledge, the present investigation represents the first study reporting histomorphometric and immunohistochemical outcomes of the use of CCXBB for regenerating atrophic alveolar bone in humans. The healing after 26 weeks was characterized in most of the samples by newly formed mineralized vital bone containing viable osteocytes, as well as bone marrow and non-mineralized connective tissue. This new bone was observed in intimate contact with the residual CCXBB. The percentages of mineralized vital bone, bone marrow, and connective tissue were 26.9, 26.2 and 25.1%, respectively. Similar proportions have been reported with the use of allogeneic blocks [23, 24]. With autogenous bone blocks the relative tissue composition attained was 25.1% of vital bone, 18.1% of connective tissue, and 56.7% of necrotic bone [25]. Similarly, [26] reported 57.75% of non-vital bone when using autogenous bone blocks. In the present investigation CCXBB was present in 21.4% of the samples after 26 weeks of healing, what is in agreement with previous studies

Table 2 Quantitative histological analysis

Tissue type	Mean	Standard deviation	Median	CI 95%
Mineralized bone	2.8×10^6	1.2×10^6	3.1×10^6	$2.0 \times 10^6 – 3.5 \times 10^6$
Connective tissue	2.7×10^6	2.7×10^6	3.1×10^6	$1.0 \times 10^6 – 4.4 \times 10^6$
Bone Marrow	2.8×10^6	2.0×10^6	2.2×10^6	$1.6 \times 10^6 – 4.1 \times 10^6$
CCXBB	2.3×10^6	1.2×10^6	2.4×10^6	$1.6 \times 10^6 – 3.1 \times 10^6$
DBBM	8.9×10^4	1.2×10^5	2.0×10^4	$1.6 \times 10^4 – 1.6 \times 10^5$

Table 3 Immunohistochemical markers proportions (i.e., TRAP, OPN, ALP, and OSC)

Patient	TRAP (%)	OPN (%)	ALP (%)	OSC (%)
1	12.36	4.86	3.73	5.79
2	11.68	14.81	0.44	11.17
3	11.01	13.01	0.16	0.72
4	2.05	8.60	4.49	0.95
5	1.81	15.71	0.34	7.63
6	3.21	11.38	1.67	2.81
7	0.22	2.92	0.515	2.92.
8	0.97	9.63	3.95	4.30
9	0.92	5.42	0.02	0.05
10	12.79	4.58	0.01	13.51
11	4.01	10.07	0.18	2.82
12	1.11	2.77	0.22	0.13
13	4.03	1.83	5.45	0.35
Mean	5.09	8.12	1.63	4.09
SD	4.91	4.73	2	4.34
95% CI	2.12;8.06	5.26;10.98	0.41;2.84	1.46;6.71

Abbreviations: *TRAP* Tartrate-resistant acid phosphatase, *OPN* Osteopontin, *ALP* alkaline phosphatase, *OSC* Osteocalcine

reporting histological outcomes of other xenogeneic bone replacement grafts placed for the regeneration of extraction sockets [27, 28]. In this indication, the percentage of residual graft was 39.8 and 33.4%, respectively.

When correlating the clinical results and the histological outcomes, there was a positive association between the presence of soft tissue dehiscence with CCXBB exposure and a diminished amount of new mineralized bone ($p = 0.06$). This lower amount of new bone within the xenogeneic graft suggests a lack of full graft integration and diminished vascular supply, what may have caused the soft tissues dehiscence. Similarly, the biopsies from patients who lost their implants had a statistical significant lower amount of MVB and a statistical significant larger proportion of connective tissue, what suggests that there is a direct relationship between the primary healing of the bone replacement graft, its integration with native bone and its healing to provide a biological base for dental implants to osseointegrate. These results corroborate the importance of minimal trauma during surgery, establishment of primary implant stability and avoidance of infection and micromotion during healing as key prerequisites for achieving dental implant osseointegration [29, 30]. In fact, the high incidence of early implant loss (29.2%) reported in this clinical study, is clearly higher when compared with epidemiological data from Sweden reporting early implant loss in 4.4% of patients and 1.4% of implants [31]. The delayed bone proliferative phase has also been described associated with other bone replacement grafts for bone regeneration [32] and with demineralized bovine bone mineral (DBBM) in the healing of fresh extraction sockets [33].

A high incidence of soft tissue dehiscence and implant failures has been reported in patients receiving fresh frozen allogeneic bone grafts for reconstructing severe alveolar atrophies (36.8% incidence of dehiscence and 31.5% incidence of implant loss) [34] and 21% of implant loss [35], respectively. With the use of a different equine

Table 4 Implant loss and tissue characteristics

Differentiated tissues	Implant lost (Yes/no)	Mean	SD	Percentage	SD (%)	Significance ($p < 0.05$)
Mineralized bone	No	*3.5×10^6	5.1×10^5	30.84	7.39	$p = 0.01^u$
	Yes	1.3×10^6	1.2×10^6	18.84	17.31	
Connective tissue	No	1.8×10^6	1.9×10^6	*15.51	16.15	$p = 0.01^t$
	Yes	4.6×10^6	3.7×10^6	46.52	19.14	
Bone marrow	No	*3.7×10^6	1.9×10^6	*31.91	15.49	$p = 0.02^t$
	Yes	1.0×10^6	9.2×10^5	13.48	11.24	
CCXBB	No	2.5×10^6	1.2×10^6	20.92	7.46	$p = 0.98^t$
	Yes	2.0×10^6	1.4×10^6	20.82	8.22	
TRAP	No	-	-	3.99	4.53	$p = 0.24^u$
	Yes			7.57	5.47	
OPN	No	-	-	6.71	4.06	$p = 0.11^t$
	Yes			11.29	5.11	
ALP	No	-	-	2.24	2.15	$p = 0.09^u$
	Yes			0.24	0.18	
OSC	No	-	-	*2	2.05	*$p = 0.02^u$
	Yes			8.78	4.65	

Abbreviations: *t* T de student, *u* Mann–Whitney, *Statistically significant

bone block, a previous publication reported total removal of the graft in 50% of the patients and in 20% of them the implants failed [36]. The high incidence of soft tissue dehiscence occurring in this clinical study may also be explained by the extreme narrow crestal defects (mean crestal width of 2.78 mm) multiple teeth absence and non-containing defects, what needed in most of the cases to use more than one block graft. In fact, there was a positive correlation between the number of blocks used and the incidence of soft tissue dehiscences. The use of large grafts or more than one graft may have hindered an appropriate blood supply or colonization of the graft material with bone-forming cells [37].

The immune-histochemical results reported expression of osteopontin mainly at the border between mineralized vital bone (MVB) with CCXBB, what coincides with findings from previous reports [38–40]. Alkaline phosphatase (ALP) is considered as an early osteoblast differentiation marker [41]. ALP-positive cells were detectable, in all specimens on the periphery of MVB, associated to areas of new bone formation. These observations were also reported on a clinical study on guided bone regeneration (GBR) [41], as well as through the evaluation of the healing of particulate xenogeneic bone grafts (DBBM) [28]. Experimental research using immune-histochemical analysis for comparing early bone remodelling between autografts and allografts has reported comparable behavior for osteoprotegerin (OPG), alkaline phosphatase (ALP), collagen 1 (COLI), osteopontin (OPN), and osteocalcin (OSC), although an increased activity of tartrate-resistant acid phosphatase (TRAP) was seen in allogenic bone grafts [42]. In this investigation TRAP, which is a specific enzyme present in large quantities at the osteoclasts edge expressing bone resorption, was present in high proportions in all the analysed samples. On the other hand, OSC (bone matrix protein), predominantly synthesized by osteoblasts, has a fundamental role in bone formation (mineralization) and resorption [43]. Experimental studies have demonstrated the role of OSC during the early healing phases of osseointegration of dental implants [44]. In the present investigation, a statistical significant correlation between higher levels of OSC and implant loss was found. This association could be explained by a greater activity of bone modelling in these situations of deficient mineralization [45].

This prospective single-arm study has clear limitations to evaluate the efficacy of this bone regenerative intervention, since there is not a control group [46]. However, this investigation has shown excellent clinical performance and histological outcomes when CCXBB were used for lateral bone augmentation and when their integration occurred without soft tissue dehiscence.

Conclusions

Within the limitations of this clinical study, we may conclude that the use of CCXBB in combination with DBBM particles and a native bilayer collagen membrane for staged lateral bone augmentation in severe atrophic alveolar crests achieved significant horizontal crestal width allowing for staged implant placement in most of the patients. Histological analysis and implant survival records indicate that special attention must be paid to prevent soft tissue dehiscence.

Abbreviations
ALP: Alkaline phosphatase; CBCT: Cone beam computed tomography; CCXBB: Collagen containing xenogeneic bone block; CM: Native collagen membrane; DBBM: Deproteinized bovine bone mineral; ETEP: Etiology and Therapy of Periodontal Diseases; OPN: Osteopontin; OSC: Osteocalcine; TRAP: Tartrate-resistant acid phosphatase

Acknowledgements
We wish to acknowledge the dedication and scientific advise of Prof. Dr. Tord Berglundh on the histological analysis as well as the diligent work in processing the histological samples to Estela Maldonado for the immunohistochemistry and Asal Shikhan and Fernando Muñoz for the histomorphometry. The work of Esperanza Gross on the statistical analysis is highly acknowledged.

Funding
This study was partially supported through a research contract between Geistlich Pharma AG and the University Complutense of Madrid.

Authors' contributions
This study has involved the direct participation of the following investigators whom we propose as authors in this manuscript. AOV contributed to the protocol design, surgical procedures, histological analysis, critical data analysis, and writing of the manuscript. SMV contributed to the immunohistochemical analysis. IS contributed to the patient's follow-up and data collection. FV contributed to the protocol design and manuscript edition. MS contributed to the protocol design, manuscript writing, and editing. All authors read and approved the final manuscript.

Competing interests
Alberto Ortiz-Vigón, Sergio Martinez-Villa, Iñaki Suarez, Fabio Vignoletti, and Mariano Sanz, declare that they have no competing interests.

Ethics approval and consent to participate
The study was conducted, recorded and reported in accordance with the Helsinki Declaration of 1975, as revised in 2000 and 2008 and prior to the commencement, the ethics committee of the Clinical San Carlos Hospital, Madrid, Spain, approved the protocol and informed consent forms under the registration number 13/404-P. This study was conducted in the ETEP (Etiology and Therapy of Periodontal Diseases) Research Group at the University Complutense of Madrid (Spain) from 11 of December 2013 to 12 of September 2016. All the investigators were trained on ISO-GCP standard before study start and on all study procedures during the site initiation visit by the sponsor. A clinical monitor of the sponsor in accordance with ISO 14155:2011 monitored this study. This study was performed in accordance with national regulations on ordinary care trials with CE marked medical devices within their intended use as well as with national regulations on data protection: Circular No. 07/2004, Decree 414/1996, DPA 15/1999, Royal Decree 1720/2007.

References

1. Sanz M, Vignoletti F. Key aspects on the use of bone substitutes for bone regeneration of edentulous ridges. Dent Mater. 2015;31:640–7.
2. Benic GI, Hammerle CH. Horizontal bone augmentation by means of guided bone regeneration. Periodontology. 2014;66:13–40.
3. Beretta M, Cicciu M, Poli PP, Rancitelli D, Bassi G, Grossi GB, et al. A Retrospective Evaluation of 192 Implants Placed in Augmented Bone: Long-Term Follow-Up Study. J Oral Implantol. 2015;41:669–74.
4. Sanz-Sanchez I, Ortiz-Vigon A, Sanz-Martin I, Figuero E, Sanz M. Effectiveness of Lateral Bone Augmentation on the Alveolar Crest Dimension: A Systematic Review and Meta-analysis. J Dent Res. 2015;94:128S–42S.
5. Berglundh T, Lindhe J. Healing around implants placed in bone defects treated with Bio-Oss. An experimental study in the dog. Clin Oral Implants Res. 1997;8:117–24.
6. Mir-Mari J, Wui H, Jung RE, Hammerle CH, Benic GI. Influence of blinded wound closure on the volume stability of different GBR materials: an in vitro cone-beam computed tomographic examination. Clin Oral Implants Res. 2016;27:258–65.
7. Jensen SS, Terheyden H. Bone augmentation procedures in localized defects in the alveolar ridge: clinical results with different bone grafts and bone-substitute materials. Int J Oral Maxillofac Implants. 2009;24(Suppl):218–36.
8. Troeltzsch M, Troeltzsch M, Kauffmann P, Gruber R, Brockmeyer P, Moser N, et al. Clinical efficacy of grafting materials in alveolar ridge augmentation: A systematic review. J Craniomaxillofac Surg. 2016;44:1618–29.
9. von Arx T, Hafliger J, Chappuis V. Neurosensory disturbances following bone harvesting in the symphysis: a prospective clinical study. Clin Oral Implants Res. 2005;16:432–9.
10. Nkenke E, Neukam FW. Autogenous bone harvesting and grafting in advanced jaw resorption: morbidity, resorption and implant survival. Eur J Oral Implantol. 2014;7 Suppl 2:S203–17.
11. Cordaro L, Torsello F, Morcavallo S, di Torresanto VM. Effect of bovine bone and collagen membranes on healing of mandibular bone blocks: a prospective randomized controlled study. Clin Oral Implants Res. 2011;22:1145–50.
12. Aloy-Prosper A, Penarrocha-Oltra D, Penarrocha-Diago M, Penarrocha-Diago M. The outcome of intraoral onlay block bone grafts on alveolar ridge augmentations: a systematic review. Med Oral Patol Oral Cir Bucal. 2015;20:e251–8.
13. Cremonini CC, Dumas M, Pannuti C, Lima LA, Cavalcanti MG. Assessment of the availability of bone volume for grafting in the donor retromolar region using computed tomography: a pilot study. Int J Oral Maxillofac Implants. 2010;25:374–8.
14. Nkenke E, Weisbach V, Winckler E, Kessler P, Schultze-Mosgau S, Wiltfang J, et al. Morbidity of harvesting of bone grafts from the iliac crest for preprosthetic augmentation procedures: a prospective study. Int J Oral Maxillofac Implants. 2004;33:157–63.
15. Cordaro L, Amade DS, Cordaro M. Clinical results of alveolar ridge augmentation with mandibular block bone grafts in partially edentulous patients prior to implant placement. Clin Oral Implants Res. 2002;13:103–11.
16. Araujo MG, Sonohara M, Hayacibara R, Cardaropoli G, Lindhe J. Lateral ridge augmentation by the use of grafts comprised of autologous bone or a biomaterial. An experiment in the dog. J Clin Periodontol. 2002;29:1122–31.
17. Schwarz F, Ferrari D, Balic E, Buser D, Becker J, Sager M. Lateral ridge augmentation using equine- and bovine-derived cancellous bone blocks: a feasibility study in dogs. Clin Oral Implants Res. 2010;21:904–12.
18. Benic GI, Thoma DS, Munoz F, Sanz Martin I, Jung RE, Hammerle CH. Guided bone regeneration of peri-implant defects with particulated and block xenogenic bone substitutes. Clin Oral Implants Res. 2016;27:567–76.
19. Schwarz F, Mihatovic I, Ghanaati S, Becker J. Performance and safety of collagenated xenogeneic bone block for lateral alveolar ridge augmentation and staged implant placement. A monocenter, prospective single-arm clinical study. Clin. Oral Impl. Res. 2016;1-7.
20. Di Stefano DA, Gastaldi G, Vinci R, Cinci L, Pieri L, Gherlone E. Histomorphometric Comparison of Enzyme-Deantigenic Equine Bone and Anorganic Bovine Bone in Sinus Augmentation: A Randomized Clinical Trial with 3-Year Follow-Up. Int J Oral Maxillofac Implants. 2015;30:1161–7.
21. Ortiz-Vigón A, Suarez I, Martinez-Villa S, Sanz-Martín I, Sanz M. Safety and performance of a novel collagenated xenogeneic bone block for lateral alveolar crest augmentation for staged implant placement. Clin Oral Implants Res. 2017.
22. Jeno L, Geza L. A simple differential staining method for semi-thin sections of ossifying cartilage and bone tissues embedded in epoxy resin. Mikroskopie. 1975;31:1–4.
23. Dias RR, Sehn FP, de Santana Santos T, Silva ER, Chaushu G, Xavier SP. Corticocancellous fresh-frozen allograft bone blocks for augmenting atrophied posterior mandibles in humans. Clin Oral Implants Res. 2016;27:39–46.
24. Nissan J, Marilena V, Gross O, Mardinger O, Chaushu G. Histomorphometric analysis following augmentation of the posterior mandible using cancellous bone-block allograft. J Biomed Mater Res A. 2011;97:509–13.
25. Spin-Neto R, Stavropoulos A, Coletti FL, Pereira LA, Marcantonio Jr E, Wenzel A. Remodeling of cortical and corticocancellous fresh-frozen allogeneic block bone grafts–a radiographic and histomorphometric comparison to autologous bone grafts. Clin Oral Implants Res. 2015;26:747–52.
26. Acocella A, Bertolai R, Colafranceschi M, Sacco R. Clinical, histological and histomorphometric evaluation of the healing of mandibular ramus bone block grafts for alveolar ridge augmentation before implant placement. J Craniomaxillofac Surg. 2010;38:222–30.
27. Carmagnola D, Adriaens P, Berglundh T. Healing of human extraction sockets filled with Bio-Oss. Clin Oral Implants Res. 2003;14:137–43.
28. Milani S, Dal Pozzo L, Rasperini G, Sforza C, Dellavia C. Deproteinized bovine bone remodeling pattern in alveolar socket: a clinical immunohistological evaluation. Clin Oral Implants Res. 2016;27:295–302.
29. Berglundh T, Abrahamsson I, Lang NP, Lindhe J. De novo alveolar bone formation adjacent to endosseous implants. Clin Oral Implants Res. 2003;14:251–62.
30. Terheyden H, Lang NP, Bierbaum S, Stadlinger B. Osseointegration–communication of cells. Clin Oral Implants Res. 2012;23:1127–35.
31. Derks J, Hakansson J, Wennstrom JL, Tomasi C, Larsson M, Berglundh T. Effectiveness of implant therapy analyzed in a Swedish population: early and late implant loss. J Dent Res. 2015;94:44S–51S.
32. Spin-Neto R, Stavropoulos A, Coletti FL, Faeda RS, Pereira LA, Marcantonio Jr E. Graft incorporation and implant osseointegration following the use of autologous and fresh-frozen allogeneic block bone grafts for lateral ridge augmentation. Clin Oral Implants Res. 2014;25:226–33.
33. Araujo MG, Linder E, Lindhe J. Bio-Oss collagen in the buccal gap at immediate implants: a 6-month study in the dog. Clin Oral Implants Res. 2011;22:1–8.
34. Chiapasco M, Colletti G, Coggiola A, Di Martino G, Anello T, Romeo E. Clinical outcome of the use of fresh frozen allogeneic bone grafts for the reconstruction of severely resorbed alveolar ridges: preliminary results of a prospective study. Int J Oral Maxillofac Implants. 2015;30:450–60.
35. Deluiz D, Santos Oliveira L, Ramoa Pires F, Reiner T, Armada L, Nunes MA, et al. Incorporation and Remodeling of Bone Block Allografts in the Maxillary Reconstruction: A Randomized Clinical Trial. Clin Implant Dent Relat Res. 2017;19:180–94.
36. Pistilli R, Felice P, Piatelli M, Nisii A, Barausse C, Esposito M. Blocks of autogenous bone versus xenografts for the rehabilitation of atrophic jaws with dental implants: preliminary data from a pilot randomised controlled trial. Eur J Oral Implantol. 2014;7:153–71.
37. Gruber R, Stadlinger B, Terheyden H. Cell-to-cell communication in guided bone regeneration: molecular and cellular mechanisms. Clin Oral Implants Res. 2016.
38. Araujo MG, Liljenberg B, Lindhe J. Dynamics of Bio-Oss Collagen incorporation in fresh extraction wounds: an experimental study in the dog. Clin Oral Implants Res. 2010;21:55–64.
39. Lindhe J, Araujo MG, Bufler M, Liljenberg B. Biphasic alloplastic graft used to preserve the dimension of the edentulous ridge: an experimental study in the dog. Clin Oral Implants Res. 2013;24:1158–63.
40. Galindo-Moreno P, Hernandez-Cortes P, Aneiros-Fernandez J, Camara M, Mesa F, Wallace S, et al. Morphological evidences of Bio-Oss(R) colonization by CD44-positive cells. Clin Oral Implants Res. 2014;25:366–71.
41. Stucki U, Schmid J, Hammerle CF, Lang NP. Temporal and local appearance of alkaline phosphatase activity in early stages of guided bone regeneration. A descriptive histochemical study in humans. Clin Oral Implants Res. 2001; 12:121–7.
42. Hawthorne AC, Xavier SP, Okamoto R, Salvador SL, Antunes AA, Salata LA. Immunohistochemical, tomographic, and histological study on onlay bone graft remodeling. Part III: allografts. Clin Oral Implants Res. 2013;24:1164–72.
43. Patti A, Gennari L, Merlotti D, Dotta F, Nuti R. Endocrine actions of osteocalcin. Int J Endocrinol. 2013;2013:846480.
44. Schwarz F, Herten M, Sager M, Wieland M, Dard M, Becker J. Histological and immunohistochemical analysis of initial and early osseous integration at chemically modified and conventional SLA titanium implants: preliminary results of a pilot study in dogs. Clin Oral Implants Res. 2007;18:481–8.

24

A novel non-surgical method for mild peri-implantitis

J. C. Wohlfahrt[1*], B. J. Evensen[2], B. Zeza[3], H. Jansson[4], A. Pilloni[3], A. M. Roos-Jansåker[5,8], G. L. Di Tanna[6], A. M. Aass[1], M. Klepp[7] and O. C. Koldsland[1]

Abstract

Aim: The aim of the present study was to evaluate the effect on peri-implant mucosal inflammation from the use of a novel instrument made of chitosan in the non-surgical treatment of mild peri-implantitis across several clinical centers.

Materials and methods: In this 6-month multicenter prospective consecutive case series performed in six different periodontal specialist clinics, 63 implants in 63 patients were finally included. The subjects had mild peri-implantitis defined as radiographic bone loss of 1–2 mm, pocket probing depth (PPD) ≥4 mm and a positive bleeding on probing (mBoP) score. The patients were clinically examined at baseline and after 2, 4, 12 and 24 weeks, and radiographs were taken at baseline and at 3 and 6 months. Treatment of the implants with the chitosan brush seated in an oscillating dental drill piece was performed at baseline and at 3 months. Reductions in the clinical parameters (PPD and mBoP) were compared between baseline and the later examination time points.

Results: Significant reductions in both PPD and mBoP were observed at all time points compared with the baseline clinical measurements ($p < 0.001$). The mean PPD and mBoP at baseline were 5.15 mm (4.97; 5.32) and 1.86 (1.78; 1.93), respectively, whereas the mean PPD and mBoP at 6 months were 4.0 mm (3.91; 4.19) and 0.64 (0.54; 0.75), respectively. Stable reductions in PPD and mBoP were evident up to 6 months after the initial treatment and 3 months after the second treatment. All 63 implants were reported to have stable radiographic levels of osseous support.

Conclusions: This case series demonstrated that an oscillating chitosan brush is safe to use and seems to have merits in the non-surgical treatment of dental implants with mild peri-implantitis. To measure the effectiveness of the method, a multicenter randomized clinical trial needs to be undertaken.

Keywords: Clinical study, Chitosan, Peri-implantitis, Dental implants, Non-surgical treatment

Background

Inflammation and loss of attachment around dental implants (i.e. peri-implantitis) has become a growing concern within the field of dental implantology [1–7]. Peri-implantitis is a microbial infection-driven soft tissue inflammation with loss of bony attachment around an implant. Peri-implant mucositis is the precursor of peri-implantitis, as gingivitis is for periodontitis [8]. It is clearly shown that daily infection control performed by the patient and regular professional maintenance of dental implants is important to prevent the progression of mucositis to peri-implantitis [9–12]. In advanced cases, peri-implantitis may lead to implant loss.

The current view is that most cases of peri-implantitis are unmanageable without surgical intervention. However, the stage of disease progression at which surgery is necessary remains undefined, and limited scientific evidence is available regarding surgical methods that hinder the progression of the disease over time. Because peri-implantitis surgery often involves a high level of patient morbidity, the development of non-surgical and less-invasive treatment methods is of interest for both patients and the dental community. Currently used methods for non-surgical implant debridement include

* Correspondence: johancw@odont.uio.no
[1]Department of Periodontology, Institute of Clinical Dentistry, University of Oslo, Pb. 1109 Blindern, 0317 Oslo, Norway
Full list of author information is available at the end of the article

titanium curettes, plastic or carbon fibre curettes, ultrasound, air-polishing and lasers. No particular non-surgical treatment for peri-implantitis resulting in superior outcomes is however supported by sufficient scientific evidence [13, 14]. Furthermore, some procedures have been suggested to cause more problems rather than improving peri-implant health [15]. The crux is to intervene and to treat the inflammation without causing further problems that may contribute to the progression of peri-implant attachment loss. For example, leaving remnants of an instrument could cause a foreign body reaction, which may accelerate disease progression and attachment loss [16]. Similarly, using an ultrasonic steel tip may induce damage to the titanium surface whereas a nylon tip may result in melted material remnants on the implant surface [17]. In a recent study by Eger et al. [15], it was reported that debridement of titanium surfaces with an ultrasonic device may release titanium particles that was shown to induce a pronounced inflammatory response which caused osteoclastogenesis. The use of ultrasonic devices on titanium surfaces may thus aggravate peri-implantitis rather than resolve the situation.

A number of other studies also report that leaving fragments of the instrument on the implant surface or scratching the surface may impede optimal peri-implant healing [17–20].

Chitosan is a marine biopolymer which is based on chitin derived from the shells of marine crustaceans. The material has been approved for use in surgical bandages, as a haemostatic agent and as a dietary supplement in a wide range of nutritional and health products. Chitosan has also been documented to be non-allergenic and may exhibit anti-inflammatory properties. The material is demonstrated to be completely biocompatible which also recently was verified in an animal experimental study [21]. In a pilot randomized split mouth clinical trial including 11 patients with mucositis, it was demonstrated that debridement with a chitosan device or titanium curettes lead to significant reduction in peri-implant mucositis. A better reduction in parameters of inflammation was however seen at 4 weeks at the implants treated with the chitosan device as compared with titanium curettes (Wohlfahrt et al. submitted for publication).

In the present study, the aim was to evaluate the effect on implant mucosal inflammation from the use of a novel instrument made of chitosan in the non-surgical treatment of mild peri-implantitis across several clinical centers.

Case presentation
Materials and methods
A 6-month multicenter prospective consecutive case series was performed in six different periodontal specialist clinics in Norway, Sweden and Italy.

Ethical approval was provided by the regional ethical review boards of each center (Norway: 2014/852/REK sør-øst; Italy: Sapienza 2011/15, 3547; and Sweden: EPN Lund 2014/695.) Fifteen patients at each center were planned to be included in the study. Patient screening, inclusions and all clinical examinations were performed by board-certified specialists in periodontology. Subjects were included in the study if they had at least one implant that had been in function for more than 12 months and had been diagnosed with mild peri-implantitis defined as 1–2-mm bone loss, pocket probing depth (PPD) ≥ 4 mm and a positive bleeding on probing score. Patients diagnosed with periodontitis were required to be finished with active periodontal treatment prior to inclusion in the study. All six surfaces of the included implants were free of supragingival visible plaque. Patients were required to have a total plaque score (dichotomous scoring) below 20% prior to inclusion, and baseline measurements were performed after careful oral hygiene instruction on an individual, as-needed basis. Radiographs were taken at baseline and at the 6 months evaluation. Endodontic lesions and dental decay should have been treated prior to inclusion. Clinical examinations were performed at baseline and at 2, 4, 12 and 24 weeks after baseline using a 0.20-N (20-g)-defined force periodontal probe (University of North Carolina, DB764R, AESCULAP, B Braun Germany). PPD and mBoP was recorded at six sites per implant. Bleeding on probing (mBoP) was recorded using a 3-graded index 30 s after probing as follows: A score of 0 represented no bleeding, 1 represented isolated minimal bleeding spots, 2 represented blood forming a confluent red line on the margin and 3 represented heavy or profuse bleeding [22]. The clinical protocol also included scoring of the height of the gingival margin relative to the crown margin.

All patient-related information and clinical recordings were recorded in a web-based clinical research form (VieDoc version 3.24, PCG solutions, Uppsala, Sweden).

Patients under 18 years of age; current smokers; patients who had undergone radiotherapy in the head and neck region, chemotherapy or systemic long-term corticosteroid treatment; patients who were pregnant or nursing; patients receiving medications known to induce gingival hyperplasia; patients with uncontrolled diabetes (HbA1c >6.5); patients who had taken systemic antibiotics less than 6 months prior to baseline; patients receiving bisphosphonate treatment; and patients with prosthetic factors that prevented clinical measurements were excluded from participation in the study. Implants with technical complications, such as loose supraconstructions, cement remnants, ill-fitted crowns with poor marginal contour or any type of prosthetic complication that according to the examiner, would be a local contributing factor to inflammation, were also excluded.

Implants that were previously treated surgically for peri-implantitis and implants with overcontoured supraconstructions obstructing access for debridement and clinical measurements of more than three surfaces were also excluded. Before agreeing to participate in this study, all patients were provided with sufficient information via a patient information sheet and a consent form, which was signed prior to final inclusion.

After clinical recordings, the implant pockets were debrided with a chitosan brush (LBC, BioClean®, LABRIDA AS, Oslo, Norway) seated in an oscillating dental drill piece (ER10M, TEQ-Y, NSK Inc., Kanuma Tochigi, Japan) for 3 min and then irrigated with sterile saline (Fig. 1). The initial debridement was performed with local anaesthesia as needed. A second debridement with the chitosan brush was performed after 3 months.

Statistical analysis

The power calculation was based on data from a pilot clinical study evaluating the same test device performed at the Department of Periodontology, University of Oslo, in 2014. Descriptive statistics were presented for continuous variables (median and interquartile range), and proportions were presented for categorical variables.

Mann-Whitney rank sum tests were used to compare changes in the clinical parameters between baseline and subsequent time points. To assess the hierarchical structure of the data (center > patient > site), a linear mixed model using the restricted maximum likelihood method (multilevel logistic models for binary outcomes) was constructed to analyse the PPD, mBoP and suppuration, adjusting for factors such as age, gender and past smoke exposure.

All statistical analyses were performed using Sigma Plot v 13.0 (Systat Software, Inc., San Jose, CA) and Stata 14 (StataCorp, College Station, TX, USA) statistical software.

Results

In total, 63 implants in 63 patients were ultimately included in the analysis. Demographic information is presented in Tables 1 and 2.

Significant reductions in both PPD and mBoP were seen at all time points relative to the baseline clinical measurements ($p < 0.001$) in both the unadjusted and adjusted models including age, gender and past smoking experience (Figs. 2 and 3). Stable reductions in PPD and mBoP were observed after 2 weeks and up to 6 months after the initial treatment. The hypothesis of no difference in PPD values between week 2 and week 4 ($p = 0.1429$) could not be rejected, but from week 4 until 3 and 6 months, statistically significant reductions with p values of 0.007 and 0.0295, respectively, were detected. A relevant cluster effect at the center level was identified with variation around the center intercepts of 0.267 and 0.117 and remaining variances of 0.432 and 0.46 for PPD and mBoP, respectively.

The mean PPD and mBoP at baseline were 5.15 mm (4.97; 5.32) and 1.86 (1.78; 1.93), respectively, whereas the

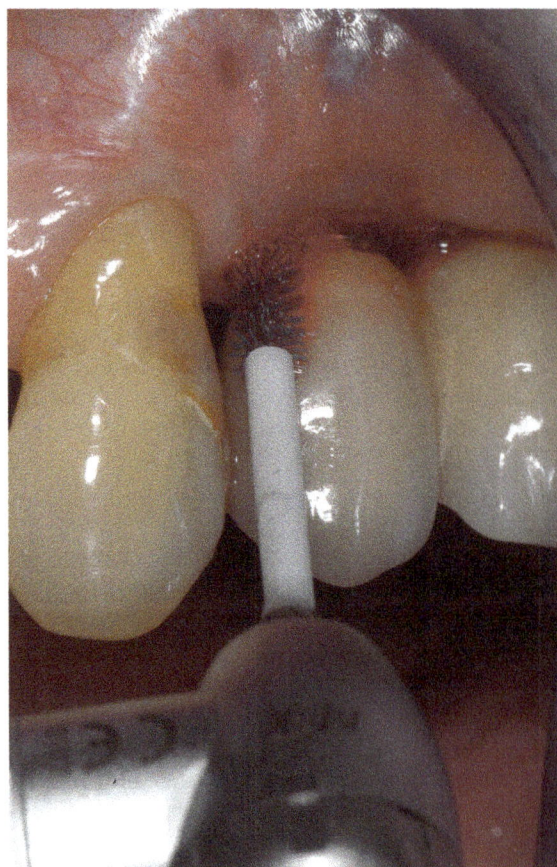

Fig. 1 A chitosan brush (LBC, BioClean®, LABRIDA AS) seated in an oscillating dental handpiece

Table 1 Demographics

Variable	Number (%)	SD	Range (min; max)
Gender (female/male)	45/18 (71.4/28.6)		
Age	58.4	14.4	23; 85
Former smokers	39 (62.1)		
Implant age	8.9	6.9	1.5; 30
Implant brand			
ASTRA	12 (19.0)		
NOBEL	27 (42.9)		
Straumann	7 (11.1)		
Sweden and Martina	2 (3.2)		
TMI	2 (3.2)		
Implandent	1 (1.6)		
Friadent	1 (1.6)		
Unknown	11 (17.5)		

Table 2 Demographics by center

Center	Oslo	Jonkoping	Rome	Stavanger	Kristianstad	Tonsberg	Total
Number of patients	12	11	12	3	11	14	63
Gender (f)	9	5	11	2	6	12	45
Age	60(26–85)	60(23–73)	55(29–77)	49(41–55)	61(36–73)	57(26–82)	63(26–85)
Implant age	12(2.3–30)	6.2(1.5–21.3)	10(2–21)	11(7.9–17)	8(1.5–23)	5.5(2.3–10.3)	8.7(1.5–30)
Tooth loss							
Agenesis	2	1	1	1	1	0	6
Caries	2	3	3	0	0	1	9
Endodontics	0	0	0	0	0	2	2
Periodontitis	4	0	4	1	3	1	13
Trauma	2	2	3	1	0	0	8
Other	2	5	1	0	7	10	25

mean PPD and mBoP at 6 months were 4.0 mm (3.91; 4.19) and 0.64 (0.54; 0.75), respectively (Figs. 2 and 3).

A mBoP index of 1 or more and PPD ≥4 mm was recorded at 35% of the sites at the final examination. At the baseline examination, PPD ≥6 mm was recorded at 31.25% (25.53; 37.59) of the sites and 17.02% (8.14; 31.35) of the implants. These numbers were reduced to 13.25% (9.31; 18.43) of the sites and 4.35% (0.76; 16.04) of the implants at the terminal examination (Fig. 4).

At the baseline visit, a mBoP index of 2 or 3 was recorded at 73.14% (67.01; 78.52) of the included sites, while this number was reduced to 28.9% (16.3; 27.1) at the final evaluation (Fig. 5).

Statistical difference in the level of the mucosal margin was recorded between baseline and all the later time points. No further change was seen after 4 weeks (Table 3).

During this study, all 63 implants were reported to have stable radiographic levels of osseous support as validated by the six different local examiners. No adverse events were reported during the study.

Discussion

Identifying peri-implant disease at an early stage and promptly treating the inflammatory condition is crucial to prevent the progression of peri-implant bone loss and ensure long-term implant survival [23–25]. After completion of active treatment and when the condition is controlled, supportive peri-implant therapy will reduce the risk of disease re-occurrence [9]. A number of scientific reports on various methods for non-surgical peri-implant therapy have been presented, but limited and short-term effects have been reported [26, 27]. Instruments for the removal of submucosal microbial deposits from implant surfaces should obviously be effective without causing damage to the implant. However, clinical devices specifically designed for this purpose are

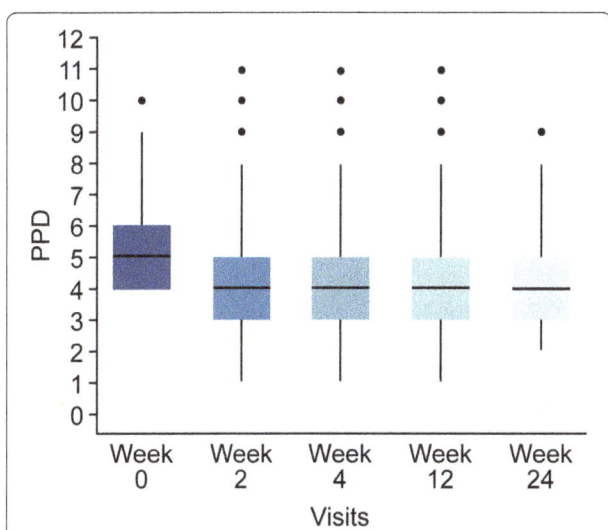

Fig. 2 Changes in PPD values between baseline and the various examination time points

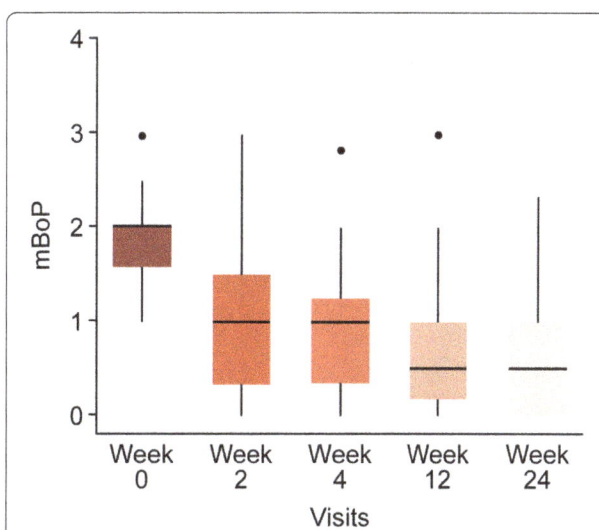

Fig. 3 Changes in BoP values between baseline and the various examination time points

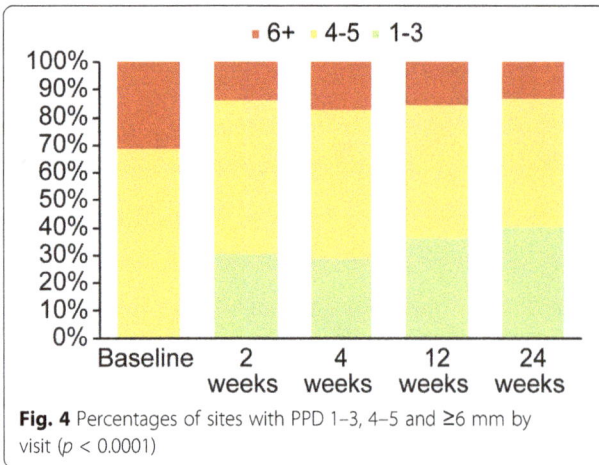

Fig. 4 Percentages of sites with PPD 1–3, 4–5 and ≥6 mm by visit ($p < 0.0001$)

experimental study demonstrated that chitosan inhibits the growth of the periodontal pathogens *Porphyromonas gingivalis* and *Aggregatibacter actinomycetemcomitans* and exerts an anti-inflammatory effect by reducing the levels of prostaglandin E-2 (PGE_2) [34]. From these perspectives, chitosan may be considered a potential candidate to be used in a device for implant debridement.

In the present study, significant reductions were observed in the clinical parameters of peri-implant inflammation at 2, 4, 12 and 24 weeks relative to baseline after debridement with the chitosan brush seated in an oscillating dental drill piece. No progression in radiographic bone loss was reported at any of the implants at the final evaluation, and the method was thus judged safe to use in cases with mild peri-implantitis.

In comparison, a randomized clinical trial by Sahm et al. [35] compared amino acid glycine powder versus mechanical debridement using carbon curettes and antiseptic therapy with chlorhexidine digluconate. At the 6-month final evaluation, PPD reductions of 0.6 and 0.5 mm, respectively, were reported. Similarly, Renvert et al. [36] performed a randomized clinical trial comparing an air-abrasive device and an Er:yttrium aluminium garnet (YAG) laser in the non-surgical treatment of peri-implantitis and reported mean PPD reductions of 0.9 and 0.8 mm, respectively, in the two groups. In the present study, a mean PPD reduction of 1.1 mm was determined at the final evaluation at 6 months which is comparable to findings reported in other studies.

A study by Riben-Grundstrom and co-workers [37] compared the use of glycine powder air-polishing and the ultrasonic treatment of peri-implant mucositis and utilized inclusion criteria comparable to those used in the present study for mild peri-implantitis. The inclusion criteria were (1) the presence of one or more sites diagnosed with peri-implant mucositis. The diagnostic criteria used were a probing depth ≥4 mm combined with bleeding with or without suppuration and (2) bone loss ≤2 mm assessed from the implant shoulder subsequent to the bone healing and remodelling process. They used dichotomous values for BoP and observed reductions of 27% in the air-polishing group and 31% in the ultrasonic group after 6 months.

scarce, and the effectiveness and safety of most such devices have rarely been scientifically validated [28]. In a review paper by Schwarz et al. [29], it was reported that mechanical debridement with, e.g. carbon fibre, titanium or plastic curettes combined with measures of oral hygiene, was effective in the management of peri-implant mucositis and that alternative or adjunctive measures such as lasers, ultrasonic devices or air abrasives with glycine powder may improve the efficacy of the treatment of sites with peri-implantitis. The same group of researchers also performed a systematic review on studies evaluating air-polishing with glycine powder of implants with peri-implantitis and reported that this method may lead to improved reduction in parameters of inflammation as compared to mechanical debridement combined with antiseptic therapy [30]. Chitosan is a completely biocompatible biopolymer which also has been demonstrated to be bacteriostatic and exhibit anti-inflammatory properties [31–33]. A recent in vitro

When pooling the index scores to dichotomous values in the present study, the mBoP score was found to have decreased from 2 or 3 to 0 or 1 in 55% of the samples. Although the complete absence of inflammation was difficult to achieve in most implants, significant and stable reductions in the parameters of inflammation were demonstrated in most sites up to 6 months after treatment with the chitosan brush. Nicotine interferes with the bleeding response in soft tissues and may, consequently, lead to false negatives for the BoP; therefore, to avoid positively skewing the results due to smoking, we

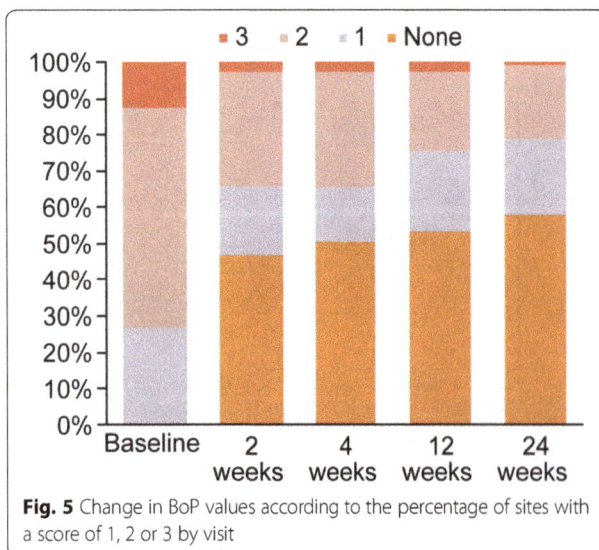

Fig. 5 Change in BoP values according to the percentage of sites with a score of 1, 2 or 3 by visit

Table 3 Level of crown margin at the different time points

	Baseline n = 306	2 weeks n = 272	4 weeks n = 267	12 weeks n = 282	24 weeks n = 294	P
Subgingival crown margins	283 (92.5%)	224 (82.4%)	224 (83.9%)	239 (84.8%)	248 (84,4%)	
Supragingival crown margins	23 (7.5%)	48(17.6%)	43 (16.1%)	43 (15.2%)	46 (15.6%)	
Baseline to 2 weeks						<0.001
Baseline to 4 weeks						0.024
Baseline to 12 weeks						0.003
Baseline to 24 weeks						0.002
4 to 12 weeks						0.668
12 to 24 weeks						0.895

decided to exclude current smokers from this study. According to the literature, bleeding on probing has low sensitivity as a predictor for active peri-implant disease because of the high frequency of false-positive responses, but it has a high level of specificity as no bleeding on probing indicates peri-implant health [38]. Due to the absence of perpendicular periodontal fibres in dental implants, a lighter probing force should be used than when probing the gingival crevice in teeth. Similarly, the standardization of the examiners' technique is critical [39]. A pressure-sensitive periodontal probe was used to record PPD and mBoP. We also used a 3-graded bleeding index to further distinguish between true disease and bleeding from the base of the pocket as the result of excessive pressure and rupture of the junctional epithelium. Scores of 1 and 0 and scores of 2 and 3 were pooled to create a more rigid, dichotomous score. This strengthens the positive results because significant differences were obtained when both the graded and dichotomous BoP scores were analysed. However, previous smokers were included but the outcomes in this patient group did not differ from finding in never smokers. Similarly, patients taking anticoagulants were excluded to avoid false-positive bleeding scores because of the increased bleeding response caused by the medication. Salvi and co-workers [40] studied the reduction in experimental peri-implant mucositis and revealed that 3 weeks of reinstituted plaque control did not yield pre-experimental levels of peri-implant health. While infection control was carefully installed prior to baseline, and the included implants were plaque free, we found significant reductions in the parameters of inflammation as early as 2 weeks after treatment with the chitosan brush. These results were stable up to 6 months after treatment, indicating a fast and stable response. More of the crown margins were exposed 2 weeks after debridement with the brush and the levels were thereafter stable. The more apical position the crown margins is most probably related to reduction in the soft tissue oedema from the inflammation.

The chitosan brush used in this study is made of a material that is soft with the aim to make a device optimized for removal of the biofilm within the implant threads. The soft bristles on the contrary make the device suboptimal for removal of hard deposits, such as calculus and cement remnants. It has been reported that such cement remnants are a common finding around dental implants [41], and in hindsight, it would have been beneficial for the analysis to record this. We did not record or analyse on cement- or screw-retained supraconstructions, and it may well be that some of the implants with cement-retained crowns and bridges had subgingival and non-visible cement remnants contributing to the mucosal inflammation. It can thus be hypothesized that combining the brush with an instrument for the removal of potential hard deposits would have yielded even better results. One such instrument for surgical use on titanium surfaces is a rotating titanium brush. The disadvantage with such a rigid metal brush is that the metal bristles may potentially cause injure to the mucosa if used non-surgically. Once active peri-implantitis treatment is finished with a positive response verified and the long-term and regular supportive treatment phase initiated, it could be argued that avoiding instruments that may damage the implant surface is preferable [15]. The consecutive case series presented here does only show the potential merits of a chitosan brush on reducing peri-implant mucosal inflammation. No control group was included in this study, and to test the clinical efficacy of this novel device in the non-surgical treatment of peri-implantitis, a randomized clinical trial will be required. It is also important with a long-term follow-up to study if the use of this novel device will prevent progression of peri-implant bone loss over time, potentially causing implant loss.

Conclusions

In this multicenter case series of implants affected by mild peri-implantitis, significant reductions in the clinical parameters of inflammation were demonstrated at all time points after the initial treatment with a chitosan brush. The use of an oscillating chitosan device appears to be safe and has potential merits for the treatment of mild peri-implantitis and for the maintenance of dental implants. To measure the effectiveness of the method, a multicenter randomized clinical trial needs to be undertaken.

Funding

This study was funded by a grant from the Norwegian Research Council FORNY Study number 234524. A short case series reporting on the results from one of the centers (Sapienza) has been accepted for publication in Minerva Stomatologica.

Authors' contributions

JCW, BJE, BZ, HJ, AP, AMR-J, AMA, MK and OCK participated in the design and undertaking of the study as well as drafting of the manuscript. GLDT carried out the statistics section and drafting of the manuscript. All authors read and approved the final manuscript.

Competing interests

J.C. Wohlfahrt is the inventor and patent holder of BioClean and is a shareholder in LABRIDA AS. B.J. Evensen, B. Zeza, H. Jansson, A. Pilloni, A.M. Roos-Jansåker, G.L. Di Tanna, A.M. Aass, M. Klepp and O.C. Koldsland state that there were no conflicts of interests during the undertaking of the study.

Author details

[1]Department of Periodontology, Institute of Clinical Dentistry, University of Oslo, Pb. 1109 Blindern, 0317 Oslo, Norway. [2]Private Practice, Tønsberg, Norway. [3]Department of Dental and Maxillofacial Sciences, Section of Periodontology, Sapienza, University of Rome, Rome, Italy. [4]Center for Oral Health, Department of Natural Science and Biomedicine, School of Health Sciences, Jönköping University, Jönköping, Sweden. [5]Department of Periodontology, Public Dental Health Service, Kristianstad, Sweden. [6]Center for Primary Care and Public Health, Queen Mary University of London, London, UK. [7]Private Practice, Stavanger, Norway. [8]Department of Periodontology, Public Specialist Dental Clinic, Karlskrona, Sweden.

References

1. Koldsland OC, Scheie AA, Aass AM. Prevalence of peri-implantitis related to severity of the disease with different degrees of bone loss. J Periodontol. 2010;81(2):231–8.
2. Roos-Jansaker AM, et al. Nine- to fourteen-year follow-up of implant treatment. Part II: presence of peri-implant lesions. J Clin Periodontol. 2006;33(4):290–5.
3. Derks J, et al. Effectiveness of implant therapy analyzed in a Swedish population: prevalence of peri-implantitis. J Dent Res. 2016;95(1):43–9.
4. Ogata Y, Nakayama Y, Tatsumi J, Kubota T, Sato S, Nishida T, Takeuchi Y, Onitsuka T, Sakagami R, Nozaki T, Murakami S, Matsubara N, Tanaka M, Yoshino T, Ota J, Nakagawa Y, Ishihara Y, Ito T, Saito A, Yamaki K, Matsuzaki E, Hidaka T, Sasaki D, Yaegashi T, Yasuda Y, Shibutani T, Noguchi K, Araki H, Ikumi N, Aoyama Y, Kogai H, Nemoto K, Deguchi S, Takiguchi T, Yamamoto M, Inokuchi K, Ito T, Kado T, Furuichi Y, Kanazashi M, Gomi K, Takagi Y, Kubokawa K, Yoshinari N, Hasegawa Y, Hirose T, Sase T, Arita H, Kodama T, Shin K, Izumi Y, Yoshie H. Prevalence and risk factors for peri-implant diseases in Japanese adult dental patients. J Oral Sci. 2017;59(1):1-11. doi:10.2334/josnusd.16-0027. Epub 2016 Oct 7.
5. Gurgel BC, et al. Frequency of peri-implant diseases and associated factors. Clin Oral Implants Res. 2016;
6. Ferreira CF, et al. Prevalence of peri-implant diseases: analyses of associated factors. Eur J Prosthodont Restor Dent. 2015;23(4):199–206.
7. Fransson C, et al. Prevalence of subjects with progressive bone loss at implants. Clin Oral Implants Res. 2005;16(4):440–6.
8. Jepsen S, et al. Primary prevention of peri-implantitis: managing peri-implant mucositis. J Clin Periodontol. 2015;42(Suppl 16):S152–7.
9. Costa FO, et al. Peri-implant disease in subjects with and without preventive maintenance: a 5-year follow-up. J Clin Periodontol. 2012;39(2):173–81.
10. Serino G, Strom C. Peri-implantitis in partially edentulous patients: association with inadequate plaque control. Clin Oral Implants Res. 2009;20(2):169–74.
11. Tonetti MS, et al. Primary and secondary prevention of periodontal and peri-implant diseases: introduction to, and objectives of the 11th European Workshop on Periodontology consensus conference. J Clin Periodontol. 2015;42(Suppl 16):S1–4.
12. Rokn A, et al. Prevalence of peri-implantitis in patients not participating in well-designed supportive periodontal treatments: a cross-sectional study. Clin Oral Implants Res. 2017;28(3):314–9.
13. Faggion CM Jr, et al. A systematic review and Bayesian network meta-analysis of randomized clinical trials on non-surgical treatments for peri-implantitis. J Clin Periodontol. 2014;41(10):1015–25.
14. Mellado-Valero A, et al. Decontamination of dental implant surface in peri-implantitis treatment: a literature review. Med Oral Patol Oral Cir Bucal. 2013;18(6):e869–76.
15. Eger M, et al. Scaling of titanium implants entrains inflammation-induced osteolysis. Sci Rep. 2017;7:39612.
16. van Velzen FJ, et al. Dental floss as a possible risk for the development of peri-implant disease: an observational study of 10 cases. Clin Oral Implants Res. 2016;27(5):618–21.
17. Mann M, et al. Effect of plastic-covered ultrasonic scalers on titanium implant surfaces. Clin Oral Implants Res. 2012;23(1):76–82.
18. Ramaglia L, et al. Profilometric and standard error of the mean analysis of rough implant surfaces treated with different instrumentations. Implant Dent. 2006;15(1):77–82.
19. Ruhling A, et al. Treatment of subgingival implant surfaces with Teflon-coated sonic and ultrasonic scaler tips and various implant curettes. An in vitro study. Clin Oral Implants Res. 1994;5(1):19–29.
20. Mengel R, et al. An in vitro study of the treatment of implant surfaces with different instruments. Int J Oral Maxillofac Implants. 1998;13(1):91–6.
21. Villa O, et al. Suture materials affect peri-implant bone healing and implant osseointegration. J Oral Sci. 2015;57(3):219–27.
22. Roos-Jansaker AM, et al. Submerged healing following surgical treatment of peri-implantitis: a case series. J Clin Periodontol. 2007;34(8):723–7.
23. Salvi GE, Cosgarea R, Sculean A. Prevalence and mechanisms of peri-implant diseases. J Dental Res. 2016;
24. Monje A, et al. Impact of maintenance therapy for the prevention of peri-implant diseases: a systematic review and meta-analysis. J Dental Res. 2016;95(4):372–9.
25. Gay IC, et al. Role of supportive maintenance therapy on implant survival: a university-based 17 years retrospective analysis. Int J Dental Hygiene. 2016;14(4):267–71.
26. Muthukuru M, et al. Non-surgical therapy for the management of peri-implantitis: a systematic review. Clin Oral Implants Res. 2012;23(Suppl 6):77–83.
27. Esposito M, Grusovin MG, Worthington HV. Treatment of peri-implantitis: what interventions are effective? A Cochrane systematic review. Eur J Oral Implantol. 2012;5(Suppl):S21–41.
28. Armitage GC, Xenoudi P. Post-treatment supportive care for the natural dentition and dental implants. Periodontol. 2016;71(1):164–84.
29. Schwarz F, Schmucker A, Becker J. Efficacy of alternative or adjunctive measures to conventional treatment of peri-implant mucositis and peri-implantitis: a systematic review and meta-analysis. Int J Implant Dent. 2015;1(1):22.
30. Schwarz F, Becker K, Renvert S. Efficacy of air polishing for the non-surgical treatment of peri-implant diseases: a systematic review. J Clin Periodontol. 2015;42(10):951–9.
31. Costa EM, et al. Evaluation and insights into chitosan antimicrobial activity against anaerobic oral pathogens. Anaerobe. 2012;18(3):305–9.
32. Choi BK, et al. In vitro antimicrobial activity of a chitooligosaccharide mixture against Actinobacillus actinomycetemcomitans and Streptococcus mutans. Int J Antimicrob Agents. 2001;18(6):553–7.
33. Sarasam AR, et al. Antibacterial activity of chitosan-based matrices on oral pathogens. Journal of materials science. Mat Med. 2008;19(3):1083–90.
34. Arancibia R, et al. Effects of chitosan particles in periodontal pathogens and gingival fibroblasts. J Dental Res. 2013;92(8):740–5.
35. Sahm N, et al. Non-surgical treatment of peri-implantitis using an air-abrasive device or mechanical debridement and local application of

chlorhexidine: a prospective, randomized, controlled clinical study. J Clin Periodontol. 2011;38(9):872–8.

36. Renvert S, et al. Treatment of peri-implantitis using an Er:YAG laser or an air-abrasive device: a randomized clinical trial. J Clin Periodontol. 2011;38(1):65–73.

37. Riben-Grundstrom C, et al. Treatment of peri-implant mucositis using a glycine powder air-polishing or ultrasonic device: a randomized clinical trial. J Clin Periodontol. 2015;42(5):462–9.

38. Lang NP, et al. Histologic probe penetration in healthy and inflamed peri-implant tissues. Clin Oral Implants Res. 1994;5(4):191–201.

39. Schou S, et al. Probing around implants and teeth with healthy or inflamed peri-implant mucosa/gingiva. A histologic comparison in cynomolgus monkeys (Macaca fascicularis). Clin Oral Implants Res. 2002;13(2):113–26.

40. Salvi GE, et al. Reversibility of experimental peri-implant mucositis compared with experimental gingivitis in humans. Clin Oral Implants Res. 2012;23(2):182–90.

41. Korsch M, Obst U, Walther W. Cement-associated peri-implantitis: a retrospective clinical observational study of fixed implant-supported restorations using a methacrylate cement. Clin Oral Implants Res. 2014;25(7):797–802.

25

Osseointegration of standard and mini dental implants: a histomorphometric comparison

Jagjit S. Dhaliwal[1*], Rubens F. Albuquerque Jr[2], Monzur Murshed[1,3] and Jocelyne S. Feine[1]

Abstract

Background: Mini dental implants (MDIs) are becoming increasingly popular for rehabilitation of edentulous patients because of their several advantages. However, there is a lack of evidence on the osseointegration potential of the MDIs. The objective of the study was to histomorphometrically evaluate and compare bone apposition on the surface of MDIs and standard implants in a rabbit model.

Methods: Nine New Zealand white rabbits were used for the study to meet statistical criteria for adequate power. Total 18 3M™ESPE™ MDIs and 18 standard implants (Ankylos® Friadent, Dentsply) were inserted randomly into the tibia of rabbits (four implants per rabbit); animals were sacrificed after a 6-week healing period. The specimens were retrieved en bloc and preserved in 10% formaldehyde solution. Specimens were prepared for embedding in a light cure acrylic resin (Technovit 9100). The most central sagittal histological sections (30–40 μm thick) were obtained using a Leica SP 1600 saw microtome. After staining, the Leica DM2000 microscope was used, the images were captured using Olympus DP72 camera and associated software. Bone implant contact (BIC) was measured using Infinity Analyze software.

Results: All implants were osseointegrated. Histologic measures show mineralized bone matrix in intimate contact with the implant surface in both groups. The median BIC was 58.5 % (IQR 8.0) in the MDI group and 57.0 % (IQR 5.5) in the control group ($P > 0.05$; Mann-Whitney test). There were no statistical differences in osseointegration at 6 weeks between MDIs and standard implants in rabbit tibias.

Conclusions: Based on these results, it is concluded that osseointegration of MDIs is similar to that of standard implants.

Keywords: Bone implant contact, Mini dental implant, Osseointegration

Background

The term "osseointegration" was first introduced to explain the phenomenon for stable fixation of titanium to bone by Brånemark et al. in the 1960s [1]. Osseointegrated implants were introduced, a new era in oral rehabilitation began, and many studies were conducted [2, 3]. A success rate of over 90% has been reported [4, 5]. Further, a success rate of 81% in the maxillary bone and 91% in the mandible can be accomplished [6]. Dental implants have been widely used for the stabilization of complete dentures and also help to maintain bone, function, esthetics, and phonetics and improve the oral health-related quality of life [7]. The dental implants are available with different surfaces and sizes. The size of the dental implants usually ranges in the diameter range of 3 mm (narrow diameter) to 7 mm (wide diameter). However, majority of the implants fall in the "standard diameter" range of 3.7 to 4.0 mm [8].

Mini dental implants or small size implants are also being widely used for stabilizing the complete dentures [9], for orthodontic anchorage [10–12], single tooth replacements [13, 14], fixing the surgical guides for definitive implant placement [15], and as transitional

---
* Correspondence: jagjitd2002@yahoo.com
[1]Faculty of Dentistry, McGill University, 2001 McGill College Avenue, Suite 500, Montreal, Quebec H3A 1G1, Canada
Full list of author information is available at the end of the article

implants for the support of interim removable prosthesis during the healing phase of final fixtures [16, 17].

The single-piece mini dental implants (MDIs) are becoming increasingly popular for the purpose of denture stabilization. There are many advantages of the MDIs over the regular implants. The surgery is minimally invasive as compared with conventional implant surgery which helps in decreased morbidity for the patient. Transmucosal placement is possible using a single pilot drill, and these can often be loaded immediately [18]. Gingival healing is typically seen in 2 to 5 days, extended healing period with MDIs is usually not necessary [19]. The insertion of MDIs needs a minimal disturbance of the periosteum, thus osseointegration process is accelerated and time needed for MDIs tends to be considerably small than that of regular implants due to less injurious insertion procedure [9]. The need for sutures or long recovery periods is eliminated [3]. The patient can walk in to the office in the morning and is out the same day with a full set of teeth, the patient is allowed to eat the same day. These can work well for patients who have significant bone loss that restrict them from being a candidate for regular dental implants. MDIs are also a solution for patients that cannot have surgery for medical reasons. MDIs are also cost effective [20]. Considerable confusion exists in the literature regarding the best method to monitor the status of a dental implant. Various methods have been used to demonstrate the osseointegration of dental implants. A common and time-tested method to evaluate biological responses to an implant is to measure the extent of bone implant contact (BIC), referred to as histomorphometry at the light microscopic level. Bone implant contact (BIC) is one of the parameters which has been used extensively to study the amount of bone apposition next to the implants [21–27]. When an implant is placed in the jaw, it is in contact with compact bone as well as cancellous bone. The different structures of the two types of bone frequently result in variation of mineralized bone-to-implant contact length along the implant surface [28, 29]. Albrektsson et al. identified the key features affecting osseointegration about 4 decades ago, e.g., implant surface and topography, surface chemistry, charge, and wettability [30]. Roughness and enhanced surface area seems to be helpful for osseointegration. Carlsson et al. reported that screw-shaped implants with a rough surface had a stronger bonding than implants with a polished surface [31]. A coarse surface seems to be more appropriate for osseointegration of implants than a relatively smoother implant surface by representing a greater degree of implant integration [32–34]. The bone contact areas of 3M ESPE MDIs are surface treated. The treatment process of these MDIs includes sandblasting with aluminum oxide particles followed by cleaning and passivation with an oxidizing acid [35].

Despite the advantages of the mini dental implants, evidence on their efficacy and long-term success is lacking. The success of these implants will depend on their union with the surrounding bone. New implant systems entering into the market have to be studied with the help of animal models first, to demonstrate the osseointegration potential for their probable success in humans. There is a limited evidence regarding the 3M ESPE MDIs. Therefore, there is a need for an animal study to explore the osseointegration of these implants to assist in better understanding of the treatment selection, prognosis, and outcomes for the patients.

Objectives of the study

The objective of this study is to compare bone apposition on the surface of mini dental implants and standard implants by means of histomorphometric methods.

Methods
Animal model

Nine clinically healthy New Zealand white rabbits weighing 3.5 kg and more were used for the study, and the animals were housed in the central animal house facility. The head of tibia/femur of the animals were used for the implantation of samples. Rabbits' tibiae and femur have been widely used as an animal model by various other authors to study osseointegration of dental implants [36–45].

Sample size

The sample size of this study has been calculated based on the results of a similar study by Bornstein et al. [22]. It was established that 88% statistical power will be achieved by using 18 mini dental implants (3M ESPE MDIs) for the experimental implants and equal number of an established regular implant (Ankylos, Dentsply Friadent GmbH) for the control. Therefore, the total number of implants used was 36. Each animal received four implants on hind limbs, i.e., right and left tibia/femur head randomly (the heads of tibia and femur have been chosen to get the maximum bulk of bone). Therefore, each animal received two experimental and two regular implants.

Surgical procedure

The procedures were approved by the institutional animals' ethics review board of McGill University, Canada. Animals were anesthetized by an intravenous injection of ketamine hydrochloride-xylazine mixture at 35–50 and 1–3 mg/kg respectively according to a method described by Green et al. [46]. Acepromazine was injected subcutaneously at dosage of 1 mg/kg. Further injections of the mixture were given to maintain anesthesia, if necessary [46]. Sterile ophthalmic ointment was put in both eyes to prevent corneal desiccation. Animals were shaved for twice the size of the expected surgical field with an electric razor. All loose hair and debris from the animal were removed. The surgical area was cleaned with gauze and 2% chlorhexidine solution to remove the majority of debris from the surgical site. Antiseptic skin preparation was done starting at the center of the surgical site and moved to the outside of the prepared area in a circular manner. Three scrubs with 2% chlorhexidine solution and three alternating rinses with alcohol were performed. The animal was draped and fixed with clamps on a sterile, impermeable covering to isolate the disinfected area. This was performed by the gloved and gowned surgical team under sterile conditions.

Surgical protocol for 3M™ESPE™ MDIs
A small longitudinal skin incision just distal to the tibia-femur joint was made. The tibia/femur head was exposed subperiosteally and an osteotomy performed with the delicately placed pilot drill over the entry point and lightly pumped up and down under copius saline irrigation just to enter the cortical bone for the MDIs. This was used for initial bone drilling to depth of 0.5 mm. The 3M™ESPE™ MDI (size 1.8 mm × 10 mm) vial was opened and the body of the implant was firmly grasped with a sterilized locking pliers. The titanium finger driver was attached to the head of the implant. The implant was transferred to the site and rotated clockwise while exerting downwards pressure. This began the self tapping process and was used until noticeable bony resistance encountered when it touched the lower cortical plate. The winged thumb wrench was used for driving the implant deeper into the bone, if necessary. All the animals received one MDI on the head of each tibia or femur. Therefore, total 18 mini dental implants were inserted.

Surgical protocol for the Ankylos® implants
Equal number of comparator implants (size 3.5 mm × 8 mm) were inserted in the other tibia/femur head of the animals after doing the osteotomy according to the manufacturer's protocol as follows. After mobilizing the mucoperiosteal flap, the 3-mm center punch was used to register a guide for the twist drill. The twist drill was used to establish the axial alignment of the implant and to assist in the guidance of the depth drill. The depth drills were sequentially used to create osteotomy to the subcrestal axial depth of 0.5 mm. The conical reamer was used to develop the conical shape of the implant body and to check the osteotomy depth. A counter-clockwise rotation was used to compress the bone in soft bone. The tap or thread cutter was used for dense bone to create the threads in the osteotomy. The thread cutter's diameter corresponds to the implant diameter.

To engage the implant into the implant placement tool, the square faces on the implant fixture mount were aligned with those on the implant placement tool, then pushed together. Using the handle (finger wheel), the implant was pulled out of inner vial and the plastic collar was discarded. The implant placement assembly was transferred to the osteotomy and the implant was secured into the osteotomy site. The implant placement was started with the handle and finally placed using the hand-ratchet. If excessive force was experienced, the osteotomy was rinsed out and the depth was checked by retapping. To disengage fixture mount from implant, the open-ended spanner was used to break the retention force of the fixture mount retention screw. The knurled top of the implant placement tool was turned by hand to fully disengage the fixture mount with the implant. Pushing down on the knurled top of the implant placement tool disengaged the fixture mount.

Suturing
Expected length of the procedure was approximately 1 h. Following placement of the implants, the wound was sutured in layers. The underlying muscle, fascia, and dermal layers were sutured with the help of Vicryl (Polyglactin 910) suture with 3/8 circle reverse cutting needle. The skin was sutured to a primary closer with the same suture material.

Radiograph
Plain X-ray images of all the rabbit tibia were taken after suturing to confirm the position of implants and to detect any injury/fracture of the bone (Fig. 1).

Post surgical treatment
After the surgical procedure, the animals were housed in a cage under the supervision of a veterinary doctor until they came out of anesthesia. The rabbit was observed every 2 h on the first day of surgery followed by once a day to check the wound for infection. The wound was protected with povidone iodine ointment. The rabbits were allowed immediate weight bearing as tolerated; therefore, they had no restraints on weight bearing.

Animals were shifted and housed together with other rabbits. The rabbit was given a dose of Cephalexin 12 mg/kg 0.5 ml I.V. once intraoperatively and a postoperative analgesic, i.e., Carprofen 2–4 mg/kg S.C. every 8 hourly for 3 days according to McGill SOP. The routine daily care was as per McGill SOP#524.01.

The feeding protocols were followed according to the university central animal house facility guidelines. The animals had a free access to water and feed. The sutures were removed after 7–10 days, and the wound was cleaned with 0.2% chlorhexidine solution.

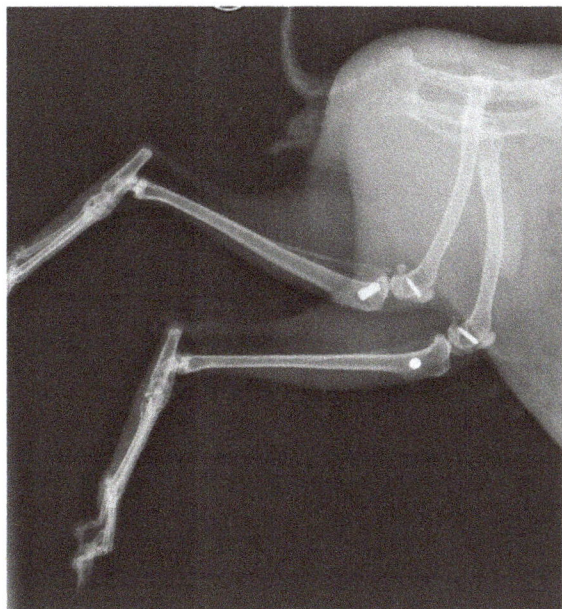

Fig. 1 Radiograph showing implants in the rabbit tibia

Euthanasia

The animals were euthanized at 6 weeks respectively. An overdose of pentobarbital sodium 1 ml/kg intravenously, under general anesthesia, was used for this purpose [47, 48].

Specimen retrieval

The implants along with their surrounding bone were excised with a surgical saw right away following the euthanasia. The excess tissue was dissected and the specimens were removed en bloc with a margin of surrounding bone of about 5–10 mm. The specimens were immediately put into the 10% formaldehyde solution.

Sample preparation for embedding

The specimens were dehydrated in the ascending graded ethanol solution and kept in a pre-filtration solution for 3 h at room temperature and then in the filtration solution at 4 °C for 17 h. The specimens were then embedded in a light curing resin Technovit 9100 NEW (Kulzer & Co., Wehrheim, Germany) polymerization system based on methyl methacrylate, specially developed for embedding mineralized tissues for light microscopy. The polymerization mixture was produced by mixing the solution A and B in the proportion of 9 parts A and 1 part of solution B directly before use. This was done in a beaker and using a glass rod to stir the mixture. The samples were then positioned in the labeled plastic moulds, completely covered in the polymerization mixture, and placed in cooled desiccators and under a partial vacuum at 4 °C for 10 min. The resulting blocks

were placed in a sealed container and left to polymerize between –8 and –20 °C. The samples were allowed to stand at 4–8 °C in the refrigerator for at least 1 h before allowing it to slowly come to room temperature. The polymerization times are dependent on the volumes of polymerization mixture used and of the constancy of the temperature at which polymerization is carried out.

Preparation of histological sections

The acrylic block was mounted into the object holder of the Leica SP 1600 saw microtome (Fig. 2). The height of the object was adjusted until the surface of the object is slightly above the upper edge of the saw blade. The surface of the block was trimmed to get a plane surface prior to producing slices of a defined thickness. During the sawing process, the water flow was adjusted so that the water jet lands on the edge of the saw blade. The built-in water cooling device prevents overheating of the object and removes saw dust from the cutting edge and thus prolongs the lift time of the saw blade. The most favorable feed rate was determined (Fig. 3). After trimming, the first undefined slice was removed from the saw blade. The desired section thickness was selected, considering the thickness of the saw blade and added to the desired thickness of final section. The section was stabilized during the sawing process. To do so, a glass cover slip was glued onto the trimmed surface of the specimen block using cyanoacrylate glue. These blocks were cut with a low speed saw under water along the lateral surface of the implant [47, 48]. The implant

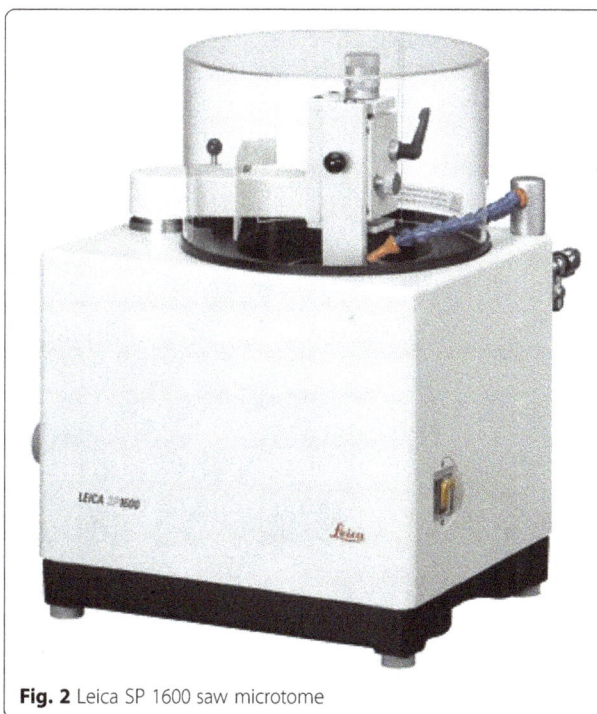

Fig. 2 Leica SP 1600 saw microtome

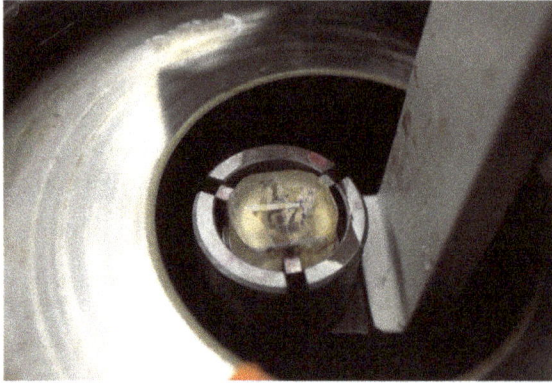

Fig. 3 Histological sections being obtained with Leica SP 1600 saw microtome

bearing blocks were cut parallel to the long axis of the implant, and 30-μm-thick specimens were obtained.

The saw blade has a thickness of 280 μm and a feed of 310 μm was selected to obtain the final section thickness of 30 μm. The knurled screw was used for the setting of the section thickness. The prepared section was finally removed from the saw blade. The specimens were prepared for histology by the method as described by Donath and Breuner [49].

Histological evaluation

Subsequently, the sections were stained with toluidine blue and basic fuchsin similar to other studies [21, 22, 50]. The specimen sections were evaluated at the most central saggital section of each implant under an optical microscope after staining. The images were photographed with a high resolution camera and interfaced to a monitor and PC, observed under the Leica DM2000 microscope, and the images were captured using Olympus DP72 camera and associated software [4, 21, 22]. Bone implant contact (BIC) was measured using Infinity Analyze software. Six images of the same implant were taken and measurements were done. The percentage of the interface contact length between implant surface and bone, i.e., bone implant contact (BIC), was calculated. The percentage of bone tissue in a 200-μm-wide zone parallel to the contour of the implant area (adjoining the implant) was measured.

Micro-computed tomography (MicroCT)

MicroCT scans of each sample of both types of implants were obtained with a Skyscan 1172 equipment (Kontich, Belgium) at 6 μm resolution with 800 ms exposure time, 70 kV electric voltage, 167 μA current, and a 0.5-mm thickness aluminum filter. The equipment was fitted with a 1.3-MP camera to capture high resolution 2D images that were assembled into 3D reconstructions using NRecon software supplied with the instrument.

Statistical methods

Mean values and standard deviations were calculated for bone implant contact (BIC). Univariate analysis was done for all the evaluations. Analysis of variance (ANOVA) was used to analyze the differences between the two implants. P value <0.05 was considered significant. Statistical analyses were carried out with the help of SPSS statistical software version 18.

Results
Clinical findings

On the whole, postoperative wound healing in all the rabbits was good. None of them exhibited any signs of wound infection or exposure. A total of 36 specimens were retrieved for histological examination.

Histological observations

All of the implants in both groups showed osseointegration and displayed a good amount of bone contact length (Figs. 4 and 5). No discernible differences were noticed between both the groups. The zone of interest was 200 μm in the peri-implant area of the implants on both sides. Due to large marrow spaces in the rabbit bone,

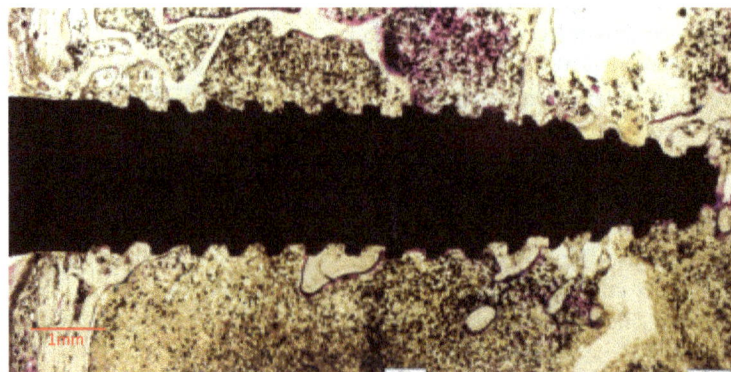

Fig. 4 Histological section of mini dental implant in rabbit tibia stained with methylene blue and basic fuchsin

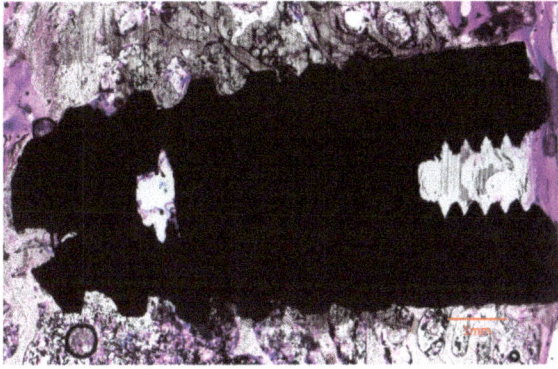

Fig. 5 Histological section of standard implant in rabbit tibia stained with methylene blue and basic fuchsin

larger volume of bone contact was mostly observed in the coronal and apical portions of the implants. The MicroCT pictures showed a three-dimensional deposition of bone in both samples (Fig. 6). It was noted that possibility of new bone formation was higher in areas adjacent to old bone. The sections of implant, which were exposed to the marrow spaces, displayed either no bone deposition or very thin bone tissue. Newly formed bone was seen with lighter staining. In the surrounding areas of both types of implants, bone fragments were noticed around the implant. These could correspond to bone fragments during the osteotomy procedure. Percentage of BIC ranged from 45 to 67% in both the groups. The median value of % BIC was 58.5 and the MDI group (IQR 7) and control group was 57.0 (IQR 5.0) (Tables 1 and 2). The mean differences of % BIC between the groups were verified through Mann–Whitney nonparametric test. There was no significant difference between the % bone implant contact (BIC) length of both the implants (P value >0.05).

Discussion

The osseointegration potential of 3M ESPE MDIs has not been studied. The MDI is a one-piece implant that

simplifies the restorative phase resulting in a reduced cost for the patient. Titanium-aluminum-vanadium alloy (Ti 6Al-4V-ELI) is used for increased strength. The success of these implants led to its use in long-term fixed and removable dental prostheses [51]. Conventional implant treatment requires adequate bone width and interdental space. Augmentation procedures are complex and can cause postoperative pain and discomfort for the patient and additional costs.

In human models, a 3–6-month period is needed to obtain osseointegration and animal models would need a shorter time (4–6 weeks) [30, 33]. Rabbit has been used extensively to examine osseointegration and appears to be an appropriate model for studying the bone healing systems [52]. The healing periods used by various authors for assessing the bone implant contact in rabbits are 2, 3, 4, 6, 8, and 12 weeks [53–57]. However, the best results have been between 6 and 12 weeks of insertion period [51, 53–55]. The 6-week healing period was carefully chosen after literature search. This was in agreement with others who have reported that a 6-week period is adequate in rabbits to develop a "rigid osseous interface" [51–60].

At the bone implant interface, woven bone starts forming after the placement of implant. Lamellar bone slowly replaces this scantily organized bone. The fully developed lamellar bone which replaces the woven bone typifies a stable and lasting osseointegration [61].

Our results are in concurrence with Balkin et al. [62]; they have also shown in their histology study in humans that the MDI undergoes osseointegration. They inserted one 3M ESPE MDI of 1.8-mm diameter in each of two patients as a transitional implant for mandibular dentures. After a period of 4 and 5 months, the implants were trephined out for histological evaluation. The results showed that there was a close apposition of bone on the implant surfaces. The bone surrounding the implant demonstrated signs of matured healing and integrated for immediate function after 4 to 5 months of healing period.

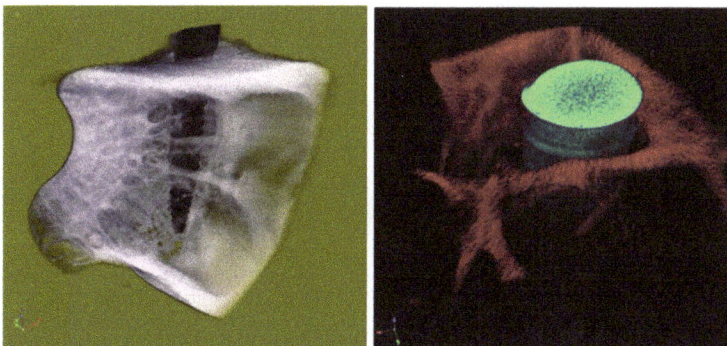

Fig. 6 Micro CT scan images of the MDIs and Ankylos® embedded in rabbit bone 6 weeks post implantation

Table 1 Comparison of % BIC in both groups

Sample	3M™ESPE™ MDIs	Ankylos®
1.	67	54
2.	59	67
3.	54	45
4.	51	58
5.	47	57
6.	64	49
7.	50	54
8.	60	56
9.	56	60
10.	61	53
11.	62	59
12.	61	55
13.	59	59
14.	45	51
15.	58	59
16.	54	62
17.	66	62
18.	56	57

Our study is also in concordance with the results of a removal torque study by Simon et al. [63] in immediately loaded "transitional endosseous implants" in humans. The percentage BIC for MDIs was similar to standard implants.

The surface topography also affects the BIC, Wennerberg et al. [32] measured and compared removal torque values on screw-shaped titanium implants with three surface types. The results showed that screws sandblasted with 25-μm particles of titanium and 75-μm particles of aluminum oxide exhibited a higher removal torque and interfacial bone contact than the machined titanium implants with smoother surface texture.

The surface of 3M™ESPE™ MDI is sandblasted with aluminum oxide and cleaned and passivized with an oxidizing acid (Technical Data Sheet, 3M ESPE) [35]. The surface of Ankylos® is sandblasted and acid etched [64]. Various authors have reported that surface roughness induces a variety of events in the course of osteoblast differentiation, spreading and proliferation, production

Table 2 Descriptive statistics of the experimental and control group

BIC	3M™ ESPE™ MDIs	Ankylos® Friadent (Dentsply)
Median	58.5	57
Mean	57	56.5
Interquartile range	8	5.5
First quartile	53.25	53.75
Third quartile	61.25	59.25

of alkaline phosphatase, collagen, proteoglycans, and osteocalcin, and synthesis of cytokines and growth factors [65–67]. Therefore, leading to bone deposition on the surface of these implants, Yan et al. [68] demonstrated that simple surface treatments can turn the titanium surface into a bone-bonding one. With the results of our in vitro study, Marulanda et al. [69] on discs of both types of implants demonstrated that surface chemistry of 3M™ESPE™ MDI is conducive to growth of osteoblasts leading to bone apposition.

One of the shortcomings of our study may be the use of rabbit tibia as a model. The tibia of the rabbit is essentially hollow except the upper and lower cortical plates. This may justify lack of bone apposition on the whole implant in both experimental as well as comparator implants. However, it provides a reliable information for human application as the human maxillary bone is also of a softer bone quality [36, 51].

Conclusions
The results of this study show that MDIs as well as regular implants osseointegrate in rabbits.

Funding
This study was funded by Ministère du Développment économique de l'Innovation et ce l'Exportation (MDEIE), Gouvernement du Québec, Indian Council of Medical Research (ICMR) and 3M ESPE IRB grant number A10-M118-9A.

Authors' contributions
JSD carried out the experiments and drafted the manuscript, RA conceived the study and helped in revising the manuscript, MM contributed to the histological preparation and data analysis, JSF participated in this study's design and overall coordination. All authors read and approved the final manuscript.

Competing interests
Jagjit Singh Dhaliwal, Rubens F. Albuquerque Jr, Monzur Murshed and Jocelyne S. Feine declare that they have no competing interests.

Author details
[1]Faculty of Dentistry, McGill University, 2001 McGill College Avenue, Suite 500, Montreal, Quebec H3A 1G1, Canada. [2]Faculty of Dentistry of Ribeirão Preto, University of São Paulo, Ribeirão Preto, SP, Brazil. [3]Department of Medicine, McGill University, Montreal, Quebec, Canada.

References
1. Branemark PI, Adell R, Breine U, Hansson BO, Lindstrom J, Ohlsson A. Intra-osseous anchorage of dental prostheses. I. Experimental studies. Scand J Plast Reconstr Surg. 1969;3(2):81–100.
2. Boerrigter EM, Stegenga B, Raghoebar GM, Boering G. Patient satisfaction and chewing ability with implant-retained mandibular overdentures: a comparison with new complete dentures with or without preprosthetic surgery. J Oral Maxillofac Surg. 1995;53(10):1167–73.
3. Del Fabbro M, Testori T, Francetti L, Taschieri S, Weinstein R. Systematic review of survival rates for immediately loaded dental implants. Int J Periodontics Restorative Dent. 2006;26(3):249–63.

4. Buser D, Mericske-Stern R, Bernard JP, Behneke A, Behneke N, Hirt HP, et al. Long-term evaluation of non-submerged ITI implants. Part 1: 8-year life table analysis of a prospective multi-center study with 2359 implants. Clin Oral Implants Res. 1997;8(3):161-72..

5. Albrektsson T, Dahl E, Enbom L, Engevall S, Engquist B, Eriksson AR, et al. Osseointegrated oral implants. A Swedish multicenter study of 8139 consecutively inserted Nobelpharma implants. J Periodontol. 1988;59(5):287-96.

6. Adell R, Lekholm U, Rockler B, Branemark PI. A 15-year study of osseointegrated implants in the treatment of the edentulous jaw. Int J Oral Surg. 1981;10(6):387-416.

7. Heydecke G, Locker D, Awad MA, Lund JP, Feine JS. Oral and general health-related quality of life with conventional and implant dentures. Community Dent Oral Epidemiol. 2003;31(3):161-8.

8. Lee JH, Frias V, Lee KW, Wright RF. Effect of implant size and shape on implant success rates: a literature review. J Prosthet Dent. 2005;94(4):377-81.

9. Bulard RA, Vance JB. Multi-clinic evaluation using mini-dental implants for long-term denture stabilization: a preliminary biometric evaluation. Compend Contin Educ Dent. 2005;26(12):892-7.

10. Buchter A, Wiechmann D, Koerdt S, Wiesmann HP, Piffko J, Meyer U. Load-related implant reaction of mini-implants used for orthodontic anchorage. Clin Oral Implants Res. 2005;16(4):473-9.

11. Fritz U, Diedrich P, Kinzinger G, Al-Said M. The anchorage quality of mini-implants towards translatory and extrusive forces. J Orofac Orthop. 2003;64(4):293-304.

12. Hong RK, Heo JM, Ha YK. Lever-arm and mini-implant system for anterior torque control during retraction in lingual orthodontic treatment. Angle Orthod. 2005;75(1):129-41.

13. Mazor Z, Steigmann M, Leshem R, Peleg M. Mini-implants to reconstruct missing teeth in severe ridge deficiency and small interdental space: a 5-year case series. Implant Dent. 2004;13(4):336-41.

14. Siddiqui AA, Sosovicka M, Goetz M. Use of mini implants for replacement and immediate loading of 2 single-tooth restorations: a clinical case report. J Oral Implantol. 2006;32(2):82-6.

15. Yeh S, Monaco EA, Buhite RJ. Using transitional implants as fixation screws to stabilize a surgical template for accurate implant placement: a clinical report. J Prosthet Dent. 2005;93(6):509-13.

16. Kwon KR, Sachdeo A, Weber HP. Achieving immediate function with provisional prostheses after implant placement: a clinical report. J Prosthet Dent. 2005;93(6):514-7.

17. Ohkubo C, Kobayashi M, Suzuki Y, Sato J, Hosoi T, Kurtz KS. Evaluation of transitional implant stabilized overdentures: a case series report. J Oral Rehabil. 2006;33(6):416-22.

18. Shatkin TE, Oppenheimer BD, Oppenheimer AJ. Mini dental implants for long-term fixed and removable prosthetics: a retrospective analysis of 2514 implants placed over a five-year period. Compend Contin Educ Dent. 2007; 28(2):92-9. quiz 100-1.

19. Campelo LD, Camara JR. Flapless implant surgery: a 10-year clinical retrospective analysis. Int J Oral Maxillofac Implants. 2002;17(2):271-6.

20. Griffitts TM, Collins CP, Collins PC. Mini dental implants: an adjunct for retention, stability, and comfort for the edentulous patient. Oral Surg Oral Med Oral Pathol Oral Radiol Endod. 2005;100(5):81-4.

21. Barros RR, Novaes Jr AB, Muglia VA, Iezzi G, Piattelli A. Influence of interimplant distances and placement depth on peri-implant bone remodeling of adjacent and immediately loaded Morse cone connection implants: a histomorphometric study in dogs. Clin Oral Implants Res. 2010;21(4):371-8.

22. Bornstein MM, Valderrama P, Jones AA, Wilson TG, Seibl R, Cochran DL. Bone apposition around two different sandblasted and acid-etched titanium implant surfaces: a histomorphometric study in canine mandibles. Clin Oral Implants Res. 2008;19(3):233-41.

23. Trisi P, Lazzara R, Rao W, Rebaudi A. Bone-implant contact and bone quality: evaluation of expected and actual bone contact on machined and osseotite implant surfaces. Int J Periodontics Restorative Dent. 2002;22(6):535-45.

24. Froum SJ, Simon H, Cho SC, Elian N, Rohrer MD, Tarnow DP. Histologic evaluation of bone-implant contact of immediately loaded transitional implants after 6 to 27 months. Int J Oral Maxillofac Implants. 2005;20(1):54-60.

25. Depprich R, Zipprich H, Ommerborn M, Naujoks C, Wiesmann HP, Kiattavorncharoen S, et al. Osseointegration of zirconia implants compared with titanium: an in vivo study. Head Face Med. 2008;4:30.

26. Novaes Jr AB, Souza SL, de Oliveira PT, Souza AM. Histomorphometric analysis of the bone-implant contact obtained with 4 different implant surface treatments placed side by side in the dog mandible. Int J Oral Maxillofac Implants. 2002;17(3):377-83.

27. Degidi M, Perrotti V, Piattelli A, Iezzi G. Mineralized bone-implant contact and implant stability quotient in 16 human implants retrieved after early healing periods: a histologic and histomorphometric evaluation. Int J Oral Maxillofac Implants. 2010;25(1):45-8.

28. Deporter DA, Watson PA, Pilliar RM, Melcher AH, Winslow J, Howley TP, et al. A histological assessment of the initial healing response adjacent to porous-surfaced, titanium alloy dental implants in dogs. J Dent Res. 1986; 65(8):1064-70.

29. Deporter DA, Friedland B, Watson PA, Pilliar RM, Howley TP, Abdulla D, et al. A clinical and radiographic assessment of a porous-surfaced, titanium alloy dental implant system in dogs. J Dent Res. 1986;65(8):1071-7.

30. Albrektsson T, Branemark PI, Hansson HA, Lindstrom J. Osseointegrated titanium implants. Requirements for ensuring a long-lasting, direct bone-to-implant anchorage in man. Acta Orthop Scand. 1981;52(2):155-70.

31. Carlsson L, Rostlund T, Albrektsson B, Albrektsson T. Removal torques for polished and rough titanium implants. Int J Oral Maxillofac Implants. 1988;3(1):21-4.

32. Wennerberg A, Albrektsson T, Andersson B, Krol JJ. A histomorphometric and removal torque study of screw-shaped titanium implants with three different surface topographies. Clin Oral Implants Res. 1995;6(1):24-30.

33. Buser D, Schenk RK, Steinemann S, Fiorellini JP, Fox CH, Stich H. Influence of surface characteristics on bone integration of titanium implants. A histomorphometric study in miniature pigs. J Biomed Mater Res. 1991;25(7):889-902.

34. Gotfredsen K, Wennerberg A, Johansson C, Skovgaard LT, Hjorting-Hansen E. Anchorage of TiO2-blasted, HA-coated, and machined implants: an experimental study with rabbits. J Biomed Mater Res. 1995;29(10):1223-31.

35. Technical Data Sheet, 3M. Literature review. St. Paul, MN: 3M ESPE Dental Products, 2009.

36. Steigenga J, Al-Shammari K, Misch C, Nociti Jr FH, Wang HL. Effects of implant thread geometry on percentage of osseointegration and resistance to reverse torque in the tibia of rabbits. J Periodontol. 2004;75(9):1233-41.

37. Faeda RS, Tavares HS, Sartori R, Guastaldi AC, Marcantonio Jr E. Biological performance of chemical hydroxyapatite coating associated with implant surface modification by laser beam: biomechanical study in rabbit tibias. J Oral Maxillofac Surg. 2009;67(8):1706-15.

38. He FM, Yang GL, Li YN, Wang XX, Zhao SF. Early bone response to sandblasted, dual acid-etched and H2O2/HCl treated titanium implants: an experimental study in the rabbit. Int J Oral Maxillofac Surg. 2009;38(6):677-81.

39. Rong M, Zhou L, Gou Z, Zhu A, Zhou D. The early osseointegration of the laser-treated and acid-etched dental implants surface: an experimental study in rabbits. J Mater Sci Mater Med. 2009;20(8):1721-8.

40. Marin C, Bonfante EA, Granato R, Suzuki M, Granjeiro JM, Coelho PG. The effect of alterations on resorbable blasting media processed implant surfaces on early bone healing: a study in rabbits. Implant Dent. 2011;20(2):167-77.

41. Yildiz A, Esen E, Kurkcu M, Damlar I, Daglioglu K, Akova T. Effect of zoledronic acid on osseointegration of titanium implants: an experimental study in an ovariectomized rabbit model. J Oral Maxillofac Surg. 2010;68(3):515-23.

42. Park YS, Yi KY, Lee IS, Han CH, Jung YC. The effects of ion beam-assisted deposition of hydroxyapatite on the grit-blasted surface of endosseous implants in rabbit tibiae. Int J Oral Maxillofac Implants. 2005;20(1):31-8.

43. Park JW, Kim HK, Kim YJ, An CH, Hanawa T. Enhanced osteoconductivity of micro-structured titanium implants (XiVE S CELLplus) by addition of surface calcium chemistry: a histomorphometric study in the rabbit femur. Clin Oral Implants Res. 2009;20(7):684-90.

44. Yang GL, He FM, Yang XF, Wang XX, Zhao SF. Bone responses to titanium implants surface-roughened by sandblasted and double etched treatments

in a rabbit model. Oral Surg Oral Med Oral Pathol Oral Radiol Endod. 2008; 106(4):516–24.

45. Le Guehennec L, Goyenvalle E, Lopez-Heredia MA, Weiss P, Amouriq Y, Layrolle P. Histomorphometric analysis of the osseointegration of four different implant surfaces in the femoral epiphyses of rabbits. Clin Oral Implants Res. 2008;19(11):1103–10.

46. Green CJ, Knight J, Precious S, Simpkin S. Ketamine alone and combined with diazepam or xylazine in laboratory animals: a 10 year experience. Lab Anim. 1981;15(2):163–70.

47. Fan Y, Xiu K, Dong X, Zhang M. The influence of mechanical loading on osseointegration: an animal study. Sci China Ser C Life Sci. 2009; 52(6):579–86.

48. Zhao L, Xu Z, Yang Z, Wei X, Tang T, Zhao Z. Orthodontic mini-implant stability in different healing times before loading: a microscopic computerized tomographic and biomechanical analysis. Oral Surg Oral Med Oral Pathol Oral Radiol Endod. 2009;108(2):196–202.

49. Donath K, Breuner G. A method for the study of undecalcified bones and teeth with attached soft tissues. The Sage-Schliff (sawing and grinding) technique. J Oral Pathol. 1982;11(4):318–26.

50. Tsetsenekou E, Papadopoulos T, Kalyvas D, Papaioannou N, Tangl S, Watzek G. The influence of alendronate on osseointegration of nanotreated dental implants in New Zealand rabbits. Clin Oral Implants Res. 2012;23(6):659–66.

51. Ahn MR, An KM, Choi JH, Sohn DS. Immediate loading with mini dental implants in the fully edentulous mandible. Implant Dent. 2004;13(4):367–72.

52. An YH, Woolf SK, Friedman RJ. Pre-clinical in vivo evaluation of orthopaedic bioabsorbable devices. Biomaterials. 2000;21(24):2635–52.

53. Klokkevold PR, Johnson P, Dadgostari S, Caputo A, Davies JE, Nishimura RD. Early endosseous integration enhanced by dual acid etching of titanium: a torque removal study in the rabbit. Clin Oral Implants Res. 2001;12(4):350–7.

54. Hayakawa T, Yoshinari M, Kiba H, Yamamoto H, Nemoto K, Jansen JA. Trabecular bone response to surface roughened and calcium phosphate (Ca-P) coated titanium implants. Biomaterials. 2002;23(4):1025–31.

55. Sul YT, Byon ES, Jeong Y. Biomechanical measurements of calcium-incorporated oxidized implants in rabbit bone: effect of calcium surface chemistry of a novel implant. Clin Implant Dent Relat Res. 2004;6(2):101–10.

56. Svanborg LM, Hoffman M, Andersson M, Currie F, Kjellin P, Wennerberg A. The effect of hydroxyapatite nanocrystals on early bone formation surrounding dental implants. Int J Oral Maxillofac Surg. 2011;40(3):308–15.

57. Breding K, Jimbo R, Hayashi M, Xue Y, Mustafa K, Andersson M. The effect of hydroxyapatite nanocrystals on osseointegration of titanium implants: an in vivo rabbit study. Int J Dentistry. 2014;2014:171305.

58. Shin D, Blanchard SB, Ito M, Chu TM. Peripheral quantitative computer tomographic, histomorphometric, and removal torque analyses of two different non-coated implants in a rabbit model. Clin Oral Implants Res. 2011;22(3):242–50.

59. Roberts WE, Smith RK, Zilberman Y, Mozsary PG, Smith RS. Osseous adaptation to continuous loading of rigid endosseous implants. Am J Orthod. 1984;86(2):95–111.

60. Slaets E, Carmeliet G, Naert I, Duyck J. Early cellular responses in cortical bone healing around unloaded titanium implants: an animal study. J Periodontol. 2006;77(6):1015–24.

61. Marco F, Milena F, Gianluca G, Vittoria O. Peri-implant osteogenesis in health and osteoporosis. Micron. 2005;36(7-8):630–44.

62. Balkin BE, Steflik DE, Naval F. Mini-dental implant insertion with the auto-advance technique for ongoing applications. J Oral Implantol. 2001;27(1):32–7.

63. Simon H, Caputo AA. Removal torque of immediately loaded transitional endosseous implants in human subjects. Int J Oral Maxillofac Implants. 2002; 17(6):839–45.

64. Krebs M, Schmenger K, Neumann K, Weigl P, Moser W, Nentwig GH. Long-term evaluation of ANKYLOS® dental implants, part i: 20-year life table analysis of a longitudinal study of more than 12,500 implants. Clin Implant Dent Relat Res. 2015;17 Suppl 1:275–86.

65. Boyan BD, Hummert TW, Dean DD, Schwartz Z. Role of material surfaces in regulating bone and cartilage cell response. Biomaterials. 1996;17(2):137–46.

66. Schwartz Z, Lohmann CH, Oefinger J, Bonewald LF, Dean DD, Boyan BD. Implant surface characteristics modulate differentiation behavior of cells in the osteoblastic lineage. Adv Dent Res. 1999;13:38–48.

67. Boyan BD, Lossdorfer S, Wang L, Zhao G, Lohmann CH, Cochran DL, et al. Osteoblasts generate an osteogenic microenvironment when grown on surfaces with rough microtopographies. Eur Cell Mater. 2003;6:22–7.

68. Yan WQ, Nakamura T, Kobayashi M, Kim HM, Miyaji F, Kokubo T. Bonding of chemically treated titanium implants to bone. J Biomed Mater Res. 1997;37(2):267–75.

69. Marulanda J DJ, Alebrahim S, Romanos G, Feine J, Murshed M..Differential growth of MC3T3-E1 and C2C12 cells on 3M™ESPE™ MDI and Ankylos®. J Dent Res 95 (Spec Iss. A) 2015. p. 4042.

Permissions

List of Contributors

Rainde Naiara Rezende de Jesus
Department of Periodontology, Faculty of Odontology, Malmö University, Carl Gustafs väg 34, 205-06 Malmö, Sweden
IBILI, Faculty of Medicine, University of Coimbra, Av. Bissaya Barreto, Bloco de Celas, 3000-075 Coimbra, Portugal

Eunice Carrilho
IBILI, Faculty of Medicine, University of Coimbra, Av. Bissaya Barreto, Bloco de Celas, 3000-075 Coimbra, Portugal

Pedro V. Antunes and Amílcar Ramalho
CEMUC, Mechanical Engineering Department, University of Coimbra, Pinhal de Marrocos, 3030-788 Coimbra, Portugal

Camilla Christian Gomes Moura
Department of Endodontics, Faculty of Odontology, Federal University of Uberlândia, Av Pará 1720, Bloco4LB, Campus Umuarama, Uberlândia, Minas Gerais 38405-900, Brazil

Darceny Zanetta-Barbosa
Department of Oral and Maxillofacial Surgery and Implantology, Faculty of Odontology, Federal University of Uberlândia, Av Pará 1720, Bloco4LB, Campus Umuarama, Uberlândia, Minas Gerais 38405-900, Brazil

H. Jansson
Center for Oral Health, Department of Natural Science and Biomedicine, School of Health Sciences, Jönköping University, Jönköping, Sweden

G. L. Di Tanna
Center for Primary Care and Public Health, Queen Mary University of London, London, UK

M. Klepp
Private Practice, Stavanger, Norway

A. M. Roos-Jansåker
Department of Periodontology, Public Dental Health Service, Kristianstad, Sweden
Department of Periodontology, Public Specialist Dental Clinic, Karlskrona, Sweden

Tobias K. Boehm
Western University of Health Sciences College of Dental Medicine, 309 E Second Street, Pomona, CA 91766, USA

Michael Dau, Bernhard Frerich and Peer Wolfgang Kämmerer
Department of Oral, Maxillofacial and Plastic Surgery, University Medical Center, Schillingallee 35, 18057 Rostock, Germany

Paul Marciak and Bial Al-Nawas
Department of Oral and Maxillofacial Surgery, Plastic Surgery, University Medical Centre, Mainz, Germany

Henning Staedt
Private Dental Praxis Dr. Rossa, Ludwigshafen, Germany

Alberto Ortiz-Vigón, Sergio Martinez-Villa, Iñaki Suarez, Fabio Vignoletti and Mariano Sanz
ETEP Research Group, Facultad de Odontología, Universidad Complutense de Madrid, Plaza Ramón y Cajal, 28040 Madrid, Spain

Jonas Lorenz, Robert A. Sader and Shahram Ghanaati
Department for Oral, FORM-Lab, Cranio-Maxillofacial and Facial Plastic Surgery, Medical Center of the Goethe University Frankfurt, Frankfurt am Main, Germany

Henriette Lerner
HL-Dentclinic, Baden-Baden, Germany

Aghiad Yassin Alsabbagh and Mohammed Monzer Alsabbagh
Department of Periodontology, Damascus University Dental School, Damascus, Syrian Arab Republic

Batol Darjazini Nahas
Department of Orthodontics, Damascus University Dental School, Damascus, Syrian Arab Republic

Salam Rajih
Temple university, Philadelphia, USA

George Furtado Guimarães and Fabiana Mantovani Gomes França
Department of Implantology, São Leopoldo Mandic Research Center, Brasília, DF, Brazil

Luís Antônio Violin Dias Pereira
Department of Biochemistry and Tissue Biology, UNICAMP – State University of Campinas, Institute of Biology, Campinas, São Paulo, Brazil

Cassio Rocha Scardueli
Department of Periodontology, UNESP – Univ. Estadual Paulista, Araraquara Dental School, Araraquara, São Paulo, Brazil
Department of Dentistry and Oral Health – Oral Radiology, Aarhus University, Aarhus, Denmark

Rubens Spin-Neto
Department of Dentistry and Oral Health – Oral Radiology, Aarhus University, Aarhus, Denmark

Andreas Stavropoulos
Department of Periodontology, Faculty of Odontology, Malmö University, Carl Gustafs väg 34, 205-06 Malmö, Sweden

James Carlos Nery
Department of Implantology, São Leopoldo Mandic Research Center, Brasília, DF, Brazil
Implant Center, SEPS 710/910, Lotes CD, Office 226, CEP: 70390-108 Brasília, DF, Brazil

Makoto Noguchi, Hiroaki Tsuno, Risa Ishizaka, Kumiko Fujiwara, Shuichi Imaue and Kei Tomihara
Department of Oral and Maxillofacial Surgery, Graduate School of Medicine and Pharmaceutical Sciences for Research, University of Toyama, 2630 Sugitani Toyama city, Toyama 9300194, Japan

Takashi Minamisaka
Department of Diagnosis Pathology, Graduate School of Medicine and Pharmaceutical Sciences for Research, University of Toyama, Toyama, Japan

Amit Dattani
Oral and Maxillofacial Surgery, Regional Maxillofacial Unit, University Hospital Aintree, Liverpool, UK

David Richardson
Maxillofacial Surgery, Regional Craniofacial Unit, Alder Hey Children's Hospital, Liverpool, UK

Chris J. Butterworth
Maxillofacial Prosthodontics, Regional Maxillofacial Unit, University Hospital Aintree, Longmoor Lane, Liverpool L9 7AL, UK

Rubens F. Albuquerque Jr
Faculty of Dentistry of Ribeirão Preto, University of São Paulo, Ribeirão Preto, SP, Brazil

Sukhbir Kaur
Department of Zoology, Panjab University, Chandigarh, India

Takaaki Tanaka
Department of Materials Science and Technology, Niigata University, Niigata, Japan

Tomoyuki Kawase
Division of Oral Bioengineering, Institute of Medicine and Dentistry, Niigata University, Niigata, Japan

Koh Nakata
Bioscience Medical Research Center, Niigata University Medical and Dental Hospital, Niigata, Japan

Miya Kanazawa, Ikiru Atsuta, Yasunori Ayukawa, Ryosuke Kondo, Yuri Matsuura and Kiyoshi Koyano
Section of Implant and Rehabilitative Dentistry, Division of Oral Rehabilitation, Faculty of Dental Science, Kyushu University, 3-1-1 Maidashi, Higashi-ku, Fukuoka 812-8582, Japan

Takayoshi Yamaza
Department of Molecular Cell and Oral Anatomy, Faculty of Dental Science, Kyushu University, Fukuoka, Japan

Rémy Tanimura
8, place du Général Catroux, 75017 Paris, France

Shiro Suzuki
Department of Clinical Community and Sciences, University of Alabama at Birmingham School of Dentistry, 1919 7th Avenue South, Birmingham, AL 35294-0007, USA

Reiner Mengel and Miriam Thöne-Mühling
Department of Prosthetic Dentistry, School of Dental Medicine, Philipps-University, Marburg/Lahn, Germany

Theresa Heim
Gruben, Brandenburg, Germany

N. A. El-Wassefy and N. S. Aref
Dental Biomaterials Department, Faculty of Dentistry, Mansoura University, 35516 El Gomhoria St., Mansoura, Egypt

F. M. Reicha
Physics Department, Faculty of science, Mansoura University, 35516 El Gomhoria St., Mansoura, Egypt

Yoshihiro Kataoka, Shinnosuke Nogami and Tetsu Takahashi
Division of Oral and Maxillofacial Surgery, Department of Oral Medicine and Surgery, Tohoku University Graduate School of Dentistry, 4-1 Seiryomachi, Aoba-ku, Sendai 980-8575, Miyagi, Japan

Kenko Tanaka
Division of Oral and Maxillofacial Surgery, Department of Oral Medicine and Surgery, Tohoku University Graduate School of Dentistry, 4-1 Seiryomachi, Aoba-ku, Sendai 980-8575, Miyagi, Japan
Division of Fixed Prosthodontics and Biomaterials Clinic of Dental Medicine, University of Geneva, 19 rue Barthélemy-Menn, CH-1205 Geneva, Switzerland

Irena Sailer
Division of Fixed Prosthodontics and Biomaterials Clinic of Dental Medicine, University of Geneva, 19 rue Barthélemy-Menn, CH-1205 Geneva, Switzerland

C. Maiorana
Oral Surgery, Center for Edentulism and Jaw Atrophies, Maxillofacial Surgery and Dentistry Unit, Fondazione IRCCS Cà Granda – Ospedale Maggiore Policlinico, University of Milan, Milan, Italy

L. Pivetti, F. Signorino and M. Beretta
Center for Edentulism and Jaw Atrophies, Maxillofacial Surgery and Dentistry Unit, Fondazione IRCCS Cà Granda – Ospedale Maggiore Policlinico, University of Milan, Via della Commenda 10, 20122 Milan, Italy

G. B. Grossi
Department of Oral Surgery, School of Dentistry, University of Milan, Milan, Italy

A. S. Herford
Department of Oral & Maxillofacial Surgery, Loma Linda University, Loma Linda, CA, USA

Abdulmonem Alshiri
Department of Biomaterial and Prosthetic Sciences, King Saud University, Riyadh, Saudi Arabia

J. C. Wohlfahrt, A. M. Aass and O. C. Koldsland
Department of Periodontology, Institute of Clinical Dentistry, University of Oslo, Pb. 1109 Blindern, 0317 Oslo, Norway

B. J. Evensen
Private Practice, Tønsberg, Norway

B. Zeza and A. Pilloni
Department of Dental and Maxillofacial Sciences, Section of Periodontology, Sapienza, University of Rome, Rome, Italy

Shamit S. Prabhu
Wake Forest School of Medicine, Winston-Salem, USA
Triangle Implant Center, 5318 NC Highway 55, Suite 106, Durham, NC 27713, USA

Kevin Fortier
Boston University Henry M. Goldman School of Dental Medicine, Boston, USA

Michael C. May
Virginia Commonwealth University School of Dentistry, Richmond, USA

Uday N. Reebye
Triangle Implant Center, 5318 NC Highway 55, Suite 106, Durham, NC 27713, USA

Daniel Wiedemeier
Statistical Services, Center of Dental Medicine, University of Zurich, Zurich, Switzerland

Enas A. Elshenawy
Dental Biomaterials Department, Faculty of dentistry, Tanta University, Tanta, Egypt

Ahmed M. Alam-Eldein and Fadel A. Abd Elfatah
Prosthodontic Department, Faculty of dentistry, Tanta University, Tanta, Egypt

Katsuhiro Tsuruta, Yasunori Ayukawa, Tatsuya Matsuzaki, Masafumi Kihara and Kiyoshi Koyano
Section of Implant and Rehabilitative Dentistry, Division of Oral Rehabilitation, Faculty of Dental Science, Kyushu University, 3-1-1 Maidashi, Higashi-ku, Fukuoka 8128582, Japan

Julia Luz, Dominique Greutmann, Claudio Rostetter, Martin Rücker and Bernd Stadlinger
Clinic of Cranio-Maxillofacial and Oral Surgery, University of Zurich, University Hospital Zurich, Zurich, Switzerland

Benedicta E. Beck-Broichsitter
Department of Oral and Maxillofacial Surgery, Charité–University Medical Center Berlin, Augustenburger Platz 1, 13353 Berlin, Germany

Dorothea Westhoff, Eleonore Behrens, Jörg Wiltfang and Stephan T. Becker
Department of Oral and Maxillofacial Surgery, Schleswig-Holstein University Hospital, Arnold-Heller-Straße 3, Haus 26, 24105 Kiel, Germany

Yutaka Kitamura, Masashi Suzuki, Tsuneyuki Tsukioka, Kazushige Isobe, Tetsuhiro Tsujino, Taisuke Watanabe, Takao Watanabe and Hajime Okudera
Tokyo Plastic Dental Society, Kita-ku, Tokyo, Japan

Shinya Homma, Yasushi Makabe and Yasutomo Yajima
Department of Oral and Maxillofacial Implantology, Tokyo Dental College, 2-9-18 Misaki-cho, Chiyoda-ku, Tokyo 101-0061, Japan

Takuya Sakai, Kenzou Morinaga and Hirofumi Kido
Section of Oral Implantology, Department of Oral Rehabilitation, Fukuoka Dental College, 2-15-1 Tamura, Sawara-ku, Fukuoka-City, Fukuoka 814-0175, Japan

Satoru Yokoue
Center for Oral Diseases, Fukuoka Dental College, 3-2-1 Hakataekimae, Hakata-ku, Fukuoka City, Fukuoka 812-0011, Japan

Jagjit S. Dhaliwal and Jocelyne S. Feine
Faculty of Dentistry, McGill University, 2001 McGill College Avenue, Suite 500, Montreal, Quebec H3A 1G1, Canada

Rubens F. Albuquerque Jr
Faculty of Dentistry of Ribeirão Preto, University of São Paulo, Ribeirão Preto, SP, Brazil

Monzur Murshed
Faculty of Dentistry, McGill University, 2001 McGill College Avenue, Suite 500, Montreal, Quebec H3A 1G1, Canada
Department of Medicine, McGill University, Montreal, Quebec, Canada

Index